1992
YEAR BOOK OF
PATHOLOGY
AND CLINICAL
PATHOLOGY®

To Allison Thomas

J.

Dr B

The 1992 Year Book® Series

Year Book of Anesthesia and Pain Management: Drs. Miller, Kirby, Ostheimer, Roizen, and Stoelting

Year Book of Cardiology®: Drs. Schlant, Collins, Engle, Frye, Kaplan, and O'Rourke

Year Book of Critical Care Medicine®: Drs. Rogers and Parrillo

Year Book of Dentistry®: Drs. Meskin, Currier, Kennedy, Leinfelder, Matukas, and Rovin

Year Book of Dermatologic Surgery: Drs. Swanson, Salasche, and Glogau

Year Book of Dermatology®: Drs. Sober and Fitzpatrick

Year Book of Diagnostic Radiology®: Drs. Federle, Clark, Gross, Madewell, Maynard, Sackett, and Young

Year Book of Digestive Diseases®: Drs. Greenberger and Moody

Year Book of Drug Therapy®: Drs. Lasagna and Weintraub

Year Book of Emergency Medicine®: Drs. Wagner, Burdick, Davidson, Roberts, and Spivey

Year Book of Endocrinology®: Drs. Bagdade, Braverman, Horton, Kannan, Landsberg, Molitch, Morley, Odell, Rogol, Ryan, and Sherwin

Year Book of Family Practice®: Drs. Berg, Bowman, Davidson, Dietrich, and Scherger

Year Book of Geriatrics and Gerontology®: Drs. Beck, Abrass, Burton, Cummings, Makinodan, and Small

Year Book of Hand Surgery®: Drs. Amadio and Hentz

Year Book of Health Care Management: Drs. Heyssel, Brock, King, and Steinberg, Ms. Avakian, and Messrs. Berman, Kues, and Rosenberg

Year Book of Hematology®: Drs. Spivak, Bell, Ness, Quesenberry, and Wiernik

Year Book of Infectious Diseases®: Drs. Wolff, Barza, Keusch, Klempner, and Snydman

Year Book of Infertility: Drs. Mishell, Paulsen, and Lobo

Year Book of Medicine®: Drs. Rogers, Bone, Cline, Braunwald, Greenberger, Utiger, Epstein, and Malawista

Year Book of Neonatal and Perinatal Medicine: Drs. Klaus and Fanaroff

Year Book of Nephrology®: Drs. Coe, Favus, Henderson, Kashgarian, Luke, Myers, and Strom

Year Book of Neurology and Neurosurgery®: Drs. Currier and Crowell

Year Book of Neuroradiology: Drs. Osborn, Harnsberger, Halbach, and Grossman

Year Book of Nuclear Medicine®: Drs. Hoffer, Gore, Gottschalk, Sostman, Zaret, and Zubal

Year Book of Obstetrics and Gynecology®: Drs. Mishell, Kirschbaum, and Morrow

Year Book of Occupational and Environmental Medicine: Drs. Emmett, Brooks, Harris, and Schenker

Year Book of Oncology: Drs. Young, Longo, Ozols, Simone, Steele, and Weichselbaum

Year Book of Ophthalmology®: Drs. Laibson, Adams, Augsburger, Benson, Cohen, Eagle, Flanagan, Nelson, Reinecke, Sergott, and Wilson

Year Book of Orthopedics®: Drs. Sledge, Poss, Cofield, Frymoyer, Griffin, Hansen, Johnson, Simmons, and Springfield

Year Book of Otolaryngology–Head and Neck Surgery®: Drs. Bailey and Paparella

Year Book of Pathology and Clinical Pathology®: Drs. Gardner, Bennett, Cousar, Garvin, and Worsham

Year Book of Pediatrics®: Dr. Stockman

Year Book of Plastic, Reconstructive, and Aesthetic Surgery: Drs. Miller, Cohen, McKinney, Robson, Ruberg, and Whitaker

Year Book of Podiatric Medicine and Surgery®: Dr. Kominsky

Year Book of Psychiatry and Applied Mental Health®: Drs. Talbott, Frances, Freedman, Meltzer, Perry, Schowalter, and Yudofsky

Year Book of Pulmonary Disease®: Drs. Bone and Petty

Year Book of Speech, Language, and Hearing: Drs. Bernthal, Hall, and Tomblin

Year Book of Sports Medicine®: Drs. Shephard, Eichner, Sutton, and Torg, Col. Anderson, and Mr. George

Year Book of Surgery®: Drs. Schwartz, Jonasson, Robson, Shires, Spencer, and Thompson

Year Book of Transplantation: Drs. Ascher, Hansen, and Strom

Year Book of Ultrasound: Drs. Merritt, Mittelstaedt, Carroll, and Nyberg

Year Book of Urology®: Drs. Gillenwater and Howards

Year Book of Vascular Surgery®: Dr. Bergan

Roundsmanship '92–'93: A Year Book® Guide to Clinical Medicine: Drs. Dan, Feigin, Quilligan, Schrock, Stein, and Talbott

Contributing Editors

James B. Atkinson, M.D., Ph.D.

Associate Professor of Pathology, Vanderbilt University School of Medicine, Nashville, Tennessee

Robert M. Austin, M.D., Ph.D.

Director of Microbiology, Charleston Pathology, P.A., Roper Hospital, Charleston, South Carolina

Eduardo Cantu, Ph. D.

Assistant Professor and Director of Cytogenetics, Department of Pathology and Laboratory Medicine, Medical University of South Carolina, Charleston, South Carolina

Paul Garen, M.D.

Professor and Director of Surgical Pathology, Department of Pathology and Laboratory Medicine, Medical University of South Carolina, Charleston, South Carolina

Russell A. Harely, M.D.

Professor and Director of the Autopsy Pathology Section, Department of Pathology and Laboratory Medicine, Medical University of South Carolina, Charleston, South Carolina

Joseph M. Harmon, M.D.

Director of Surgical Pathology and Immunology, Charleston Pathology, P.A., Roper Hospital, Charleston, South Carolina

Roy A. Jensen, M.D.

Assistant Professor of Pathology, Vanderbilt University School of Medicine, Nashville, Tennessee

Mahlon Johnson, M.D., Ph.D.

Assistant Professor of Neuropathology, Vanderbilt University School of Medicine, Nashville, Tennessee

Elizabeth A. Manci, M.D.

Associate Professor and Director of Pediatric Pathology, University of South Alabama Children and Women's Hospital, Mobile, Alabama

John S. Metcalf, M.D.

Associate Professor and Director of Surgical Pathology, Department of Pathology and Laboratory Medicine, Medical University of South Carolina, Charleston, South Carolina

James R. Stubbs, M.D.

Assistant Professor of Pathology; Director of Blood Bank, University of South Alabama, Mobile, Alabama

J. Allan Tucker, M.D.

Associate Professor of Pathology, University of South Alabama, Mobile, Alabama

David J. Wells, Ph.D.

Associate Professor of Pathology, University of South Alabama, Mobile, Alabama

Song W. Wong, M.D.

Assistant Professor of Pathology, University of South Alabama, Mobile, Alabama

1992
The Year Book of PATHOLOGY AND CLINICAL PATHOLOGY®

Editor-in-Chief
William A. Gardner, Jr., M.D.
Professor and Chair, Department of Pathology, University of South Alabama, Mobile, Alabama

Editors
Betsy D. Bennett, M.D., Ph.D.
Professor and Vice Chair, Department of Pathology, University of South Alabama, Mobile, Alabama

John B. Cousar, M.D.
Associate Professor of Pathology and Director of Laboratories, Vanderbilt University School of Medicine, Nashville, Tennessee

A. Julian Garvin, M.D.
Professor and Chair, Department of Pathology, Medical University of South Carolina, Charleston, South Carolina

G. Fred Worsham, M.D.
Chief of Pathology, Charleston Pathology, P.A., Roper Hospital, Charleston, South Carolina

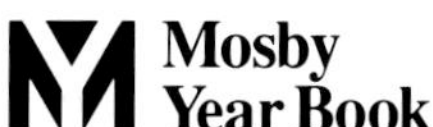

St. Louis Baltimore Boston Chicago London Philadelphia Sydney Toronto

Editor-in-Chief, Year Book Publishing: Kenneth H. Killion
Sponsoring Editor: Kristine Antens
Manager, Literature Services: Edith M. Podrazik
Senior Information Specialist: Terri Santo
Senior Medical Writer: David A. Cramer, M.D.
Assistant Director, Manuscript Services: Frances M. Perveiler
Associate Managing Editor, Year Book Editing Services: Elizabeth Fitch
Production Coordinator: Max F. Perez
Proofroom Manager: Barbara M. Kelly

Mosby–Year Book, Inc.
11830 Westline Industrial Drive
St. Louis, MO 63146

Editorial Office:
Mosby–Year Book, Inc.
200 North LaSalle St.
Chicago, IL 60601

International Standard Serial Number: 0084-3946
International Standard Book Number: 0-8151-1247-5

Table of Contents

The material in this volume represents literature reviewed up to July 1991.

Journals Represented

Mosby–Year Book subscribes to and surveys nearly 900 U.S. and foreign medical and allied health journals. From these journals, the Editors select the articles to be abstracted. Journals represented in this YEAR BOOK are listed below.

Acta Cytologica
American Journal of Clinical Pathology
American Journal of Dermatopathology
American Journal of Gastroenterology
American Journal of Law and Medicine
American Journal of Obstetrics and Gynecology
American Journal of Ophthalmology
American Journal of Pathology
American Journal of Perinatology
American Journal of Surgical Pathology
American Journal of the Medical Sciences
American Review of Respiratory Disease
American Surgeon
Annals of Clinical Biochemistry
Annals of Internal Medicine
Annals of Rheumatic Diseases
Archives of Dermatology
Archives of Internal Medicine
Archives of Otolaryngology—Head and Neck Surgery
Archives of Pathology and Laboratory Medicine
Archives of Surgery
Arthritis and Rheumatism
Biology of the Neonate
Blood
British Journal of Cancer
British Journal of Haematology
British Journal of Obstetrics and Gynaecology
British Journal of Surgery
British Medical Journal
Cancer
Cancer Research
Cell
Chest
Circulation
Clinica Chimica Acta
Clinical Chemistry
Diabetic Medicine
Diagnostic Microbiology and Infectious Disease
Diseases of the Colon and Rectum
European Journal of Cancer
Experimental and Molecular Pathology
Gastroenterology
Gut
Gynecologic Oncology
Hepatology
Histopathology
Human Pathology
International Journal of Cancer

International Journal of Gynecological Pathology
Journal of Clinical Investigation
Journal of Clinical Microbiology
Journal of Clinical Oncology
Journal of Clinical Pathology
Journal of Cutaneous Pathology
Journal of Experimental Medicine
Journal of Infectious Diseases
Journal of Laboratory and Clinical Medicine
Journal of Neurology, Neurosurgery and Psychiatry
Journal of Neurosurgery
Journal of Oral and Maxillofacial Surgery
Journal of Pathology
Journal of Pediatrics
Journal of the American College of Cardiology
Journal of the American Geriatrics Society
Journal of the American Medical Association
Klinische Wochenschrift
Laboratory Investigation
Lancet
Mayo Clinic Proceedings
Medicine, Science and the Law
Modern Pathology
Nature
New England Journal of Medicine
Obstetrics and Gynecology
Oral Surgery, Oral Medicine, Oral Pathology
Pathology, Research and Practice
Pediatric Pathology
Pediatrics
Quality Assurance and Utilization Review
Radiology
Reviews of Infectious Diseases
Scandinavian Journal of Clinical and Laboratory Investigation
Scandinavian Journal of Thoracic and Cardiovascular Surgery
Science
Surgery
Surgical Neurology
Surgical Pathology
Transfusion
Transplantation
Ultrastructural Pathology
Urology
Virchows Archiv A: Pathological Anatomy and Histopathology
Virchows Archiv B: Cell Pathology

Standard Abbreviations

The following terms are abbreviated in this edition: acquired immunodeficiency syndrome (AIDS), central nervous system (CNS), cerebrospinal fluid (CSF), computed tomography (CT), electrocardiography (ECG), human immunodeficiency virus (HIV), and magnetic resonance (MR) imaging (MRI).

Publisher's Preface

We are delighted to welcome William A. Gardner, Jr., M.D., and his associates, Betsy D. Bennett, M.D., Ph.D, John B. Cousar, M.D., A. Julian Garvin, M.D., Ph.D., and G. Frederick Worsham, M.D., as editors of the YEAR BOOK OF PATHOLOGY AND CLINICAL PATHOLOGY. This team is carrying on the tradition of distinguished editorial direction for this YEAR BOOK, commencing with the 1992 edition. We congratulate them and extend our appreciation for their superb work with the YEAR BOOK.

As publishers, we feel challenged to seek ways of presenting complex information in a clear and readable manner. To this end, the 1992 YEAR BOOK OF PATHOLOGY AND CLINICAL PATHOLOGY now provides structured abstracts in which the various components of a study can easily be identified through headings. These headings are not the same in all abstracts but, rather, are those that most accurately designate the content of each particular journal article. We are confident that our readers will find the information contained in our abstracts to be more accessible than ever before. We welcome your comments.

Introduction

This volume represents the 44th YEAR BOOK OF PATHOLOGY AND CLINICAL PATHOLOGY. It follows more than a decade of distinguished effort on the part of Dr. Kenneth Brinkhous and his colleagues at the University of North Carolina. The current Editorial Board represents a diversification of editorial effort. Moreover, the inclusion of Dr. G. Fred Worsham and his colleagues engaged in the community practice of pathology reflects a wish to underscore the perspective of applicability in daily practice. For all editors (while reviewing 2,000+ manuscripts) the essential criteria have remained the same. Does the paper provide new information or fresh perspective? Does it illustrate a distinctive histologic pattern? Does it challenge accepted dogma? And, in some cases, does it simply have the intangible quality of attracting the interest of pathologists?

The extraordinary breadth of medical literature that relates to pathology could not possibly be encompassed in a single survey volume. Therefore, the major focus has been on human disease, restricting comments on animal experimentation to those studies that have clear implications for human practice. The vast amount of literature dealing with techniques such as antibodies, probes, and the like that "show promise" of application in clinical medicine has also largely been eschewed in favor of that demonstrated applicability.

The Editors particularly wish to acknowledge the cheerful support and encouragement of Nancy Gorham, especially in the initial phases of this effort.

William A. Gardner, Jr., M.D.

PART ONE
PATHOLOGY

1 General Pathology

Capillary Leakage in Inflammation: A Study by Vascular Labeling

Joris I, Cuénoud HF, Doern GV, Underwood JM, Majno G (Univ of Massachusetts)

Am J Pathol 137:1353–1363, 1990 1–1

Background.—It has long been recognized that the "inflammatory tumor" is best explained by increased permeability of the vascular wall. Vascular labeling studies give evidence that local injury—whether mechanical, thermal, or toxic—causes leakage from all segments of the microcirculation. Vasoactive mediators, in contrast, produce a "histamine type" of leakage from venules. Aseptic necrosis was used as a model in which a mass of dying or dead tissue lies adjacent to an intact vascular network that acted as the target tissue.

Methods.—Samples of rat liver and kidney were implanted in the cremasteric sac of recipient animals under aseptic conditions. Control rats received boiled tissues and spheres of glass or Teflon. Carbon black was injected intravenously at different intervals, and the animals were killed an hour later for vascular labeling studies.

Findings.—Vascular labeling was exclusively venular for up to 8 hours; between 12 and 24 hours it was associated with capillary labeling. At 48 hours, labeling was totally or at least mainly of capillaries. Labeled areas exhibited an acute inflammatory infiltrate, with neutrophils predominating in the early stages and mononuclear cells subsequently. Control specimens showed weaker labeling and less marked inflammatory changes.

Conclusions.—This study of aseptic inflammation distinguishes between an initial venular phase of vascular leakage, a capillary phase, and the inflammatory reaction itself. Immediate leakage from all vessels may result from a direct injury, whereas venular leakage is caused by chemical mediators. Leakage from regenerating capillaries in granulation tissue occurs in the repair phase. The cellular component of the exudate might be chiefly responsible by producing cytokines or other mediators. Alternatively, the hemodynamic changes leading to acute inflammation could induce endothelial mitosis, thereby triggering capillary leakage.

▶ It is remarkable that in these days of refined techniques of molecular biology, there continue to be new light microscopic observations of the basic reaction to injury. Recognition of a more complex involvement of capillaries in this process should lead to reevaluation of pathogenetic mechanisms in multiple disease states and to what Majno (1) has referred to as a neglected field, i.e., the pathology of the capillary.—W.A. Gardner, Jr., M.D.

Reference

1. Majno G: The capillary: Then and now: An overview of capillary pathology. *Mod Pathol* 5:9–22, 1992.

A Proinflammatory Mediator With Potential Relevance in Aging

Beutler B (Univ of Texas, Dallas)
J Am Geriatr Soc 38:1027–1036, 1990 1–2

Introduction.—Tumor necrosis factor (TNF), or cachectin, is a macrophage-derived protein that protects the host against various invasive agents. At the same time, it mediates many of the adverse effects of an invader. Findings that the factor can produce cachexia in chronically ill patients and can act as a central mediator of shock in septic patients suggest that it may contribute to the immune deficit associated with aging.

Pathophysiology.—The primary structure of cachectin/TNF is strongly conserved among diverse mammalian forms. Secreted cachectin interacts with a plasma membrane receptor widely present on mammalian cells and tissues. The factor induces a shock syndrome when given to rats and dogs (Fig 1–1). Agents that sensitize animals to the lethal effect of lipopolysaccharide also make them vulnerable to cachectin/TNF. Chronic

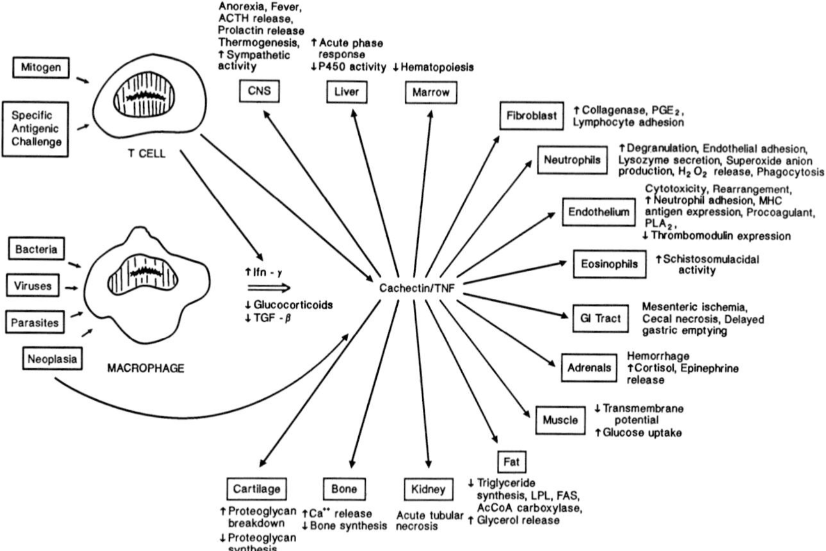

Fig 1–1.—Effect of cachectin/tumor necrosis factor (TNF) on various cells in the mammal. Both T cells and macrophages produce cachectin when approximately stimulated. The widespread effects of cachectin in various cells produce the final picture of anorexia, fever, inflammation, hyperlipidemia, tissue necrosis, cachexia, and shock. *ACTH,* adrenocorticotrophic hormone; *PGE2,* prostaglandin E_2; *MHC,* major histocompatibility complex; *PLA_2,* phospholipase A_2; *LPL,* lipoprotein lipase; *FAS,* fatty acid synthetase; *Ifn-γ,* interferon-γ; *TGF-β,* transforming growth factor-β. (Courtesy of Beutler B: *J Am Geriatr Soc* 38:1027–1036, 1990.)

administration of cachectin/TNF can produce marked wasting, supporting the supposition that chronic exposure might lead to cachexia.

Disease States.—Cachectin/TNF has been found in sera from patients with meningococcal septicemia; high levels correlate with a fatal outcome. Cerebral malaria also has been associated with secretion of cachectin/TNF. Conflicting data have been reported on the association of cachectin/TNF with cancer.

Aging.—Cachectin/TNF might help to remove advanced glycosylation end-products that accumulate in the extracellular matrix in the course of aging. Much more study is needed to determine whether the anorexia and wasting often seen in older persons might be related to production of cachectin//TNF, or whether dysregulation of the factor increases susceptibility to infection.

▶ The panoply of effects of the cachectins is still unfolding, and this paper by one of the leading investigators in the field succinctly reviews these diverse influences (see Fig 1–1).—W.A. Gardner, Jr., M.D.

Genetic and Molecular Diagnostics

The Molecular Genetic Analysis of Hemophilia A: A Directed Search Strategy for the Detection of Point Mutations in the Human Factor VIII Gene

Pattinson JK, Millar DS, McVey JH, Grundy CB, Wieland K, Mibashan RS, Martinowitz U, Tan-Un K, Vidaud M, Goossens M, Sampietro M, Mannucci PM, Krawczak M, Reiss J, Zoll B, Whitmore D, Bowcock S, Wensley R, Ajani A, Mitchell V, Rizza C, Maia R, Winter P, Mayne EE, Schwartz M, Green PJ, Kakkar VV, Tuddenham EGD, Cooper DN (Haemostasis Research Group, MRC Clinical Research Centre, Harrow, England; Thrombosis Research Inst, London)

Blood 76:2242–2248, 1990 1–3

Background.—It is important to characterize the point mutations occurring in the factor VIII gene in patients with hemophilia A, not only to understand the basis of CpG hypermutability but to relate the structure of factor VIII protein to its function.

Methods.—A systematic screening technique was used to describe CpG sites in the factor VIII gene in DNA samples from patients with hemophilia A. The DNA was isolated for investigation in blood samples from 793 unrelated patients with hemophilia A. A directed search strategy was used to screen for point mutations in 8 potentially hypermutable CpG dinucleotides at sites that were thought to be functionally important. These sites were codons −5, 336, 372, 427, 583, 795, 1,689, and 1,696. The DNA samples were amplified by polymerase chain reaction and screened by oligonucleotide hybridization.

Findings.—Samples from 16 patients showed point mutations consistent with a model of 5-methylcytosine (5mC) deamination. New current mutations were shown at codons 336 (CGA → TGA), 372 (CGC → TGC and CGC → CAC), and 1,689 (CGC → TGC). The sites were thought to be as important as cleavage sites for activated protein C or thrombin. The remaining arginine codons screened showed further novel

C → T transitions that resulted in the creation of TGA termination codons. Within and among different ethnic groups and CpG sites, differing mutation frequencies were found. The differences probably resulted from differing levels of cytosine methylation, although there is no direct evidence of this.

Discussion.—New examples of recurrent mutation of CpG dinucleotides have been found in the factor VIII gene that causes hemophilia A. These mutations are consistent with a model of 5mC deamination. If CpG mutability is shown to correlate with methylation status, the methylation status of specific CpG sites in a given gene should be established before labor-intensive screening is done.

▶ This analysis of hemophilia A patients provides valuable insight into the role of the CpG dinucleotide as a "hot spot" for point mutations that cause the expression of genetic diseases. A total of 16 point mutations were found, including 5 previously undescribed mutations and 4 new examples of recurrent mutations. The mutations also appear to play a critical role in the phenotypic expression of disease. Disease phenotype is affected through changes in a critical genetic location or through significant codon alteration. The concept of deamination of 5-methylcytosine leading to these mutations is presented. In addition, there is a discussion regarding the variable methylation of CpG sites as an explanation for differences in mutation rates within specific genes and, on a broader scale, between races.—J.R. Stubbs, M.D.

Gene Rearrangements in the Diagnosis of Lymphoma/Leukemia: Guidelines for Use Based on a Multiinstitutional Study

Cossman J, Zehnbauer B, Garrett CT, Smith LJ, Williams M, Jaffe ES, Hanson LO, Love J (Georgetown Univ; Johns Hopkins Univ; George Washington Univ; Univ of Florida; Univ of Virginia; et al)

Am J Clin Pathol 95:347–354, 1991 1–4

Background.—Rearrangement of antigen receptor genes in various human lymphoproliferative diseases is increasingly supported by research. Tests for rearrangement of the antigen receptor genes, however, require further validation as to these assays' specificity, sensitivity, and reproducibility before they can be used routinely in a diagnostic laboratory. The accuracy and reproducibility of gene rearrangement analysis was quantified by a random, blinded, multisite study of 275 patient tissue samples.

Methods.—Tissue samples were collected from 275 patients with malignant lymphomas and leukemias (173 patients), nonmalignant lymphoproliferative disorders (35), malignant tumors other than lymphoma (23), and normal peripheral blood lymphocytes (44). Immunophenotyping was performed on frozen sections for solid samples and flow cytometry for fluid-phase cell suspensions. Analysis of DNA was done on fresh or snap frozen samples.

Findings.—The table summarizes the results of 240 tissue sample analyses. Five samples were too degraded for DNA analysis. Of the 151 spec-

Interpretation

	Clinical Diagnosis		
DNA Probe Results	***Positive (malignant Dx)***	***Negative (benign or normal)***	***Indeterminate***
Positive	136	2	14
Negative	15	60	13
Total	151	62	27

(Courtesy of Cossman J, Zehnbauer B, Garrett CT, et al: *Am J Clin Pathol* 95:347–354, 1991.)

imens from malignant disorders, 136 showed gene rearrangements, yielding a false negative rate of 9.9%. Of these 15 false negative cases, 6 occurred in patients with follicular lymphoma in which the B cells were fewer in number for phenotypic analysis, and 7 occurred in individuals with large cell lymphomas. Among the 62 patients with a negative diagnosis who would not be expected to have gene rearrangement based on histologic testing and phenotyping, 4 samples had evidence of gene rearrangement. Of the 23 other malignancy samples tested, none showed any gene rearrangement based on the 3 DNA probes used. Of the 100 cases phenotyped as either B cell or pre-B cell, 97 demonstrated B cell rearrangement, whereas 32 of the 36 cases phenotyped as T cell showed rearrangement, thus producing a 97% concurrence with phenotypic analysis. Based on data from 50 cases randomly selected for repeat testing in 2 separate laboratories, the reproducibility rate was 94% for the C_T β probe and 98% for the J_H and the J_K probes. The overall agreement for reproducibility of interpretation for the gene rearrangement assay was 95.4% among the 11 interpreters.

Conclusions.—The application of gene rearrangement analysis in the diagnosis of lymphoproliferative disorders appears very reproducible based on the highly defined nature of the restriction fragments used in the assay.

▶ This study is important for anyone who uses molecular genetics data in the diagnosis of hematopoietic/lymphoid neoplasms or is considering the development of these techniques in his or her laboratory.—J.B. Cousar, M.D.

Utility of Molecular Genetic Analysis for the Diagnosis of Neoplasia in Morphologically and Immunophenotypically Equivocal Hematolymphoid Lesions

Davis RE, Warnke RA, Dorfman RF, Cleary ML (Stanford Univ)

Cancer 67:2890–2899, 1991 1–5

Objective.—The utility of molecular genetic analysis in the diagnosis of neoplasia was assessed in a retrospective review of 175 hematolymphoid lesions.

Comparison of Genotyping With Favored Impression by Conventional Analysis in 81 Problem Cases

Favored impression	Ig and/or β-TCR genes	Consensus diagnosis	Genotyping contribution	No. of cases
Benign	Germline	Benign	Confirmatory	9
		Benign	Essential	1
		Uncertain	—	1
	Rearranged	Malignant	Essential	6
		Benign	Discrepant/overruled	1
		Uncertain	—	3
Malignant	Germline	Benign	Essential	3
		Malignant	Discrepant/overruled	13
		Uncertain	—	2
	Rearranged	Malignant	Confirmatory	24
		Malignant	Essential	15
		Uncertain	—	2
Uncertain	Rearranged	Uncertain	—	1

Abbreviations: Ig, immunoglobulin; β-*TCR,* beta chain T cell receptor.
(Courtesy of Davis RE, Warnke RA, Dorfman RF, et al: *Cancer* 67:2890–2899.)

Methods.—Based on the presence or absence of diagnostic uncertainty remaining after conventional morphological and immunophenotypic analysis, 85 cases were assigned to the problem group and 90 to the control group. All cases were analyzed for immunoglobulin (Ig) or beta chain T cell receptor gene rearrangements. The results were compared with the diagnosis and lineage established by conventional analysis.

Results.—All 90 controls had unequivocal morphological features diagnostic for non-Hodgkin's lymphoma (NHL), and all had appropriate lineage-specific gene rearrangements. However, immunostaining was almost as sensitive in demonstrating abnormal phenotypes. These findings indicate that genotyping is of little or no diagnostic worth in cases with NHL that are unequivocal by conventional analysis. Genotyping, however, was diagnostically useful in problem cases, which included cases of NHL and other hematolymphoid neoplasia and various reactive hematolymphoid lesions. Excluding the 4 cases of Hodgkin's disease, genotyping was helpful in arriving at a consensus diagnosis in 58 of 81 (72%) cases, including 25 (35%) in which genotyping was considered essential to the diagnosis (table). Genotyping did not contribute positively to the diagnosis in the remaining problem cases. In no case, however, did genotyping lead to an incorrect diagnosis when findings were cautiously interpreted with primary reliance on conventional analysis and with knowledge of known causes of potentially misleading results, both positive and negative. For the 58 cases with a diagnosis of malignancy, genotyping gave a positive result in 45, for a sensitivity of 78%; only 1 of 14 cases judged to be benign or nonneoplastic showed gene rearrangements, for a specificity of 93%.

Conclusion.—Genotyping is highly sensitive and specific for hematolymphoid neoplasia, but it is noncontributory in cases that are unequivocally malignant on conventional analysis, in cases of suspected Hodgkin's disease, or for the sole purpose of lineage assignment. Genotyping should be reserved for cases whose diagnosis is uncertain after conventional analysis.

▶ Although most malignant lymphomas can be diagnosed correctly using conventional morphology and immunophenotypic studies, molecular genetic analysis has a definite role in a significant number of cases.—J.B. Cousar, M.D.

Genotypic Analysis of Diffuse, Mixed Cell Lymphomas: Comparison With Morphologic and Immunophenotypic Findings

Medeiros LJ, Lardelli P, Stetler-Stevenson M, Longo DL, Jaffe ES (Natl Cancer Inst, Bethesda, Md)

Am J Clin Pathol 95:547–555, 1991 1–6

Background.—As defined in the Working Formulation, malignant lymphoma with diffuse, mixed small and large cells is heterogeneous both morphologically and immunophenotypically. Clonality may be difficult to determine. Twenty diffuse, mixed cell lymphomas were genotyped, and the results were compared with histologic and immunophenotypic findings.

Methods.—After exclusion of lymphomas that were not entirely diffuse, the remainder were subdivided into follicular center cell and

Table 1.—Histologic Subclassifications and Immunophenotypic Findings in Diffuse Mixed Cell Lymphomas

Case No.	*Histologic Classification*	*Immunophenotype*	*Monoclonal B Cells (%)*	*T Cells (%)*
1	Non-FCC	Uncertain	—	75% (ER)
2	Non-FCC	Uncertain	—	48% (ER)
3	Non-FCC (E)	Uncertain	—	61% (F)
4	Non-FCC	Uncertain	—	74% (F)
5	Non-FCC	Uncertain	—	77% (ER)
6	Non-FCC (E)	Uncertain	—	>50% (FS)
7	Non-FCC (E)	Uncertain	—	>50% (FS)
8	Non-FCC	Uncertain	—	65% (F)
9	Non-FCC	Uncertain	—	70% (F)
10	Non-FCC (E)	Uncertain	—	65% (F)
11	Non-FCC (E)	Uncertain	—	68% (F)
12	Non-FCC (E)	Uncertain	—	>50% (FS)
13	FCC	Ig-CD20+	—	81% (F)
14	Non-FCC	IgM kappa	<10% (FS)	90% (F)
15	Non-FCC (E)	IgM lambda	45% (F)	44% (F)
16	Non-FCC	IgM kappa	35% (F)	55% (F)
17	Non-FCC (E)	IgM kappa	19% (F)	65% (F)
18	FCC	IgM kappa	16% (F)	63% (F)
19	Non-FCC	Aberrant T*	—	>50% (FS)
20	Non-FCC	Aberrant T†	—	91% (F)

Abbreviations: FCC, follicular center cell; *(E),* epithelioid histiocytic reaction present; *Ig,* immunoglobulin; *M,* mu; *(ER),* E-rosette; *(F),* flow cytometry; *(FS),* frozen section estimate.

*CD2+, CD3−, CD5−, CD7+.

†CD2+, CD3+, CD5+, CD7−.

(Courtesy of Medeiros LJ, Lardelli P, Stetler-Stevenson M, et al: *Am J Clin Pathol* 95:547–555, 1991.)

Table 2.—Summary of Genotypic Results in Diffuse Mixed Cell Lymphomas

	Genotype					
Case No.	***J_H (% Clone*)***	*J_K*	*C_β*	*J_γ*	*Bcl-2*†	Bcl-2/J_H‡
1	G	G	G	ND	G	ND
2	R1 (10–25%)	G	R1 (10–25%)	ND	G	–
3	R1 (<10%)	ND	R1 (<10%)	P	ND	+
4	G	G	R2 (<10%)	P	G	–
5	G	G	R1 (25–50%)	R (25–50%)	G	–
6	G	G	G	P	ND	ND
7	G	G	G	P	G	–
8	G	G	G	P	G	+
9	R1 (10–25%)	R	G	P	G	–
10	R1 (<10%)	R	G	P	G	–
11	G	ND	R2 (<10%)	P	ND	–
12	G	G	G	R (<10%)	G	–
13	R2 (10–25%)	R	G	P	R	+
14	R1 (10–25%)	ND	G	ND	ND	+
15	R1 (25–50%)	R	G	ND	R	+
16	R2 (25–50%)	R	G	P	R	+
17	R2 (10–25%)	R	G	ND	G	–
18	R1 (10–25%)	R	R1 (10–25%)	P	R	+
19	G	G	G	P	G	–
20	G	G	R1 (10–25%)	R (10–25%)	G	ND

Abbreviations: R1, allele rearranged; *R2,* alleles rearranged; *G,* germline configuration; *ND,* not done or DNA insufficient for analysis; *P,* polyclonal T cells present.
*Percentage of clonal cells estimated by comparing rearranged band with germline band.
†By Southern blot analysis.
‡By polymerase chain reaction.
(Courtesy of Medeiros LJ, Lardelli P, Stetler-Stevenson M, et al: *Am J Clin Pathol* 95:547–555, 1991.)

nonfollicular center cell subtypes. Immunophenotypic and gene rearrangement analyses and polymerase chain reaction amplification were done.

Results.—All lesions were composed predominantly of T cells. There were 5 lesions with a monoclonal B cell population, 2 with an aberrant T cell immunophenotype, and 1 with an aberrant B cell immunophenotype. These findings support the diagnosis of malignancy. Of these 8 lymphomas, genotypic analysis confirmed the presence of a population of clonal cells in 7, 1 with an abnormal T cell phenotype having a germline configuration. In 12 samples, no clonal population or abnormal immunophenotype was identified (Table 1). Evidence of clonality was provided by genotypic analysis (Table 2) in 8 of these. Southern blot analysis also could not identify a clonal population in 4 samples with uncertain immunophenotypic results. The major breakpoint region of the *bcl*-2 protooncogene on chromosome 18 was analyzed by Southern blot analysis, polymerase chain reaction, or both. The t(14;18)(q32;q21) translocation was identified in 7 B cell lymphomas. Five of these were not classified as follicular center cell type by morphological findings.

Conclusions.—In the study of diffuse mixed cell lymphomas, gene rearrangement analysis is a valuable complement to immunophenotypic studies. The histologic spectrum of follicular center cell lymphomas may be greater than has been suggested previously.

▶ Diffuse mixed cell lymphoma is a "wastebasket" category of non-Hodgkin's lymphomas and contains a mix of B and T cell neoplasms. Sometimes, molecular genetic analysis is necessary to precisely categorize these lymphomas.—J.B. Cousar, M.D.

Diagnostic Relevance of Clonal Cytogenetic Aberrations in Malignant Soft-Tissue Tumors

Fletcher JA, Kozakewich HP, Hoffer FA, Lage JM, Weidner N, Tepper R, Pinkus GS, Morton CC, Corson JM (Brigham and Women's Hosp; Children's Hosp; Massachusetts Gen Hosp, Boston)

N Engl J Med 324:436–442, 1991 1–7

Background.—The diagnosis of malignant soft tissue tumors may be a challenging problem. In some tumors, possibly diagnostic chromosomal aberrations have been identified. The overall frequency and diagnostic relevance of these aberrations were investigated.

Methods.—Attempts were made to determine karyotypes in cells from 62 consecutive, unselected malignant spindle cell or small round cell soft tissue tumors after direct harvesting or short-term culture. The 46 adults and 16 children from whom samples were taken were seen during a 14-month period. In addition to routine light microscopic evaluation, all tumors were examined independently by immunohistochemical staining. Electron microscopy was done on cells from all but 2 tumors.

Results.—Metaphases were successfully obtained from 61 tumors. In 89% of these, clonal chromosome aberrations were identified (Figs 1–2, 1–3, and 1–4). In the remaining tumors, nonneoplastic stro-

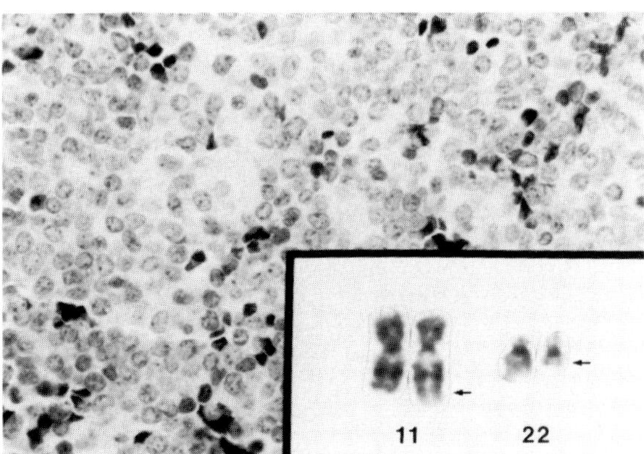

Fig 1–2.—Undifferentiated small round cell neoplasm arising in the pharynx of a 7-month-old boy. **Inset,** translocation (11;22) supporting a diagnosis of peripheral primitive neuroectodermal tumor. *Arrows* indicate translocation breakpoints. (Courtesy of Fletcher JA, Kozakewich HP, Hoffer FA, et al: *N Engl J Med* 324:436–442, 1991.)

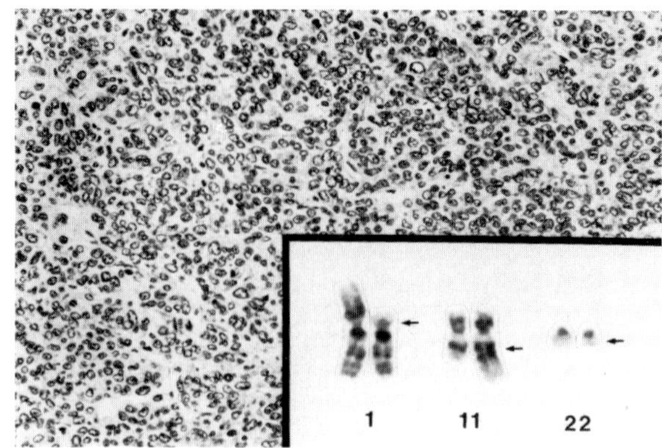

Fig 1–3.—Undifferentiated round cell neoplasm arising from the pelvis in a 21-year-old man. **Inset,** the translocation (1;11;22) supporting a diagnosis of atypical Ewing's sarcoma. *Arrows* indicate translocation breakpoints. (Courtesy of Fletcher JA, Kozakewich HP, Hoffer FA, et al: *N Engl J Med* 324:436–442, 1991.)

mal elements within the specimens were found to be the source of the normal metaphases. A clonal chromosomal aberration suggesting or confirming a specific diagnosis was found in 65% of tumors. The aberration was important in establishing the final diagnosis in 24% of all tumors. Cytogenetic abnormalities were particularly useful in diagnosing small round cell neoplasms in children; the information was diagnostically important in 8 of 14 such tumors. An unambiguous diagnosis was established for 60 of the 62 tumors by the combination of light and electron microscopy, immunohistochemistry, and cytogenetics.

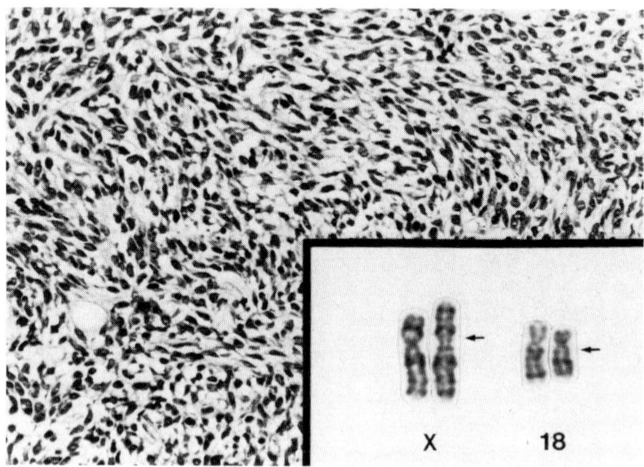

Fig 1–4.—Spindle cell neoplasm arising in the abdomen of a 52-year-old women. **Inset,** the translocation (X;18) supporting a diagnosis of monophasic synovial sarcoma. *Arrows* indicate translocation breakpoints. (Courtesy of Fletcher JA, Kozakewich HP, Hoffer FA, et al: *N Engl J Med* 324:436–442, 1991.)

Conclusions.—Clonal chromosome aberrations may be found in almost all malignant soft tissue tumors by cytogenetic analysis. These aberrations are often diagnostically relevant, especially for small round cell tumors in children.

▶ Numerous karyotypic abnormalities of solid tumors have been described, and many of these are specific for a particular type of tumor. In this series, the karyotype was important for diagnosis in 24% of cases. Additional series of solid soft tissue tumors are essential to test the validity and establish the karyotype of other soft tissue tumors.—A.J. Garvin, M.D., Ph.D.

Postmortem Chorionic Villus Sampling Is a Better Method for Cytogenetic Evaluation of Early Fetal Loss Than Culture of Abortus Material

Johnson MP, Drugan A, Koppitch FC III, Uhlmann WR, Evans MI (Hutzel Hosp, Detroit; Wayne State Univ)

Am J Obstet Gynecol 163:1505–1510, 1990 1–8

Background.—The poor success rate of obtaining viable cells for culture and successful karyotyping has hindered the cytogenetic evaluation of embryonic or fetal loss. The usefulness of amniocentesis with cultured fetal skin, products of conception, or aminocytes was compared to that of in utero chorionic villus sampling for diagnosis of intrauterine fetal death.

Methods.—In all, 102 specimens from early fetal losses were evaluated. There were 33 skin biopsy specimens, 19 from spontaneous abortions and 14 from fetal tissues obtained after evacuation for intrauterine fetal death. Thirty-six specimens contained products of conception; 7 came from amniocentesis, and 26 from chorionic villus sampling. All of the villus specimens were obtained by the transcervical approach. Specimens were processed by either a direct or a long-term culture method.

Results.—All of the chorionic villus specimens grew, compared to failure rates of 36.1% to 85.7% for the other types of specimens. Of the chorionic villus samples, 95.7% were abnormal. The overall rate of successful growth and karyotyping was 58.6%. Of these, 56.9% were chromosomally abnormal. Of the abnormal karyotypes, 71% were trisomies, 12.9% were 45,X, 9.6% were triploid, and 3.2% each were mosaics and multiple trisomies. The mean maternal ages were 29.25 for normal karyotypes and 36.67 for abnormal karyotypes.

Conclusions.—Postmortem chorionic villus sampling offers the best chance of a cytogenetic result in early fetal loss. Long after the embryo has died, the extraembryonic component appears to remain viable and continues to grow. The greatest chance of a successful karyotype is in samples obtained when fetal death is diagnosed.

▶ The degree of embryonic and fetal wastage is high in humans, with studies suggesting that 50% to 80% of fertilized ova are lost before the second trimester. Chromosomal abnormalities are a significant factor in fetal loss but are difficult to determine in cultures of aborted material. In this study, patients in whom fetal death was found by ultrasound had either a transcervical biopsy of the placenta or a culture of the aborted material for karyotyping. Successful karyotyping and a high percentage of abnormal karyotypes are more likely to be obtained by chorionic villus sampling than in postmortem cultures.—A.J. Garvin, M.D., Ph.D.

Cytogenetic Profile of 109 Lipomas

Sreekantaiah C, Leong SPL, Karakousis CP, McGee DL, Rappaport WD, Villar HV, Neal D, Fleming S, Wankel A, Herrington PN, Carmona R, Sandberg AA (Cancer Ctr of Genetrix, Scottsdale, Ariz; Univ of Arizona; Roswell Park Mem Inst, Buffalo; Cigna Healthplan of Arizona, Tucson; Tucson Med Ctr; et al)

Cancer Res 51:422–433, 1991 1–9

Background.—Recent studies have identified cytogenetic subtypes in lipomas that may have probable implications in the biology and behavior of these tumors.

Methods.—Cytogenetic analysis of short-term cultures was undertaken on 109 lipomas from 92 patients. Results were also correlated with clinicopathologic data.

Results.—Clonal chromosomal abnormalities were present in 50% of tumors. Of these tumors with clonal abnormalities, 70.5% contained cytogenetically normal cells; only 12% had abnormalities in all of the cells. Three main groups of tumors were identified based on their cytogenetic characteristics: tumors with normal karyotypes; tumors with abnormalities involving region q13–15 on chromosome 12; and tumors with other clonal aberrations. Rearrangement of chromosome 12 at bands q13–15 was the most consistent change, accounting for 64% of the tumors. These tumors included subgroups with t/ins(1;12)(p32–33;q13–15), t(2;12)(p21–22;q13–14), t(3;12)(q28;q14), t(12;21)(q13;q21), complex, and nonrecurrent aberrations. The tumors with heterogeneous clonal abnormalities included subgroups with del(13)(q12q22), der(6)(p21–23), der(11)(q13), and nonspecific aberrations. Structural rearrangements in lipomas preferentially involved chromosome bands 1p36, 1p32–33, 2p21–22, 3q27–28, 6p21–23, 11q13, 12q13–15, 13q12, 13q22, 17p13, 17q21, and 21q21–22. There was a significant correlation between abnormal karyotype and age and sex of the patient, as well as depth, size, and site of the tumor.

Implications.—These results confirm the nonrandom involvement of chromosomal regions 12q13–15, 3q27–28, 6p21–23, and 13q12–22, and identify new cytogenetic subtypes involving specific regions on chromosomes 1, 2, 11, and 21. The identification and establishment of these specific chromosomal abnormalities may allow characterization of the biology and behavior of lipomas.

▶ The karyotype of many soft tissue tumors is diagnostically important. Although lipomas are rarely a diagnostic problem, the karyotype of tumors in this series was related to the age, sex, depth, size, and site of the tumor. These results suggest that altered gene function may give rise to these benign tumors.—A.J. Garvin, M.D., Ph.D.

Diagnostic Value of DNA Analysis in Effusions by Flow Cytometry and Image Analysis: A Prospective Study on 102 Patients as Compared With Cytologic Examination

Rijken A, Dekker A, Taylor S, Hoffman P, Blank M, Krause JR (Univ of Pittsburgh)

Am J Clin Pathol 95:6–12, 1991 1–10

Introduction.—Although cytologic examination often detects malignant disease in patients with effusions, the method does not diagnose all neoplasms. Ancillary methods for detecting cancer in effusions (e.g., chromosome analysis and tissue culture) have not been entirely successful. Chromosome abnormalities are strong evidence for neoplasia, and DNA content can be detected by flow cytometry and image analysis. The value of DNA analysis of effusions by flow cytometry combined with image analysis was compared with that of the more conventional cytologic technique.

Materials.—Cytology and flow cytometry were used to examine 126 effusion samples from 102 consecutive patients. Thirty-one fluid samples, 26 malignant and 5 benign, were also examined by image analysis. The samples were from 75 pleural, 46 peritoneal, and 5 pericardial effusions.

Results.—The overall correlation between cytologic and flow cytometry results was 84%. Among 36 malignant neoplasms determined by cytologic examination, flow cytometry revealed an aneuploid peak in 20. When image analysis was performed on the malignant cytologic cells with a diploid flow pattern, 2 additional aneuploid peaks were detected. Three neoplasms initially interpreted as benign by cytologic examination were found by flow cytometry to be aneuploid. Twenty-three of the 24 aneuploid cases detected by flow cytometry were associated with malignancy, yielding a predictive value of 96%.

Conclusion.—The use of flow cytometry is advantageous when moderate to large numbers of tumor cells are present. Specimens containing smaller numbers of malignant cells can be directly analyzed with image analysis. If an aneuploid peak is found, suggesting malignancy, an initially negative cytologic screen should be reviewed. When tumor cells are diploid, neither flow cytometry nor image analysis will aid in tumor detection. Thus cytologic examination remains the definitive technique in some cases.

▶ The sensitivity of the cytologic detection of malignancy in effusions is low. Ancillary techniques have been proposed to increase the sensitivity, including cytogenetics, tissue culture, electron microscopy, and immunohistochemistry. This prospective study compares the use of flow cytometry and image analysis to aid in the diagnosis of malignancy in effusions. The detection of an aneuploid population of cells was synonymous with the detection of malignancy. However, 25% of all tumors are diploid and 10% to 15% are near diploid (1). Therefore, this technique would provide for a maximum sensitivity of 60%.—A.J. Garvin, M.D., Ph.D.

Reference

1. Barlogie B, et al: *Cancer Res* 43:3982, 1983.

Improved Flow Cytometric Determination of Proliferative Activity (S-Phase Fraction) From Paraffin-Embedded Tissue

Weaver DL, Bagwell CB, Hitchcox SA, Whetstone SD, Baker DR, Herbert DJ, Jones MA (Maine Cytometry Research Inst, Portland; Maine Med Ctr, Portland; Univ of Vermont)

Am J Clin Pathol 94:576–584, 1990 1–11

Introduction.—Recent studies indicate that the S-phase fraction (SPF) may be a better prognostic indicator than total nuclear DNA content in various neoplasms. Little work has been done, however, on SPF from paraffin-embedded tissue specimens because of contamination by debris.

Methods.—Cell cycle analysis was performed on 124 matched tissue specimens. One part of each fresh tissue specimen was frozen and the other was processed and embedded in paraffin. It was possible to estimate the S-phase in both frozen and paraffin-embedded specimens in 81 instances.

Findings.—When 2 new subtraction algorithms were used to subtract debris from the histograms, the coefficient of correlation between SPF values for frozen tissues and those for paraffin-embedded tissues was .80. Use of a standard exponential debris subtraction algorithm rather than the multicut and single-cut algorithms (which relate to the magnitude and position of histogram peaks) gave a correlation of .67. Correlation for aneuploid cases was closest when the SPF was calculated as a percentage of the aneuploid cell population.

Conclusions.—The S-phase fraction can be reliably estimated from paraffin-embedded tissues, and this fact should widen the use of SPF as a prognostic indicator. In studies of the prognostic value of SPF, it may be necessary to set different S-phase cut-off values for diploid and aneuploid tumors.

▶ The proliferative activity of some solid tumors is an important prognostic factor. One method of measuring proliferative activity is to measure the SPF of a tumor by flow cytometry. This technique generally requires fresh tissue and is not possible when tissue cannot be spared or for retrospective studies. Previous attempts to measure the SPF of paraffin-embedded tissue have been difficult and unreliable because of measurable debris. In this study, 2 algorithms were used to subtract the debris allowing correlation of SPFs from frozen and paraffin-embedded tissue. This will allow for reliable measurement of the SPF on the paraffin-embedded material.—A.J. Garvin, M.D., Ph.D.

Effects of Various Fixatives and Fixation Conditions on DNA Ploidy Analysis: A Need for Strict Internal DNA Standards

Esteban JM, Sheibani K, Owens M, Joyce J, Bailey A, Battifora H (City of Hope Natl Med Ctr, Duarte, Calif)

Am J Clin Pathol 95:460–466, 1991 1–12

Background.—Cell cycle and DNA ploidy analyses are used increasingly as supplemental, but sometimes independent, predictors of the biological behavior of various malignancies. Studies have been mostly retrospective, using archival paraffin-embedded tissues likely to have been fixed and processed differently. The effects of various fixatives and fixation conditions on DNA ploidy analysis were evaluated in a prospective study.

Study Design.—Five contiguous pieces from 26 fresh tissue samples were fixed in formalin for 8, 24, and 48 hours; in B5 for 4 hours; and in ethanol-based fixative (Omnifix) for 2–6 hours. The samples were prepared and stained by Hedley's method. Cell cycle and DNA studies were performed with a flow cytometer, and the resulting histograms were interpreted with Multicycle software (Phoenix Flow Systems). The mean channels and the coefficients of variation (CVs) of G_0/G_1 peaks and DNA indices were compared.

Findings.—The mean channels of the G_0/G_1 peaks varied with increasing fixation times in formalin, producing a left-shifted histogram with differences up to 13 channels. Omnifix induced similar but more remarkable changes, with maximal shifting of 51 channels. Tissues fixed in B5 produced right-shifted histograms with differences up to 22 channels. The CVs worsened progressively with increasing fixation times with formalin. Omnifix and B5 yielded the poorest histograms. With a CV cut-off value of 8, about half of the tissues fixed in Omnifix and one third of those fixed in B5 would have been considered uninterpretable.

Conclusions.—Fixatives and fixation conditions are critical in the evaluation of DNA ploidy from paraffin blocks. The wide variations in DNA content after different fixations may explain some of the controversies about the clinical significance of DNA ploidy analysis. Internal DNA standards and more stringent criteria are needed to define aneuploidy in paraffin-embedded tissues. Samples obtained from adjacent nonmalignant tissue that has been fixed and processed simultaneously with the tumor may provide a more accurate and reliable internal standard for DNA analysis of paraffin-embedded tissues.

▶ This paper provides solid documentation of what many have suspected in their own laboratories and in interpreting the literature on DNA ploidy analysis. This is the kind of study that can help to bring about more reasonable expectations of ploidy analysis on the part of both clinicians and pathologists.—W.A. Gardner, Jr., M.D.

Analysis of Antigen Receptor Gene Rearrangements in Ethanol and Formaldehyde-Fixed, Paraffin-Embedded Specimens

Wu AM, Ben-Ezra J, Winberg C, Colombero AM, Rappaport H (City if Hope Natl Med Ctr, Duarte, Calif)
Lab Invest 63:107–114, 1990 1–13

Background.—Neoplastic cell lineage has been studied by molecular hybridization analysis of DNA prepared from frozen specimens or from fresh cells. A study was undertaken to determine whether high-molecular weight DNA suitable for nucleic acid hybridization studies can be obtained from paraffin-embedded material.

Methods.—For 9 representative lymphoid lesions, DNA was extracted from frozen sections by standard methods and from ethanol-fixed tissue in paraffin blocks. The extracted DNA was subjected to Southern blot hybridization and probed for rearrangements of immunoglobulin genes and of the T cell receptor beta-chain gene.

Findings.—Yields of DNA from ethanol-fixed blocks and from frozen tissue were comparable. Similar probing results were obtained in each case regardless of the source of DNA, and identical results were obtained with DNA extracted from ethanol-fixed blocks and stored for 2 years. Five of 6 formaldehyde-fixed, paraffin-embedded tissue specimens yielded spoolable DNA, but the DNA was degraded more than that obtained from frozen or ethanol-fixed specimens. Many hybridization studies based on formaldehyde-treated DNA were not interpretable.

Conclusion.—Ethanol-fixed, paraffin-embedded tissues are an excellent source of DNA for use in nucleic acid hybridization studies. Such tissues are easily handled and can be stored for long periods.

▶ The application of molecular techniques for diagnostic purposes requires the optimal preservation of DNA and/or RNA. The authors compare the DNA obtained from frozen sections with DNA from ethanol and formaldehyde-fixed, paraffin-embedded tissue. The extracted DNA was probed by Southern blot hybridization for markers of B and T cell clonality. Formalin-fixed, paraffin-embedded tissue was less than optimal compared to freezing or ethanol fixation.—A.J. Garvin, M.D., Ph.D.

In Situ Hybridization of Immunoglobulin Light Chain mRNA in Paraffin Sections Using Biotinylated or Hapten-Labelled Oligonucleotide Probes

Pringle JH, Ruprai AK, Primrose L, Keyte J, Potter L, Close P, Lauder I (Univ of Leicester, England; Univ of Cape Town, South Africa)
J Pathol 162:197–207, 1990 1–14

Introduction.—The demonstration of specific mRNAs in tissue section by in situ hybridization may be used to determine patterns of gene expression at the cellular level. A technique was developed for detecting immunoglobulin light-chain mRNAs in routine pathology specimens using specific hapten-labeled oligonucleotide probes; these were compared with RNA probes derived from the same recombinant sequences.

Methods.—The method detects κ- or λ-constant region sequences using synthetic oligonucleotide probes labeled with biotin or fluorescein 5-isothiocyanate (FITC) as a reporter molecule. The probes are labeled chemically at flanking sites by primary amine-directed acylation and by "homopolymer tailing" with terminal deoxynucleotidyl transferase. The mRNA is unmasked in formalin-fixed tissue sections by digestion with proteinase K. Hybrids are demonstrated using alkaline phosphatase and either a streptavidin-biotin-based 4-stage system or an anti-FITC antibody-based detection system. Alkaline phosphatase is visualized by the Fast Red naphthol-capture method.

Results.—Specific mRNAs may be detected using these nonradioactive methods, and good morphology is retained. Compared with immunocytochemical studies for light-chain immunoglobulin, this approach does not stain extracellular immunoglobulin and nonspecific background staining is virtually absent.

Summary.—This method has been applied to non-Hodgkin's lymphoma, Hodgkin's disease, and multiple myeloma. It is especially advantageous in studying the site of gene expression where the gene product is rapidly transferred from cells into tissue.

▶ The immunohistochemical demonstration of cytoplasmic immunoglobulin (Ig) has been possible for some time (1). However, the presence of cytoplasmic Ig can be related either to its production by the cell or the uptake of exogenous Ig by way of Fc receptors. The technique described in this study eliminates this background staining, in addition to extracellular Ig. This should be an improvement in the demonstration of cytoplasmic Ig.—A.J. Garvin, M.D., Ph.D.

Reference

1. Garvin AJ, et al: *Am J Pathol* 82:457, 1976.

Identification of Mutations in the COL4A5 Collagen Gene in Alport Syndrome

Barker DF, Hostikka SL, Zhou J, Chow LT, Oliphant AR, Gerken SC, Gregory MC, Skolnick MH, Atkin CL, Tryggvason K (Univ of Utah; Univ of Oulu, Finland; Univ of Rochester)

Science 248:1224–1227, 1990 1–15

Introduction.—X-linked Alport's syndrome, a hereditary glomerulonephritis, is characterized by progressive loss of kidney function and is frequently accompanied by progressive loss of hearing. Ultrastructural defects in glomerular basement membranes (GBMs) in patients with this syndrome suggest that the cause of nephritis is an altered structural protein. An attempt was made to identify mutations in the COL4A5 collagen gene in Alport's syndrome.

Results.—The product of COL4A5, the α5(IV) collagen chain, is a specific component of GBM in the kidney. The gene maps to the same X chromosomal region as that for Alport's syndrome. Three structural aberrations were identified in COL4A5. These were an intragenic deletion, a Pst I site variant, and an uncharacterized abnormality. These structural aberrations appeared to cause nephritis and deafness, with allele-specific severity, in 3 kindreds with Alport's syndrome seen in Utah.

Conclusions.—The demonstration of 3 different mutations in the COL4A5 gene in 3 kindreds with Alport's syndrome supports the hypothesis that mutations in this gene account for at least some, and possibly all, X-linked Alport's syndrome. It is likely that a wide range of mutations will eventually be found on the COL4A5 gene in patients with Alport's syndrome.

▶ This report identifies mutations in a gene for a collagen component of GBM. This gene was mapped to the X chromosome in the same region as Alport's syndrome, a hereditary glomerulonephritis with associated deafness. Mutations in this gene may account for the pathogenesis of this rare syndrome.—A.J. Garvin, M.D., Ph.D.

A Major Segment of the Neurofibromatosis Type 1 Gene: cDNA Sequence, Genomic Structure, and Point Mutations

Cawthon RM, Weiss R, Xu G, Viskochil D, Culver M, Stevens J, Robertson M, Dunn D, Gesteland R, O'Connell P, White R (Howard Hughes Med Inst, Salt Lake City; Univ of Utah)

Cell 62:193–201, 1990 1–16

Background.—A new gene, the translocation breakpoint region (TBR) gene, found at the neurofibromatosis type 1 (NF1) locus, is interrupted by deletions and a translocation breakpoint. The TBR gene may be the NF1 gene, but the rearrangements could actually be compromising the relationship between some other gene and its regulatory elements.

Methods.—Overlapping cDNA clones were sequenced from the TBR gene, and a 4-Kb sequence was compared with sequences of genomic DNA.

Findings.—Identification of splice junctions and of a large open reading frame indicated that the TBR gene is oriented with its 5′ end toward the centromere, in contrast to the 3 known active genes in this region. Polymerase chain reaction amplification of a subset of exons and electrophoresis of the denatured product demonstrated 6 variant conformers specific to patients with NF1. This indicates the occurrence of base pair changes in the gene. One mutant allele contained a T-to-C transition that altered a leucine to a proline, and another exhibited a C-to-T transition that changed an arginine to a stop codon.

Conclusion.—These findings establish the TBR gene as the gene of NF1. A basic molecular pathophysiologic understanding of the disease may allow effective intervention.

▶ Neurofibromatosis type 1 is one of the most frequent and important of the inherited autosomal dominant disorders. Affected individuals have peripheral neurofibromas and café-au-lait spots, as well as an increased risk of learning disabilities, renal hypertension, and malignancies. This study identified the gene on chromosome 17 that gives rise to these clinical manifestations and discovered mutations in the gene in 6 patients. As the gene becomes more fully characterized, the molecular biology and molecular pathophysiology associated with gene mutations should begin to emerge.—A.J. Garvin, M.D., Ph.D.

Identification of the Primary Gene Defect at the Cytochrome P_{450} *CYP2D* Locus

Gough AC, Miles JS, Spurr NK, Moss JE, Gaedigk A, Eichelbaum M, Wolf CR (Clare Hall Labs, Potters Bar, England; Univ Dept of Biochemistry, Edinburgh; Dr Margarete Fischer-Bosch Inst of Clinical Pharmacology, Stuttgart, Germany)

Nature 347:773–776, 1990 1–17

Background.—The mammalian cytochrome P_{450}-dependent monooxygenase system is involved in drug metabolism. There is an autosomal recessive polymorphism at the cytochrome P_{450} *CYP2D6* debrisoquine hydrolyase locus that results in the "poor-drug-metabolizer" phenotype. Reportedly, this polymorphism is associated with an altered cancer risk. The primary mutation responsible for this polymorphism was identified and used to develop a DNA-based assay to identify at-risk persons. The association of this polymorphism with lung and bladder cancer also was explored.

Method.—To develop a genetic assay for the poor metabolizer phenotype, cDNA associated with normal *(db1)* and "a" and "b" variants was isolated. Variant "a" contained a base pair deletion, which introduces a frameshift that leads to a premature stop codon. Variant "b" contained a frameshift caused by an insertion. Of the 40 poor metabolizers analyzed, 2 contained no *db1* (deletion) and 38 contained both variants, indicating that variant "b" is irrelevant to the phenotype. By using the variant "a" sequence, the phenotype of 44 normal metabolizers and 89% of 42 poor metabolizers could be predicted.

Results.—An analysis of the frameshift site of the "a" variant indicated that no normal individuals were homozygous for this mutation; however, 79% of poor metabolizers were homozygous for this frameshift. Therefore, the variant "a" frameshift mutation appears to be the predominant mutation associated with the poor metabolizer phenotype. The association of this mutation with cancer was examined in 140 patients with lung cancer and 117 with bladder cancer. In both types of cancer the mutant phenotype appeared to be associated with a reduced risk of cancer.

Conclusions.—The primary mutation responsible for the poor metabolizer phenotype can be used in a genetic test to identify those at risk. If the association between this mutant phenotype and cancer is real, the normal product of this locus may be directly involved in the initiation of cancer by chemical carcinogens, e.g., those found in cigarette smoke.

▶ The development of this DNA-based genetic assay offers the exciting prospect of a simple test to those at risk of drug side effects. This assay should also allow resolution of the continuing question of whether there is a genetically based susceptibility to environmental carcinogens.—W.A. Gardner, Jr., M.D.

Automation of Specific Human Gene Detection

Mayrand PE, Hoff LB, McBride LJ, Bridgham JA, Cathcart R, Corcoran KP, Golda GS, Keith DH, Lachenmeier EW, Madden DE, Mordan W, Recknor MW, Shigeura J, Ting C-H, Whiteley NW, Ziegle JS, Kronick MN (Applied Biosystems Inc, Foster City, Calif)
Clin Chem 36:2063–2071, 1990 1–18

Background.—Automation is greatly needed in molecular biology. A system was developed that automates a chemical procedure functionally equivalent to Southern blotting.

Procedure.—Samples are produced by a prototype liquid-handling instrument that automates a solution-phase hybridization/solid-phase capture chemistry for DNA analysis. A fluorescence gel scanner that detects migrating DNA fragments in real-time analyzes the samples. This chemistry, combined with the gel scanner and robotic automation, eliminates the tedium involved in traditional techniques for specific gene detection. It also reduces the time needed for analysis from days to hours. The measurement of restriction fragment lengths is made more precisely using in-lane standards to minimize effects attributable to migration anomalies.

Conclusions.—This automated, fluorescent, gel-scanning instrument, combined with robotic liquid handling, can be used successfully to automate specific human gene detection. It yields results similar to those produced by Southern blotting. The procedure is simpler and quicker than the manual techniques currently used and does not involve radioactivity.

▶ As more genetic defects related to human disease are identified, widespread availability of their mechanisms of diagnosis will be required. Automation of the labor-intensive laboratory processes now used for gene analysis will be crucial for the incorporation of this methodology into routine laboratory procedures. This paper describes an initial attempt at such automation that can produce results equivalent to those of Southern blotting.—D.J. Wells, Ph.D.

Neoplasia

Cancer-Associated Carbohydrates Identified by Monoclonal Antibodies
Sell S (Univ of Texas, Houston)
Hum Pathol 21:1003–1019, 1990 1–19

Background.—"New" carbohydrate antigens have been found on the surface of, or are secreted by, cancer cells. The structure of these antigens, identified by monoclonal antibodies as epitopes, was examined, with special attention to clinically useful markers.

Review.—These carbohydrate structures may result from the accumulation of precursor chains with deletion of more complex structures. This process could occur because of decreased synthesizing enzyme activity, increased or aberrant glycosylation of carbohydrate chains resulting in production of new oligosaccharides, changed density of cell surface carbohydrates, or exposure of chains that are usually covered by other structures. Glycolipid synthesis alterations may include aberrant sialyation and fucosylation of the type 1 or type 2 lacto series, sialyation or fucosylation of the globo series, or increased sialyation of the ganglio series. Important markers in this series include CA 15.3, CA 19.9, CA 50, CA 125, CA 242, MCA, and SLEX, among others. None of the globo series oligosaccharides is clinically useful. The important cancer antigen, B72.3, which is sialyated Tn, results from incomplete glycosylation of O-linked mucin oligosaccharide. Some of the glycoproteins with complex carbohydrate components include α-fetoprotein, whose level of glycosylation determines the binding ability of lectins; carcinoembryonic antigen, whose weight may be up to 60% different carbohydrates; and epidermal growth factor receptor, which includes several type 1 and type 2 lacto chain structures. Other cell surface glycoproteins contribute to lectin and monoclonal antibody binding by altering the cell surface expression of mannose of sialic acid. Many of the glycosylation patterns of cancer cells or their products reflect those seen during normal development; therefore, oligosaccharides associated with cancer are oncodevelopmental in nature.

Conclusions.—Many of the carbohydrate markers are not diagnostically useful because they are not specific for cancer. The useful markers may give information on prognosis or monitoring of patients with various types of cancer. Carbohydrates on cell surfaces may play a role in cell to cell recognition, intracellular glycoprotein processing, and cell activation, and in the ability of cancer cells to metastasize.

▶ The author comprehensively, yet succinctly, reviews cancer-associated molecules with carbohydrate epitopes that can be detected by monoclonal antibodies. Many alterations in carbohydrate moieties have been identified in cancer cells, and carbohydrate structures are typically preserved in formalin-fixed, paraffin-embedded tissue, whereas protein epitopes may be destroyed. These structures, then, have important potential as tumor markers. The author reviews the metabolic pathways leading to the formation of the glycolipids, mucins, and glycoproteins that have a known association with cancer. The relationship to normal products (e.g., blood group antigens) is illustrated. In addition to monoclonal antibody probes against these antigens, there is also a brief discussion of lectins. Some of these tumor markers have a proven role in monitoring patients and, to a lesser extent, in establishing prognosis. Continued progress may yield diagnostic and therapeutic roles. Although the elaborate and complex metabolism of these carbohydrate moieties suggests an important biological role, the function of most of these structures in both normal and neoplastic cells remains largely speculative.—J.A. Tucker, M.D.

Altered Expression of the Retinoblastoma Gene Product in Human Sarcomas

Cance WG, Brennan MF, Dudas ME, Huang C-M, Cordon-Cardo C (Mem Sloan-Kettering Cancer Ctr, New York: PharMingen, San Diego)

N Engl J Med 323:1457–1462, 1990 1–20

Background.—The retinoblastoma (Rb)-susceptibility gene is the prototype tumor suppressor gene that can promote tumor growth when both alleles are inactivated. The Rb gene encodes a nuclear phosphoprotein, the expression of which is altered in several human tumors.

Methods.—Expression of the Rb gene product was studied in 44 primary and 12 metastatic high-grade human sarcomas by immunohistochemical and Western blot techniques. Computerized image analysis quantified the level of Rb gene product in individual tumor cells.

Results.—Thirteen primary sarcomas (30%) exhibited normal expression of Rb protein in nearly all of the tumor cells. In 40%, the protein was heterogeneously expressed, and in 30% it was present in fewer than 20% of tumor cells. Expression of Rb protein was altered in all metastatic sarcomas. In patients with primary sarcoma, survival was significantly better among those whose tumors expressed Rb protein homogeneously.

Conclusions.—Expression of the Rb gene product may be a useful prognostic indicator in patients with sarcoma. Those whose tumors express the protein in an altered manner might be candidates for investigational treatments.

▶ Human sarcomas comprise a spectrum of tumors of mesenchymal origin. The most important factors predicting their clinical behavior are their size and grade. The grade of a sarcoma is based on the histologic assessment of differentiation, cellularity, necrosis, and number of mitotic figures. The histologic type of sarcoma (e.g., liposarcoma, leiomyosarcoma, or malignant fibrous histiocytoma) is not an independent prognostic factor (1). The high incidence of sarcomas in patients who survive Rb suggested that this suppressor gene may be associated with sarcomas as well. Indeed, deletions and mutations in the Rb gene have been found in some sporadic sarcomas (2). Decreased expression of the gene product correlated with a more aggressive clinical behavior. The quantitation of this protein may be an important prognostic factor in the behavior of sarcomas.—A.J. Garvin, M.D., Ph.D.

References

1. Collins C, et al: *J Clin Oncol* 5:601, 1987.
2. Reissmann PT, et al: *Oncogene* 4:839, 1989.

Lineage-Restricted Clonality in Biphasic Solid Tumors

Fletcher JA, Pinkus GS, Weidner N, Morton CC (Brigham and Women's Hosp; Children's Hosp, Boston)

Am J Pathol 138:1199–1207, 1991 1–21

Introduction.—Occasional tumors are characterized by the proliferation of both epithelial and mesenchymal elements, e.g., the chondroid hamartoma of the lung and the adenofibroma of the breast. The histogenesis of these biphasic tumors remains controversial. A combined immunohistochemical/cytogenetic analysis was made of 2 biphasic solid tumors that enabled the simultaneous determination of the neoplastic nature of each component.

Findings.—In 1 of the 2 pulmonary hamartomas studied, the neoplastic proliferation was limited solely to the mesenchymal component, and the epithelial cells appeared to be reactive. The same was true for 2 of the 9 breast adenofibromas. The remaining pulmonary hamartoma and 1 of the breast adenofibromas consisted entirely of mesenchymal tissue. Four adenofibromas were mosaics, containing cells with clonal cytogenetic aberrations and others without chromosomal abnormality. Five adenofibromas lacked chromosomal aberrations altogether.

Conclusions.—Because the mesenchymal component is the only neoplastic element of a pulmonary chondroid hamartoma, it should be redesignated as a "pulmonary chondroma." Carcinoma within a breast fibroadenoma appears to arise from reactive epithelial proliferation and not from a neoplastic epithelium. A combined immunohistochemical and cytogenetic analysis may prove helpful in assessment of additional new biphasic solid tumors.

▶ This study describes a new approach to determining the neoplastic nature of a biphasic tumor. Are both components neoplastic, or has one component proliferated as the result of the proliferation of another? This technique provides a way to answer this question.—A.J. Garvin, M.D., Ph.D.

Ki-67 Labeling Index Is a More Reliable Measure of Solid Tumor Proliferative Activity Than Tritiated Thymidine Labeling

Deshmukh P, Ramsey L, Garewal HS (Univ of Arizona; Tucson VA Med Ctr)

Am J Clin Pathol 94:192–195, 1990 1–22

Introduction.—Ki-67 is a monoclonal antibody directed against a proliferation-related nuclear antigen. It recognizes cells in all phases of the cycle except G_0. It should therefore identify most proliferative cells from a tumor. The tritiated thymidine labeling index identifies only S-phase cells.

Methods.—Seven solid tumor specimens were obtained from surgical resections. Portions were halved, and each half was processed for thymidine labeling or Ki-67 labeling.

Findings.—In all 7 solid tumors examined, the Ki-67 labeling index exceeded the thymidine labeling index. Thymidine indices ranged from 4% to 17%, and Ki-67 labeling indices ranged from 26% to 41%. Variations between different sections of a given specimen were substantially less with the Ki-67 method.

Conclusion.—The Ki-67 labeling index may be more reliable than the tritiated thymidine labeling index for assessing the proliferative activity of tumors. Consistently more tumor cells are labeled with the Ki-67 technique.

▶ The proliferative activity of some solid tumors is an important prognostic factor. This has been demonstrated in breast carcinoma in several series (1,2). In this study, measurement of proliferative activity was compared by the classic method of ^{3}H-thymidine labeling versus immunostaining for a nuclear antigen, Ki-67. The Ki-67 activity was greater and demonstrated less variability than with the classic method.—A.J. Garvin, M.D., Ph.D.

References

1. Gentili C, et al: *Cancer* 48:974, 1981.
2. Meyer JS, et al: *Cancer* 57:1879, 1983.

Tumor Infiltrating Leukocytes (TILs) During Progressive Tumor Growth and BCG-Mediated Tumor Regression

Steerenberg PA, De Jong WH, Elgersma A, Burger R, Poels LG, Claessen AME, Den Otter W, Ruitenberg EJ (Natl Inst of Public Health and Environmental Protection, Bilthoven, The Netherlands; Robert Koch Inst, Berlin; Univ of Nijmegen, The Netherlands; Free Univ Hosp, Amsterdam)

Virchows Arch [B] 59:185–194, 1990 1–23

Background.—Immune response mediation of tumor regression is poorly understood. Light and electron microscopy have been used to study the regression of hepatocellular carcinoma induced by bacille Calmette-Guerin (BCG). The role of tumor-infiltrating leukocytes (TILs) and the expression of major histocompatibility complex (MHC) class I and II antigens on TILs and tumor cells have not been studied during tumor regression. An immunohistochemical study was made of the inflammatory reaction in progressively growing and BCG-treated line 10 tumors.

Methods.—Hepatocellular carcinoma cells were injected into strain 2 guinea pigs. Seven days later, intralesional injection of BCG was done to induce tumor regression. At day 12, during the induction phase of immunity, and at day 28, during immune-mediated tumor regression, TILs were characterized by immunohistochemical methods using 11 monoclonal antibodies (MoAbs).

Results.—At day 12, no major differences were seen between TIL subpopulations of treated and untreated tumors. Most of the TILs were T cells, as shown by MoAbs against Pan-T cells, T cytotoxic/suppressor cells, and T helper/inducer cells. Some macrophages also were seen. At day 28, the fibrous stroma was dramatically increased in most of the tumors treated with BCG. Thus the tumor cell islets were smaller than those in untreated tumors. Increased numbers of T cells and macrophages were present in BCG-treated tumors, and MHC antigens were strongly expressed in TILs and tumor stroma in growing and regressing tumors. The tumor cells showed no MHC antigens before inoculation, and they were not expressed in the centers of the tumor islets at days 12 and 28. Tumor cells expressed MHC class I and II antigens at sites where they lay close to the fibrous stroma or TILs, especially in BCG-treated tumors.

Conclusions.—After BCG treatment to induce immunity, increased numbers of macrophages and expression of MHC class I antigen are seen. Immune-mediated regression is clear by day 28. The total amount of MHC antigens is increased by their presence on almost all TILs, on the fibrous stroma, and on some tumor cells.

▶ The immune-mediated regression of this model system was studied by immunohistochemical analysis of tumor leukocytes and the MHC antigens. Antigens I and II probably have a crucial role in the interaction between tumor cells and the immune system. Within this model system, immunohistochemical studies demonstrated increased MHC antigens during tumor regression.—A.J. Garvin, M.D., Ph.D.

Reexcision Perineural Invasion: Not a Sign of Malignancy

Stern JB, Haupt HM (Dermatopathology Consultation Services, Damascus, Md; Pennsylvania Hosp, Philadelphia)

Am J Surg Pathol 14:183–185, 1990 1–24

Introduction.—Perineural invasion occurs occasionally in various malignancies. It can be an ominous finding in squamous cell cancers of the head and neck, but it also has been associated with several benign disorders. Epithelial perineural invasion was encountered in 2 reexcision specimens removed because a melanocytic lesion was found at initial biopsy.

Case 1.—Man, 26, had reexcision of a pigmented spindle cell nevus from his lower back 6 days after initial biopsy. Zones of apparently benign epithelial cells infiltrated perineurally in the midreticular dermis (Fig 1–5). No neoplasia was observed.

Case 2.—Woman, 82, who had reexcision of a lentigo maligna from her cheek also had apparently benign epithelial cells in a perineural distribution without evidence of malignancy.

Discussion.—In distinguishing between reexcision perineural invasion and perineural invasion from a primary epithelial neoplasm, the former is

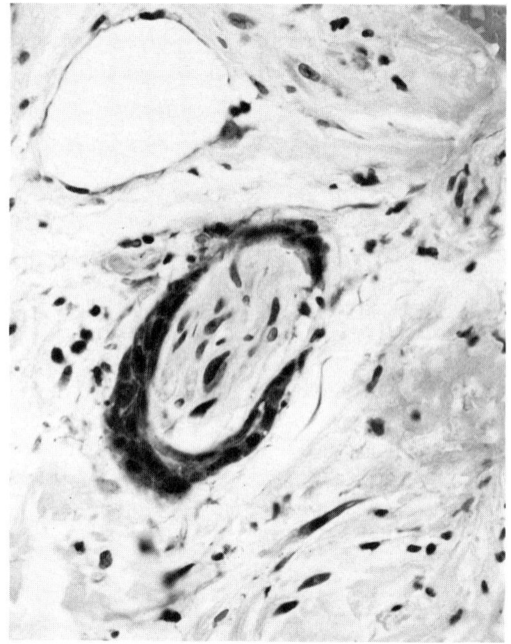

Fig 1–5.—High-power view of nerve showing perineural invasion by apparently benign epithelial cells. (Courtesy of Stern JB, Haupt HM: *Am J Surg Pathol* 14:183–185, 1990.)

favored by the absence of perineural spread beyond the immediate biopsy site and by a benign appearance of the perineural epithelial cells. In addition, the absence of residual epithelial tumor helps to exclude neoplastic invasion.

▶ Implantation of squamous epithelial cells into the perineural lymphatics can occur from surgical excision. A caveat for the surgical pathologist!—A.J. Garvin, M.D., Ph.D.

Influence of Cigarette Smoking on the Levels of DNA Adducts in Human Bronchial Epithelium and White Blood Cells

Phillips DH, Schoket B, Hewer A, Bailey E, Kostic S, Vincze I (Inst of Cancer Research, London; Natl Inst of Hygiene, Budapest; Med Research Council Labs, Carshalton, Surrey, England; Korányi Natl Inst of Pulmonology, Budapest)

Int J Cancer 46:569–575, 1990 1–25

Purpose.—The ^{32}P-postlabeling assay for detection of carcinogen-DNA adducts is well suited for evaluating smoking-induced DNA damage. This assay has been used to demonstrate a linear relationship between cigarette consumption and levels of aromatic DNA adducts in human peripheral lung. The presence of these adducts may be an indication of cancer risk.

Methods.—Deoxyribonucleic acid was isolated from nontumorous bronchial tissue obtained from 8 nonsmokers, 8 former smokers, and 37 cigarette smokers. It was also isolated from peripheral white blood cells in blood samples obtained from 31 heavy smokers and 20 nonsmokers. By using the ^{32}P-postlabeling assay, the presence of aromatic or hydrophobic DNA adducts, or both, was investigated.

Findings.—Adducts were detected as diagonal bands of radioactivity, which were generally more intense in the samples from smokers than in those from former or nonsmokers. The distribution of adduct levels in the 3 groups did not differ significantly from normal distributions; however, adduct levels were significantly higher in smokers than in either nonsmokers or former smokers. Differences between nonsmokers and former smokers were not significant. There was a linear correlation between levels of adducts and number of cigarettes smoked daily, and a similarly significant correlation between the cumulative lifetime intake of cigarette smoke and levels of adducts, but the correlation coefficient was lower. There was no significant difference between DNA from white blood cells of smokers and nonsmokers in either levels or patterns of aromatic-hydrophobic adducts.

Discussion.—Aromatic-hydrophobic DNA adducts appear to be found more frequently in the respiratory tracts of smokers than in those of nonsmokers. Such damage is associated with early events in carcinogenesis; therefore, the findings support epidemiologic evidence that correlates smoking with lung cancer. Because there was no observable effect in white blood cell DNA, there are limits to the extent to which nontarget sources of DNA can be used as surrogate markers for determining exposure.

▶ For years, tobacco apologists and those rationalizing the overwhelming evidence for a relationship between tobacco use and neoplasia have pointed to the absence of a "smoking gun," i.e., direct cause and relationship. This paper takes us a step nearer to that evidence. Such direct evidence is likely to come with the demonstration of tobacco-specific DNA adducts similar to the tobacco-specific hemoglobin adduct that has been demonstrated (1) in tobacco users, especially snuff dippers.—W.A. Gardner, M.D.

Reference

1. Carmella SG, et al: *Cancer Res* 50:5438, 1990.

Perinatal Pathology

The Association of Single Umbilical Artery With Cytogenetically Abnormal Pregnancies

Saller DN Jr, Keene CL, Sun C-CJ, Schwartz S (Univ of Maryland)

Am J Obstet Gynecol 163:922–925, 1990 1–26

Introduction.—The occurrence of a single umbilical artery in the umbilical cord is among the most common umbilical cord abnormalities of clinical significance. Several early descriptions of autosomal trisomies mention a single umbilical artery as an occasional feature in anecdotal cases. A possible association between a single umbilical artery and aneuploidy was examined.

Karyotypes Found in Association With Single Umbilical Artery

Karyotype	*No.*
47,XY,+13	2
47,XX,+18	2
46,XX,del(5)(qter→p14:)	1
46,XX/47,XX,+9	1

Courtesy of Saller DN Jr, Keene CL, Sun C-CJ, et al: *Am J Obstet Gynecol* 163:922-925, 1990.)

Findings.—Between 1982 and 1989, of 109 cytogenetically abnormal pregnancies identified from amniocentesis specimens and tissue culture specimens, the number of umbilical cord vessels could be documented in only 53 cases. Six (11.3%) of these 53 pregnancies had a single umbilical artery. A single umbilical artery was noted in 2 of 9 fetuses with trisomy 18, in 2 of 6 fetuses with trisomy 13, and in 2 fetuses with other unusual chromosomal constitutions (table). None of the 18 fetuses with trisomy 21 and none of the 11 with sex chromosome abnormalities had a single umbilical artery.

Conclusion.—The presence of a single umbilical artery is associated with anatomical and karyotypic abnormalities. Trisomy 21 does not appear to be associated with a single umbilical artery.

▶ Diagnosis of a single umbilical artery must be confirmed by microscopic examination of a section taken more than 2 cm from the placental insertion site where the 2 arteries sometimes fuse to form 1 vessel. The single umbilical artery may arise either by failure of development or by remodeling or obliteration of 1 of the 2 umbilical arteries. Other associations with the single umbilical artery include twinning (usually, the smaller twin), preterm delivery, fetal growth retardation, maternal diabetes mellitus, seizure disorders, toxemia of pregnancy, antepartum hemorrhage, polyhydramnios, and oligohydramnios (1,2).—E.A. Manci, M.D.

References

1. Leung AKC, et al: *Am J Dis Child* 143:108, 1989.
2. Some H: *Curr Top Pathol* 66:159, 1979.

Separation of the Umbilical Cord: Histological Findings

Oudesluys-Murphy AM, den Hollander JC (Zuiderziekenhuis, Rotterdam; Erasmus Univ, Rotterdam)

Biol Neonate 58:54–56, 1990 1–27

Background.—There is great interest in how the umbilical cord separates, but the process has not been described in the literature. A histologic study of the umbilical area was conducted in 25 infants who died within 7 days after birth.

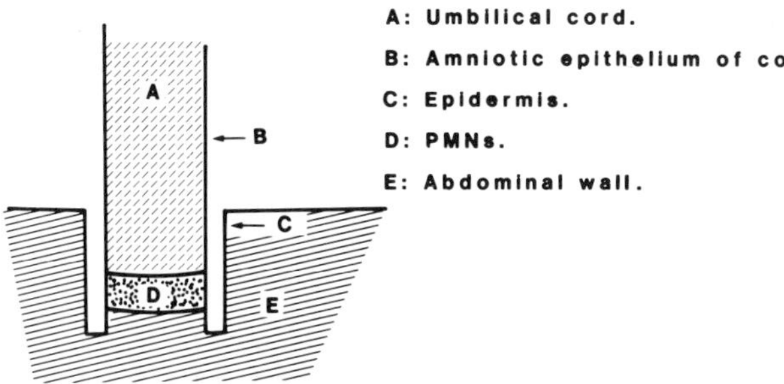

Fig 1–6.—Schematic representation of the junction between the umbilical cord and the epidermis at the time of cord separation. (Courtesy of Oudesluys-Murphy AM, den Hollander JC: *Biol Neonate* 58:54–56, 1990.)

Methods.—The infants' mean age at death was 3 days (mean gestational age, 33 weeks). Autopsies were done within 72 hours of death. Transverse blocks of tissue were removed 1 cm cranially and 1 cm caudally from the center of the umbilicus, and a longitudinal section was taken between these 2 blocks.

Findings.—In all cases except those in which the cord had recently separated, the transition from epidermis to amniotic epithelial covering was

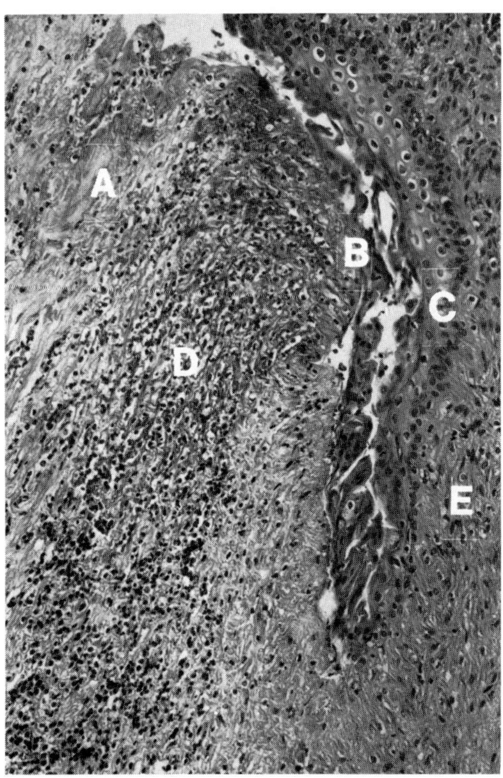

Fig 1–7.—Photograph of the area delimited by the square in Figure 1–6, showing the junction between the amniotic epithelium covering of the cord and the epidermis, with infiltration of PMNs; original magnification, ×120. (Courtesy of Oudesluys-Murphy AM, den Hollander JC: *Biol Neonate* 58:54–56, 1990.)

visible. The cord stump became dried and mummified, with no bacteria or leukocytes in it. Infiltrating polymorphonuclear leukocytes (PMNs) were seen in all sections at the junction of the umbilicus and the epidermis. The band of PMNs progressed from the edge toward the center (Figs 1–6 and 1–7) and formed a demarcation zone between the cord stump and the umbilical area. The PMNs were the only cells in this zone.

Conclusions.—Separation of the umbilical cord appears to involve mummification of the stump and infiltration of the area of separation with PMNs. This zone of demarcation is found superficially in the plane of the epidermis. Its extent of development varied among the preparations studied.

▶ Delayed separation of the umbilical cord has been associated with widespread infections, defective neutrophil mobility, and a genetically determined deficiency of leukocyte adherence glycoproteins.—E.A. Manci, M.D.

The Clinical Significance of Absent Subchorionic Fibrin in the Placenta

Naeye RL (Pennsylvania State Univ)

Am J Clin Pathol 94:196–198, 1990 1–28

Background.—Fibrin is usually found on the undersurface of the chorionic plate of the placenta. To determine whether this fibrin is the consequence of fetal movements that strike the placenta, data from a large prospective study were analyzed to learn whether conditions associated with fetal activity are associated with increased or decreased amounts of placental subchorionic fibrin.

Methods.—Data on 31,622 full-term placentas and children from the Collaborative Perinatal Study were evaluated. The amount of subchorionic fibrin in the placentas was analyzed, and individual clinical outcomes chosen to reflect normal and abnormal fetal motor activity were studied. Neonatal hypotonia or lethargy, Down's syndrome, and a short umbilical cord were the markers of fetal hypoactivity. The tension applied to the umbilical cord strongly influences its length; shorter cords are associated with fewer movements.

Results.—Fibrin was absent in 11% of placentas, patchy in 64%, and diffuse in 25%. It was often absent when the child had neonatal hypotonia or lethargy, CNS malformations, Down's syndrome, breech presentation at delivery, quadriplegic cerebral palsy, or a low IQ score in later childhood. Cord length was abnormally short in 5% of the placentas, normal in 85%, and abnormally long in 10%. Short cords were also associated with markers of fetal hypoactivity. Subchorionic fibrin was increased in the placentas of mothers whose children were hyperactive at 1 year of age, suggesting that these children were hyperactive before birth.

Conclusions.—Normal fetal movements may traumatize the placenta, leading to fibrin deposits beneath its surface. There apparently is an association between reduced fetal activity and the absence of subchorionic fibrin. In conjunction with other findings, this finding may help to establish whether a child's psychomotor abnormalities originated before labor and delivery.

▶ This important observation suggests that absence of subchorionic fibrin belongs to the spectrum of the fetal akinesia syndrome as an indicator of decreased intrauterine fetal activity. This gross placental finding identifies infants who require frequent follow-up for evaluation of psychomotor development and who may benefit by early intervention.—E.A. Manci, M.D.

The Association of Maternal Floor Infarction of the Placenta With Adverse Perinatal Outcome

Andres RL, Kuyper W, Resnik R (Univ of California, San Diego)

Am J Obstet Gynecol 163:935–938, 1990 1–29

Introduction.—Maternal floor infarction of the placenta is fairly rare. On gross examination this disorder is characterized by a thickened yellow placental floor. There is histologic evidence of massive deposition of fibrin involving the decidua basalis and contiguous villi. This lesion is thought to be recurrent and has been linked to fetal death and intrauterine growth retardation. The association between this disorder and an adverse perinatal outcome was investigated.

Findings.—Forty-eight women had maternal floor infarction a total of 60 times. Fetal death occurred in 24 of the 60 cases (40%). Twenty-one of 36 liveborn infants (58.3%) were born preterm. Nineteen of 35 liveborn infants whose birth weight was known had evidence of intrauterine growth retardation (54%). Five of the 41 multiparous women in this series had documented recurrences. The reproductive histories of these 48 women, which included a total of 196 pregnancies, revealed a significant incidence of fetal death (24.1%), intrauterine growth retardation (31.3%), and preterm death (35.4%).

Discussion.—The association between maternal floor infarction and fetal death stresses the importance of a placental examination in all cases of fetal death and infants with intrauterine growth retardation. Because there is a risk of recurrence, identification of maternal floor infarction should alert clinicians to the potential for fetal death, preterm birth, and growth retardation in subsequent pregnancies.

▶ Maternal floor infarction is misnamed because ischemic changes are not features of the areas of fibrin deposition or of the surrounding viable chorionic villi. It is recognized as a cause for elevation of maternal serum α-fetoprotein (1). In addition to these adverse perinatal associations, a long-term follow-up study indicates that infants who survive a maternal floor infarction are at increased risk for mental retardation with motor abnormalities (2). Close monitoring of subsequent pregnancies has been beneficial (3).—E.A. Manci, M.D.

References

1. Katz VL, et al: *Am J Perinatol* 4:225, 1987.
2. Naeye RL: *Disorders of the Placenta, Fetus and Neonates. Diagnosis and Clinical Significance.* St Louis, Mosby—Year Book, 1992, pp 148–154.
3. Clewell WH, et al: *Am J Obstet Gynecol* 147:346, 1983.

Can One Make a Diagnosis of Intrauterine Pregnancy in the Absence of Chorionic Villi?

Daya D, Sabet L (McMaster Univ; Univ of Western Ontario, London)
Surg Pathol 3:205–210, 1990 1–30

Background.—The identification of chorionic villi in uterine curettings provides a positive diagnosis of intrauterine pregnancy. It has been established that intermediate trophoblast (IT) is present routinely in the decidual cells at the implantation site. Although decidual cells and IT cells are morphologically different, they may not be distinguishable using routine stains. The feasibility of using certain immunohistochemical markers to more specifically identify IT cells was evaluated.

Methods.—A total of 57 cases of uterine curettings with chorionic villi (ranging from 4 to 17 weeks of gestation) were included. Three slides from each specimen were analyzed. Immunohistochemistry studies included cytokeratin (AE_1/AE_3), another low-molecular-weight cytokeratin (CAM 5.2), and human placental lactogen (hPL), using the peroxidase antiperoxidase (PAP) method to evaluate these markers. A control representing "pure decidual tissue" without trophoblast also was tested.

Findings.—All 15 control samples of "pure" decidua were totally negative for the 3 immunohistochemical markers tested. Intermediate trophoblast, however, appeared strongly positive for both cytokeratin markers AE_1/AE_3 and CAM 5.2. These IT cells resided in sheets of decidua that had enlarged hyalinized vessels (Fig 1–8). The hPL marker was

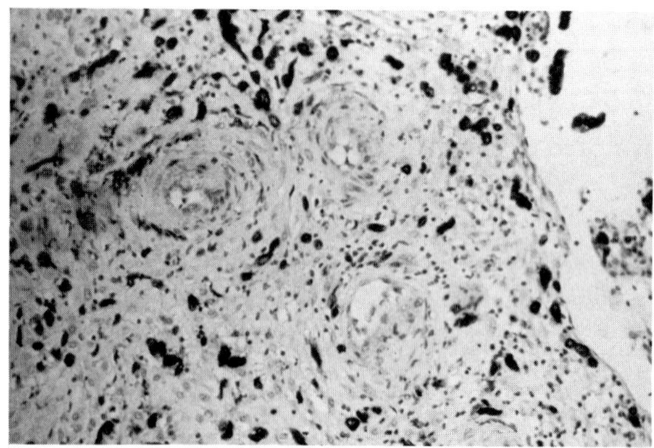

Fig 1–8.—Individually scattered intermediate trophoblastic cells within decidua stain with cytokeratin AE_1/AE_3. Similar results were obtained with cytokeratin CAM 5.2. (Courtesy of Daya D, Sabet L: *Surg Pathol* 3:205–210, 1990.)

slightly positive in 30% of IT cells. The endometrial glands were positive for both cytokeratin markers, but the stain pattern of the glands could be seen easily, whereas the IT cells appeared scattered among the decidual cells.

Conclusion.—These results support the use of cytokeratin markers, but not hPL, for IT cells in decidual cells associated with intrauterine pregnancy. Such markers can aid in the diagnosis of intrauterine pregnancy even when chorionic villi are absent in the tissue sample.

▶ These authors provide evidence that one can diagnose intrauterine pregnancy using immunohistochemical stains for cytokeratin to identify IT. This procedure may be very useful in solving a common diagnostic problem in surgical pathology.—A.J. Garvin, M.D., Ph.D.

Rapid Prenatal Diagnosis of Congenital *Toxoplasma* Infection by Using Polymerase Chain Reaction and Amniotic Fluid

Grover CM, Thulliez P, Remington JS, Boothroyd JC (Stanford Univ; Institut de Puericulture, Paris)

J Clin Microbiol 28:2297–2301, 1990 1–31

Background.—Congenital *Toxoplasma* infection can be treated in the fetus, or therapeutic abortion can be performed if the condition is diagnosed prenatally. However, attempts at in utero diagnosis are rare because the process is time consuming; also, many infected mothers do not transmit the infection to their offspring. A prospective study was done to determine the feasibility of in utero diagnosis using a recently developed polymerase chain reaction (PCR).

Methods.—The study sample comprised 43 pregnant women in whom *Toxoplasma* infection acquired during pregnancy was detected by serologic screening. Another 5 positive women were later selected, along with 5 patients with other indications for amniocentesis to serve as a negative control group. Mouse inoculation or cell culture was used to establish the diagnosis of fetal infection. Polymerase chain reaction was performed by direct lysis of pelleted amniotic fluid cells, followed by amplification of a gene sequence specific for *Toxoplasma gondii.*

Results.—*Toxoplasma gondii* was correctly identified by PCR in 5 of 5 samples from 4 patients with proven congenital infection. In the nonprospective group, PCR detected 3 of 5 positive cases. Detection of specific IgM and inoculation of amniotic fluid into tissue culture, although comparable in speed to PCR, correctly identified 3 and 4 of 10 positive samples, respectively. Seven of 10 positive samples were correctly identified by mouse inoculation of amniotic fluid and fetal blood, a process that takes considerably longer. No method yielded a false positive diagnosis.

Conclusions.—Congenital *T. gondii* infection can be detected rapidly and sensitively prenatally by PCR. The diagnosis might be made as early as 15–19 weeks of gestation, although 20 weeks was the earliest time of amniocentesis in the present study. Such timely diagnosis could allow early treatment with pyrimethamine and sulfonamides, which is usually restricted to documented cases of fetal infection.

▶ The exquisite sensitivity of this technology is again demonstrated in the context of an immediate clinical application. As with other potential diagnostic applications of PCR, uncertainties about patent rights, licensing fees, and so on cloud the future of this entire field. This is another area in which technology is well ahead of legal, commercial, and administrative practices.—W.A. Gardner, Jr., M.D.

Amniotic Fluid Glucose Concentration: A Rapid and Simple Method for the Detection of Intraamniotic Infection in Preterm Labor

Romero R, Jimenez C, Lohda AK, Nores J, Hanaoka S, Avila C, Callahan R, Mazor M, Hobbins JC, Diamond MP (Yale Univ)

Am J Obstet Gynecol 163:968–974, 1990 1–32

Background.—Intra-amniotic infection appears to be associated with preterm labor and delivery.

Methods.—The value of amniotic fluid glucose concentrations in the rapid diagnosis of intra-amniotic infection was determined in 168 patients with preterm labor and intact membranes who underwent amniocenteses. Amniotic fluid was cultured for aerobic and anaerobic bacteria and *Mycoplasma* species.

Findings.—Cultures of amniotic fluid were positive in 13.6% of women studied. Patients with positive cultures had significantly lower median amniotic fluid glucose levels than those with negative cultures. Amniotic fluid glucose levels of less than 14 mg/dL had a sensitivity of 86.9%, a specificity of 91.7%, a positive predictive value of 62.5%, and a negative predictive value of 97.8% in detecting positive amniotic fluid culture.

Discussion.—Amniotic fluid glucose determination proved to be a sensitive test for detecting intra-amniotic infection in women with preterm labor and intact membranes. Amniotic fluid glucose determination is also fast, simple, and inexpensive.

▶ The fact that a concept is simple does not mean that all of its applications have been determined. A low glucose concentration in body fluid has long been an indicator of inflammation/infection. The mechanisms that produce this finding in the CSF, pleural fluid, and the like appear to work equally well in amniotic fluid and allow an earlier suspicion of infection than might otherwise be possible. A subsequent study (1) confirms the utility of this technique and demonstrates an improved specificity (at the expense of sensitivity) by use of a lower cut-off level.—B.D. Bennett, M.D., Ph.D.

Reference

1. Kirshon B, et al: *Obstet Gynecol* 164:818, 1991.

Detection of Phenylketonuria in the Very Early Newborn Blood Specimen
Doherty LB, Rohr FJ, Levy HL (Children's Hosp, Boston)
Pediatrics 87:240–244, 1991 1–33

Introduction.—The standard filter paper blood specimen test for phenylketonuria (PKU) and other neonatal disorders is usually performed 2–3 days after birth before discharge from the nursery. Early hospital discharge of the mother and infant, however, has prompted screening the neonate during the first day of life. Some physicians have voiced concern that this may lead to overlooking some infants who have PKU but do not manifest the condition until several days post partum. The level of phenylalanine concentrations in newborns at risk for PKU was determined.

Methods.—The pregnancies of women who had previous children with PKU or with non-PKU mild hyperphenylalaninemia were reviewed. Their newborns were tested for phenylalanine via heel puncture at 4, 12, and 24 hours of age and at nursery discharge. The medical records for each affected neonate and the feeding history were examined.

Results.—During the 6 years of the study, 23 neonates at risk for hyperphenylalaninemia were assessed. Six of the 23 had PKU and 1 had non-PKU mild hyperphenylalaninemia, each similar to a metabolic defect found in a sibling. The 6 PKU neonates had blood phenylalanine levels of 3 mg/dL or higher at 4 hours or 6 hours of age. At 12 hours post partum, these infants had phenylalanine levels ranging from 3 to 7 mg/dL and, at 24 hours of age, 6–10 mg/dL. At discharge after 2–4 days, their phenylalanine concentrations were 8 mg/dL or higher. Unaffected neonates had early phenylalanine levels of less than 2 mg/dL. Evaluation of the relationship between early protein ingestion and early blood phenylalanine levels demonstrated that the relatively high content of protein and phenylalanine in colostrum produced a higher calculated protein and phenylalanine intake for breast-fed as opposed to formula-fed infants during the first 3 days of life.

Implications.—A cut-off level of 4 mg/dL for serum phenylalanine would have missed the 2 infants with PKU who had a blood phenylalanine concentration of 3 mg/dL during the first 12 hours of life. By causing a cut-off level of 2 mg of phenylalanine per dL, all neonates with PKU would have been identified in this study population. In addition, breast-feeding did not delay the increase in the serum phenylalanine level in those infants with PKU during the first 24 hours of life.

▶ Newborn screening programs require major efforts by personnel responsible for the collection and distribution of screening specimens. Such efforts are largely negated if the samples are handled or obtained inappropriately. Emphasis on cost-efficient medical care has resulted in a significant number of discharges from the neonatal nursery within the first 24 hours of life. The policy makes blood samples that would previously have been considered inappropriate now the only available specimens for analysis in many cases. This paper discusses the effect of early analysis on detection of PKU and suggests that, in these early samples, standard reference levels may need to be changed.

As screening techniques for inherited metabolic diseases become more sophisticated, their use will expand and screens for additional diseases will become available. Current methods of screening will also undoubtedly be revised to include gene analysis techniques (1,2). As with other laboratory tests, results are only as good as the specimen provided. If less than adequate specimens must be used for evaluation, the precise effects on results must be known and taken into consideration.—B.D. Bennett, M.D., Ph.D.

References

1. Prior TW, et al: *Clin Chem* 36:1756, 1990.
2. Ranieri E, et al: *Br Med J* 302:1237, 1991.

Clinical Biochemistry of Preeclampsia and Related Liver Diseases of Pregnancy: A Review

Freund G, Arvan DA (Univ of Rochester)

Clin Chim Acta 191:123–152, 1990 1–34

Background.—Pregnancy is associated with substantial changes in metabolic and biochemical processes. The pathophysiologic mechanisms of certain syndromes unique to pregnancy—preeclampsia, eclampsia, HELLP syndrome, and fatty liver of pregnancy—were reviewed.

Discussion.—In preeclampsia and related liver diseases of pregnancy, the disease mechanisms are largely unknown. Thus multiple markers and sequential test analysis must be done to characterize and follow the disease. Laboratory studies reported to date have rarely been systematic and are not uniform enough to allow data pooling. In all liver disease there is sometimes discordance between the severity of symptoms and the degree of serum enzyme abnormality. Women with severe preeclampsia may have normal or slightly raised levels of transaminases at first, with the same tests becoming markedly abnormal within hours as the patient's clinical status changes. Frequent sampling may be needed to confirm rapid changes in biochemical abnormalities and to monitor the development of complications. Initial laboratory findings may also be normal or only slightly abnormal in women with hemolysis, elevated liver enzymes, and low platelet count (HELLP) syndrome and with fatty liver of pregnancy. Rapid deterioration of clinical status appears to be associated with, or followed by, equally fast changes in laboratory values. However, asynchrony may also occur. The concentration or activity of plasma enzymes or other relevant analytes at any point in time indicates the net effect of several variables.

Conclusions.—Evidence suggests that preeclampsia and eclampsia, the HELLP syndrome, and fatty liver of pregnancy comprise a spectrum of the same disease. Currently, delivery is the treatment of choice for any of these conditions. Further research on pathogenetic mechanisms is clearly needed.

▶ This article gives an excellent review of the "normal" changes that occur in pregnancy and their impact on routine laboratory testing. Having thus established a different frame of reference for this patient population, the authors describe deviations that occur in patients with diseases unique to pregnancy and with the disseminated intravascular coagulation that may accompany such diseases. The paper brings to our attention the fact that laboratory abnormalities associated with these important conditions would be misinterpreted without knowledge of the basic laboratory changes occurring in all pregnancies. The progression of increased activation of the coagulation system (occurring in normal pregnancy) to a state of chronic consumptive coagulopathy (in hypertensive disorders of pregnancy) discussed in this article is supported by Reinthaler et al. (1). The latter authors describe enhanced activation of the coagulation cascade as indicated by measurement of thrombin and antithrombin complexes occurring in chronic hypertensive disorders of pregnancy.

Another recent study emphasizes the use of laboratory testing to identify a patient population at risk for the development of preeclampsia. Sanchez-Ramos et al. (2) describe decreased levels of urinary calcium excretion in a patient who later became preeclamptic. This finding encourages prospective laboratory testing to identify at-risk patients and stimulates interest in the role of altered calcium metabolism in the development of preeclampsia. In this regard, other common laboratory tests should be evaluated as "flags" for early identification of patients with potentially serious complications of pregnancy.—B.D. Bennett, M.D., Ph.D.

References

1. Reinthaller A, et al: *Br J Obstet Gynaecol* 97:506, 1990.
2. Sanchez-Ramos L, et al: *Obstet Gynecol* 77:685, 1991.

Human Placenta Expresses Endothelin Gene and Corresponding Protein Is Excreted in Urine in Increasing Amounts During Normal Pregnancy

Benigni A, Gaspari F, Orisio S, Bellizzi L, Amuso G, Frusca T, Remuzzi G (Mario Negri Inst for Pharmacological Research, Bergamo, Italy; Ospedali Riuniti di Bergamo; Univ of Brescia, Italy)

Am J Obstet Gynecol 164:844–848, 1991 1–35

Background.—The systemic and renal hemodynamic changes that occur in normal pregnancy are believed to be partly a result of changes in the vascular synthesis of vasodilatory prostaglandins. In addition to vasodilatory substances, endothelium generates vasoconstrictors, including endothelin. The ability of placental tissue from normal pregnant women to express endothelin gene and to generate endothelin was explored.

Methods.—Three groups of normotensive women were included: 9 women in their first trimester, 7 women in their second trimester, and 8 women admitted for routine delivery at 28–40 weeks of gestation. The possible influence of placental endothelin production on plasma levels of the peptide also was studied.

Results.—Placental tissue expressed a single 2.3-kb preproendothelin mRNA. It produced comparable amounts of endothelin 3, Big endothelin 1, and endothelin 1, as well as a minor amount of endothelin 2. Plasma endothelin levels, measured at delivery, were numerically higher than those in nonpregnant women. Urinary excretion of endothelin tended to increase, although nonsignificantly, in the first 14 weeks of pregnancy. This trend continued throughout pregnancy and resulted in a significant rise from the second trimester to delivery.

Conclusions.—Normal placental tissue expresses the endothelin gene and generates endothelin, a 21-amino-acid peptide originally isolated from porcine aorta that induces hypertension in rats when infused intravenously. There was a numerical tendency for endothelin plasma levels to rise in pregnancy.

▶ These data are consistent with the concept of endothelin as a local regulator of blood supply to the tissues. Vascular endothelium generates endothelin as well as vasodilator substances, which must be in appropriate balance. The role of endothelin biosynthesis and/or metabolism in the hypertensive disorders of pregnancy and in maternal tobacco use needs further study.—E.A. Manci, M.D.

Pediatric Pathology

Children Born to Women With HIV-1 Infection: Natural History and Risk of Transmission

Ades AE, Newell ML, for the European Collaborative Study (Inst of Child Health, London)

Lancet 337:253–260, 1991 1–36

Background.—Knowledge of the natural history of vertically acquired HIV-1 comes primarily from analysis of children with symptoms seen in specialist centers. The European Collaborative Study, a prospective investigation of children born to HIV-infected mothers, was conducted.

Methods.—A total of 600 children born to infected mothers in 10 European centers were examined every 3 months after birth to 18 months of age. Thereafter, they were examined every 6 months.

Findings.—At the last follow-up, 64 children were considered HIV infected, and 353 had lost antibody and were presumed to be uninfected. In infected children the initial clinical feature was usually a combination of persistent lymphadenopathy, splenomegaly, and hepatomegaly. However, 30% of the children had AIDS or oral candidiasis rapidly followed by AIDS. About 83% of infected children had laboratory or clinical signs of HIV infection by 6 months of age. By 12 months, 26% had AIDS and 17% had died of HIV-related disease. The disease subsequently progressed more slowly, with most children remaining stable or even improving in the second year. Based on results in 372 children born at least 18 months before the analysis, the vertical transmission rate was 12.9%. Virus has been isolated repeatedly in an additional small percentage of children who lost maternal antibody and who remain normal clinically and immunologically. Without a definitive virologic diagnosis, the monitoring of immunoglobulins, CD4/CD8 ratio, and clinical signs was able to identify HIV infection in 48% of infected children by 6 months, with a greater than 99% specificity.

Conclusions.—In the absence of a definitive diagnosis, immunologic and clinical signs can serve as predictors of HIV infection in children younger than 18 months. These findings have implications for management and the design of clinical trials.

▶ The broad spectrum of HIV-1 infection recognized in adults, including minor complaints and even "healthy carriers," has recently been described among pediatric patients. Early detection of HIV infection is increasingly important because antiretroviral treatment is now available. In the absence of HIV-defining symptoms, laboratory diagnosis has been complicated by the persistence of passively acquired maternal antibodies in infants up to 15 months of age, the delay/absence of HIV antibody production in some infected children, the low sensitivity of viral culture, and the variable expression of p24 antigen during the course of the HIV infection (1).—E.A. Manci, M.D.

Reference

1. McKinney, RE, et al: *J Pediatr* 116:640, 1990.

Prostate Development in Prune Belly Syndrome (PBS) and Posterior Urethral Valves (PUV): Etiology of PBS—Lower Urinary Tract Obstruction or Primary Mesenchymal Defect?

Popek EJ, Tyson RW, Miller GJ, Caldwell SA (Armed Forces Inst of Pathology, Washington, DC; Univ of Louisville; Univ of Colorado; Children's Hosp, Denver)

Pediatr Pathol 11:1–29, 1991 1–37

Background.—Prune belly syndrome (PBS) is characterized by the absence of abdominal wall musculature, undescended testes, and urinary tract anomalies. The etiology remains unclear. Some authors have proposed theories of mesenchymal maldevelopment, obstruction, and genetic origin. The role of lower urinary tract obstruction as it relates to prostatic development and PBS was assessed.

Methods.—The autopsy files of 3 institutions were reviewed (dating back to 1976). Fifteen cases of PBS were identified. These patients were compared with 8 patients with posterior urethral valves (PUV) and 34 age-matched controls.

Results.—After assessment of the mesenchymal and epithelial differentiation and relationships, distinctly different and consistent abnormalities between PBS and PUV were found. In PBS, prostatic growth and development appeared to be hindered because of destruction or absence of the appropriate primitive mesenchyme.

Conclusions.—This is a detailed study of the lower urinary tract in infants with PBS and PUV compared to normal controls. The lack of normal development of the prostate appears to be the etiologic mechanism in the development of PBS. Differentiating between the 2 disorders may be important for surgical treatment in utero or neonatally. A detailed level 3 ultrasound of the fetal urinary system or a neonatal-voiding cystourethrogram may help clinicians to identify the abnormalities that distinguish PBS and PUV.—A.J. Garvin, M.D., Ph.D.

Pediatric Fine-Needle Aspiration Biopsy

Silverman JF, Gurley AM, Holbrook CT, Joshi VV (East Carolina Univ)
Am J Clin Pathol 95:653–659, 1991 1–38

Objective.—A total of 135 fine-needle aspiration (FNA) biopsies were performed in 123 children aged 1 day to 18 years during a 5-year period. All but 5 of the biopsy specimens were suitable for evaluation. The most frequent biopsy sites were superficial lymph nodes, the abdomen, breast, and thyroid gland. Clinical and/or histopathologic follow-up was available in 120 cases.

Findings.—No false positive diagnoses were made in the patients followed up. There were 4 false negative diagnoses, for a sensitivity of 90.6%; 3 of them involved aspirates from the CNS. Fifty neoplasms were diagnosed, 28 malignant. The positive and negative predictive values of FNA biopsy were 100% and 94%, respectively.

Discussion.—Fine-needle aspiration biopsy is an accurate, safe, rapid, and inexpensive way of assessing superficial and deep masses in children that can be done in the outpatient setting. The procedure has allowed treatment of unresectable malignancies, provided material for culture of infectious lesions, avoided operating on benign lesions, and helped surgeons to plan the extent of surgery for resectable malignant tumors.

▶ The authors review their experience with the use of FNA in the pediatric population. The most valuable use was in the evaluation of lymphadenopathy. Whereas the aspiration of tumors can be helpful in identification of recurrence, the diagnosis of primary tumors in children often requires the ancillary techniques of immunohistochemistry, electron microscopy, tissue culture, and cytogenetics. The FNA specimen can be used for each of these, but usually an insufficient quantity of material is obtained for all of these techniques. In addition, there are no data on the potential risk of seeding childhood tumors with aspiration. Fine-needle aspiration is suboptimal in recognizing the definite histologic type of neoplasm. Verdeguer et al. reported 12 unsatisfactory specimens among 70 FNAs in children (1). Lymph nodes, which are most frequently reactive, can easily be aspirated and cultured for diagnostic purposes.—A.J. Garvin, M.D., Ph.D.

Reference

1. Verdeguer A, et al: *Med Pediatr Oncol* 16:98, 1988.

Metachronous Soft-Tissue Masses in Children and Young Adults With Cancer: Correlation of Histology and Aspiration Cytology

Wakely PE Jr, Powers CN, Frable WJ (Med College of Virginia)

Hum Pathol 21:669–677, 1990 1–39

Introduction.—Twenty-eight fine-needle aspiration biopsy specimens of soft tissue were taken from 22 children and young adults (younger than age 30 years) with masses in the peripheral soft tissues or breast that appeared 1 day to 17 years after the diagnosis of a primary malignancy. The mean interval was 39 months.

Findings.—Twenty of the 28 specimens yielded a malignant diagnosis on aspiration cytology, usually sarcoma. Benign diagnoses included gynecomastia, fibroadenoma, and fat tissue necrosis. The overall accuracy of aspiration biopsy was 96%, its specificity was 88%, and its sensitivity was 100%. There was 1 false positive cytologic diagnosis, but there were no false negative diagnoses.

Conclusions.—Fine-needle aspiration biopsy is a useful means of determining the cause of soft tissue masses in children and young adults with cancer. A new primary neoplasm may be found or a benign and unrelated condition may be diagnosed.

▶ Fine-needle aspiration (FNA) can be useful in the assessment of soft tissue masses in adults with a history of cancer. A high degree of accuracy may be obtained and ancillary techniques may be used. The role of FNA in the pediatric population appears to be more in the identification of recurrence than in the primary diagnosis (1).—A.J. Garvin, M.D., Ph.D.

Reference

1. Silverman JF: *Am J Clin Pathol* 95:653, 1991.

Trends in Survival for Childhood Cancer in Britain Diagnosed 1971–85

Stiller CA, Bunch KJ (Univ of Oxford, England)

Br J Cancer 62:806–815, 1990 1–40

Introduction.—To date, the only detailed analysis of childhood cancer survival rates using population-based data from all of Great Britain covered children registered from 1962 to 1970, with a brief addendum for 1971–1974. The survival rates for the whole of Britain for children with cancer diagnosed between 1971 and 1985 were examined.

Findings.—The series analyzed included more than 15,000 childhood cancers. Highly significant improvements in survival were noted for many major diagnostic groups. Between 1971 and 1973 and 1983 and 1985, the actuarial 5-year survival rate rose from 37% to 70% for children with acute lymphoblastic leukemia, from 4% to 26% for those with acute nonlymphoblastic leukemia, from 76% to 88% for those with Hodgkin's disease, from 22% to 70% for those with non-Hodgkin's lymphoma, from 61% to 72% for those with astrocytoma, and from 24% to 42% for medulloblastoma. Also, the actuarial 5-year survival increased from 15% to 43% for neuroblastoma, 58% to 79% for Wilms' tumor, 17% to 54% for osteosarcoma, 26% to 61% for rhabdomyosarcoma, 59% to 94% for malignant testicular germ cell tumors, and 43% to 77% for malignant ovarian germ cell tumors. The 2 main diagnostic groups for which there was no evidence of any trend were retinoblastoma and Ewing's sarcoma. Retinoblastoma already bore an excellent prognosis, with a 5-year survival rate of more than 85%. For Ewing's sarcoma, the survival rate remained below 45%.

Conclusions.—The increases observed in population-based survival rates for many major diagnostic groups reflect the substantial advances since 1970 in treatment of a wide range of childhood cancers. These improvements occurred at a time when increasing numbers of children were treated at specialist centers participating in national and international clinical trials and studies. This centralization of care may provide the opportunity for further improvements in the prognosis of many childhood cancers.

▶ This large clinical study documents the advances in the diagnosis and treatment of 15,000 children with cancer. Noteworthy advances in survival during a 12-year period were made with acute lymphoblastic leukemia, malignant lymphoma, Wilms' tumor, rhabdomyosarcoma, and germ cell tumors of the ovary and testis. Patients with other tumors (e.g., neuroblastoma, medulloblastoma, acute nonlymphoblastic leukemia, and Ewing's sarcoma) did not have the survival rates associated with the other pediatric tumors. Great strides in treatment have also been made in this area by large centers and cooperative study groups, e.g., the Pediatric Oncology Group and the Children's Cancer Study Group in the United States.—A.J. Garvin, M.D., Ph.D.

Follicular Lymphomas in Pediatric Patients

Pinto A, Hutchison RE, Grant LH, Trevenen CL, Berard CW (St Jude Children's Research Hosp, Memphis; Univ of Calgary, Alta)

Mod Pathol 3:308–313, 1990 1–41

Background.—Making the correct diagnosis of follicular lymphoma in children is difficult, as it must be distinguished from follicular hyperplasia. The appearance of follicular lymphoma in the faucial tonsils of 2 children prompted a review of the occurrence of this disease in children.

Patients and Findings.—Follow-up information was available for 20 children with follicular lymphoma. The 15 males and 5 females ranged in age from 2 to 20 years at the time of diagnosis. The lymphoma was localized to lymph nodes in 10 patients and to extranodal sites in 10. At presentation, 15 patients were in stage I, 2 in stage II, and 3 in stage III; the primary tumor sites were the faucial tonsils in 7 patients, other sites in the head and neck in 5, the inguinal lymph nodes in 4 or 5, and the abdomen in 2. There were 6 cases of follicular small cleaved cell type

(FSCC), 5 of follicular mixed small cleaved and large cell, and 9 of follicular large cell. A purely follicular architectural pattern was seen in 5 patients, a predominantly follicular pattern in 6, and a predominantly diffuse pattern in 3. The follicular large cell type progressed from a predominantly follicular to a predominantly diffuse pattern in 1 child.

Outcome.—Complete remission was achieved in all 20 patients. At follow-up of 6 months to 16 years (median, 4 years) 19 patients were alive and disease free. There was 1 death from acute lymphoblastic leukemia 7 years after the diagnosis of FSCC non-Hodgkin's lymphoma. Therapy was initially deferred in 3 patients, which had no apparent adverse influence.

Conclusions.—Follicular lymphoma in children is a rare disorder distinct from follicular lymphoma in adults and from the usual high-grade lymphomas in children. Pediatric follicular lymphoma typically presents with localized disease in the head, neck, or inguinal area, and the outcome is generally favorable.

▶ Follicular lymphomas account for approximately half of the non-Hodgkin's lymphomas in adults. In general, these lymphomas are indolent, high-stage neoplasms that persist or recur after treatment. In contrast, follicular lymphomas in children are so rare (approximately 30 reported cases) that the diagnosis should be viewed with skepticism. In this review, of one of the largest number of reported cases of follicular lymphoma in children, there is direct contrast with the adult form. The tumors were localized and responded to therapy, with a good outcome. This suggests that, in children, follicular lymphoma may be identical morphologically to that in adults but is a biologically different disease.—A.J. Garvin, M.D., Ph.D.

Cellular Peripheral Neural Tumors (Neurofibromas) in Children and Adolescents: A Clinicopathological and Immunohistochemical Study

Coffin CM, Dehner LP (St Paul-Ramsey Med Ctr and Ramsey Clinic, St Paul; Univ of Minnesota)

Pediatr Pathol 10:351–361, 1990 1–42

Background.—Peripheral nerve sheath or neural neoplasms have certain histologic features qualifying them as atypical but not malignant. In a recent review of soft tissue neoplasms in children, 9 lesions initially thought to be neurofibromas were pathologically borderline because of their marked cellularity and focal mitotic activity. The clinicopathologic and immunohistochemical features of these cellular peripheral neural tumors (CPNTs) were compared with those of classic neurofibromas and malignant peripheral nerve sheath tumors (MPNSTs) in other children.

Patients.—The 9 CPNTs were found among 139 peripheral nerve sheath neoplasms in children. There were 60 neurofibromas and 16 MPNSTs in this series. The 9 patients with CPNT had a mean age of 7 years at diagnosis. Four CPNTs were discovered at birth. The ratio of boys to girls was 1:2. The tumors were located on the extremities in 4 children, in the head and neck region in 3, and on the trunk in 2. Four patients had manifestations of von Recklinghausen's neurofibromatosis.

Findings.—Seven children were well after initial resection, but 2 had recurrences. In 1 case the histology was identical to that of the original tumor. In the second, overt malignant transformation had occurred. This second child was the only one to die of tumor-related causes. The CPNTs were circumscribed but not encapsulated, measuring 1.8–7.5 cm. They involved the dermis, the subcutis, and deep soft tissues. The cells had a compact spindle pattern, occasional mitoses, and minor foci of typical neurofibroma. On immunohistochemical staining, immunoreactivity for vimentin was noted in 7 of 7 lesions, that for Leu-7 in 6, that for myelin basic protein and S-100 protein in 5, and that for desmin in 1. Actin was expressed in none. Compared with neurofibroma and MPNSTs, CPNT tended to occur earlier in childhood and slightly more commonly in girls. These tumors had an anatomical distribution and immunoreactivity pattern similar to neurofibroma. The cellularity and mitotic activity of the CPNTs, however, raised concern about prognosis.

Conclusions.—Evidently, CPNT is a variant of neurofibroma and, in this series, represented 15% of those tumors. When a CPNT is found in a child with von Recklinghausen's neurofibromatosis, it may be a low-grade MPNST or nothing more than a disturbing morphological phenomenon without serious implications.

▶ These reviewers of a large series of peripheral nerve sheath tumors in children identified a small number (15%) with marked cellularity and focal mitotic activity. Only 1 tumor demonstrated overt malignant behavior. Thus the morphological features of cellularity and focal mitotic activity rarely identify tumors with malignant potential.—A.J. Garvin, M.D., Ph.D.

Chondrosarcoma of Bone in Children

Young CL, Sim FH, Unni KK, McLeod RA (Mayo Clinic and Found, Rochester, Minn)

Cancer 66:1641–1648, 1990 1–43

Background.—Because chondrosarcoma rarely occurs in children, few reports of the clinicopathologic features and behavior of chondrosarcoma have included patients younger than 20 years. The prognosis in children is reported to be worse than that in adults. The clinicopathologic features of conventional chondrosarcoma in childhood were reviewed.

Patients.—Forty-seven patients younger than 17 years of age were studied. Most lesions were located on the trunk and upper ends of the long bones. The humerus was the most common skeletal site. Twelve tumors were secondary.

Findings.—The radiographic results were similar to those described in series of adults with chondrosarcoma. On pathologic assessment, the tumors were found to be low grade. En bloc resection was the preferred treatment because of the high incidence of local recurrence associated with lesser surgical margins. The prognosis in this series was no worse than that reported for adult chondrosarcoma. None of the children followed had metastasis.

Conclusions.—The prognosis for children with chondrosarcoma appears to be no different from that for adults. Childhood chondrosarcoma seems to be essentially a locally aggressive tumor, with metastasis occurring infrequently and late.

▶ This large series of a rare bone tumor in children demonstrates diagnostic features and clinical behavior identical to that in adults.—A.J. Garvin, M.D., Ph.D.

Intraabdominal Desmoplastic Small-Cell Tumors With Divergent Differentiation: Observations on Three Cases of Childhood

Gonzalez-Crussi F, Crawford SE, Sun C-CJ (Children's Meml Hosp, Chicago; Northwestern Univ; Univ of Maryland)

Am J Surg Pathol 14:633–642, 1990 1–44

Background.—Rarely, an intra-abdominal tumor grows to large size and disseminates widely with no apparent primary site. The peritoneum is usually judged to be the primary site by exclusion, although the tumor conforms to no recognized pattern of peritoneal tumor. In 3 pediatric cases the histopathology was sufficiently repetitive from case to case as to suggest a distinctive clinicopathologic entity.

Patients.—The 2 girls were aged 6 years and 12 years; and the boy was aged 8 years. All 3 were previously healthy. Fever, vomiting, and pain developed in 1; 1 was operated on for appendicitis; and in 1 a mass was discovered on a routine screening examination. All had an intra-abdominal mass attached to the peritoneum and histologic findings of a metastatic epithelial tumor. After follow-up of 1–6 years, however, no evidence of a primary neoplasm was found. Children were treated with chemotherapy and surgery. The boy was alive at 4 years; the 2 girls died after 1 year and 6 years.

Findings.—Histologically, all 3 tumors had discrete islands of compact epithelial-like cells surrounded by fibrous stroma. The nuclei showed 1–3 small nucleoli against the nuclear envelope, and the cell masses were mostly without structure. Nearly all cells stained positive for cytokeratin, and 30% to 50% were immunoreactive to desmin antibodies. On electron microscopy the nuclei were irregular with prominent Golgi apparatus. Intercellular appositions were poorly formed, scanty, and made up of segments of increased subplasmalemmal electron density in adjacent cells.

Conclusions.—These 3 intra-abdominal tumors with no apparent primary site in children appeared to be primitive neoplasms of uncertain histiogenesis that might simultaneously express epithelial, mesenchymal, and sometimes neural phenotypes. Embryonic neoplasms, including nephroblastoma in atypical sites, may be difficult to exclude in children.

▶ To the expanding group of pediatric and adult neoplasms with "small cell" features is added the rare neoplasm described above. The 3 patients presented with intra-abdominal tumors without definite involvement of a parenchymal organ. In each case, the differential diagnosis of metastatic neoplasm from another well-known tumor of childhood, often Wilms' tumor, was entertained. The authors called attention to a similar group of cases described in 1988 at the Pediatric Pathology Society of North America (1) and one additional case (2). As noted in the case histories, most of these tumors have pursued an aggressive course. The description of this neoplasm emphasizes a common problem in surgical pathology: to predict the origin of a primary tumor from its differentiation when there is no obvious parenchymal organ primary site. Clarification of whether this entity is related to other better known pediatric neoplasms, specifically extrarenal Wilms' tumor, awaits further study.— G.F. Worsham, M.D.

References

1. Gerald WL, Rosai J: *Pediatr Pathol* 9:177, 1989.
2. Ordonez NG: *Am J Surg Pathol* 13:413, 1989.

Cytopathology

Cervical Screening Revisited

van der Graaf Y, Vooijs GP, Zielhus GA (Univ of Nijmegen, The Netherlands)
Acta Cytol 34:366–372, 1990 1–45

Background.— Routine screening for cervical cancer has shown its effectiveness in reducing morbidity and mortality only in the later years of its practice. Effectiveness has been shown mainly in studies comparing incidence rates in regions before and after the introduction of screening, or between regions with varying intensities of screening. Some of these results were reviewed, including specific aspects of cervical cancer screening programs.

Review.— Although the potential benefits of screening are evident, there is controversy as to the most efficient and effective organization. A collaborative study of programs in 8 countries suggested that relative protection was substantially lower in areas with no centralized mass screening program. Protection appears to remain high for the first 3 years after the first negative screening and then to decline steadily. However, protection probably remains substantial for 6–9 years, in agreement with the concept that many lesions can remain preinvasive for at least 10 years. The best approach to false negative results is probably thoroughly supervised quality control, although some reports have recommended yearly screening. The consequences of false negative diagnoses could probably be reduced significantly by obtaining a repeat smear 1 year after a first negative smear, then extending the interval to 5 years. Women aged 30–34 years might be included because of the high number of in situ carcinomas in this age group.

Discussion.— Screening appears to be effective if the compliance rate is high, increasing the likelihood that women at increased risk are included, the quality of the sample and the cytologic diagnosis are high, proper follow-up is ensured, and treatment is adequate. Less radical treatment is often required by women whose invasive cervical cancers are diagnosed after the introduction of screening. One disadvantage of screening is the inevitable inclusion of nonprogressive cervical intraepithelial neoplasias in treatment, leading to overtreatment. The large number of false positive diagnoses is another concern. The burden of these diagnoses and the amount of unnecessary damage has been reduced by the introduction of colposcopy. A well-organized screening program, although expensive, should decrease future hospital expenses for the treatment of malignancies.

Conclusions.—Cervical screening programs can be a cost-effective way of dealing with the problem of cervical cancer if they are centrally organized and cautiously executed. All involved parties must cooperate closely. The cost effectiveness of various policies can be compared on computer simulation models.

▶ Modest additional protection against cervical cancer mortality has been reported with every-other-year and annual screening when compared to the every-3-year screening endorsed in this article (1). Annual screening also has theoretical advantages in the presence of rapidly developing cervical carcinomas not associated with preexisting dysplastic cytologic changes (2) and among partially compliant patient groups.—R.M. Austin, M.D., Ph.D.

References

1. Koss LG: *JAMA* 261:737, 1989.
2. Kurman RJ, et al: *Am J Obstet Gynecol* 159:293, 1988.

Significance of Anucleated Squames in Papanicolaou-Stained Cervicovaginal Smears

Kern SB (Medical Arts Lab, Oklahoma City)

Acta Cytol 35:89–93, 1991 1–46

Background.—When anucleated squames are found in Papanicolaou-stained cervicovaginal smears, hyperkeratosis may be suspected. Detec-

Histologic or Cytologic Follow-Up Diagnosis in Patients With Anucleated Squames on Papanicolaou Smears

	Cases	
Diagnosis	**No.**	**%**
Histology		
Condyloma or more serious lesion	9	3.0
Benign hyperkeratosis	25	8.2
Chronic cervicitis without hyperkeratosis	23	7.5
Cytology		
Condyloma or more serious lesion	4	1.3
Persistent anucleated squames	47	15.4
Negative follow-up smear without anucleated squames	196	64.6

(Courtesy of Kern SB: *Acta Cytol* 35:89–93, 1991.)

tion of true hyperkeratosis appears to be an important part of routine evaluation of these smears. Anucleated squames were evaluated as markers of hyperkeratosis with significant underlying atypia.

Methods.—Of 168,215 cervicovaginal smears screened in a 2-year period, 785 (.47%) had anucleated squames and no other abnormality. Laboratory files were searched to find cytologic or histologic follow-up material, which was found for 304 patients (42%).

Results.—Condyloma or some more significant lesion was found in 4.3% of patients (table). The most common finding was a negative follow-up smear. Overall, condyloma or a more significant lesion was found in 1.69% of samples.

Conclusions.—In the absence of any other abnormalities, anucleated squames appear to be of marginal value in screening for significant lesions. Their presence should continue to be noted in patients with known condyloma or dysplasia. The finding of anucleated squames may have low predictive value because of the lack of standardization among pathologists in recognizing them.

▶ Hyperkeratosis or anucleate squamous cells are commonly reported by cytopathology laboratories because of the association of abnormal keratinization of the cervix with underlying human papillomavirus effect and dysplasia/cervical intraepithelial neoplasia. This study identified a group of women with this finding, slightly less than half of whom had follow-up. It provides quantitative information regarding the number of patients who had significant lesions on follow-up and shows that this is a finding with low predictive value. Quantitative information such as provided in this study will be useful in communicating with physicians and justifying laboratory reporting procedures, particularly in light of increasing federal regulation of this part of pathology practice as a result of CLIA'67 and CLIA'88.—G.F. Worsham, M.D.

Longitudinal Study of Women With Negative Cervical Smears According to Endocervical Status

Mitchell H, Medley G (Victorian Cytology Service, Melbourne, Australia)

Lancet 337:265–267, 1991 1–47

Background.—An early repeat test is often recommended for women whose Papanicolaou smears lack an endocervical component. It is assumed that the rate of abnormalities will be higher than normal in later smears with an endocervical component if the first smear lacked these cells. A large longitudinal study was done to examine abnormality rates according to endocervical status.

Methods.—The study sample comprised 20,222 women who had a negative cytology report during 1987 and a subsequent smear. A cytology report of cervical intraepithelial neoplasia (CIN) on the exit smear was the outcome of interest. The incidence of reported CIN was determined in women for whom both smears contained an endocervical component (group A), in those whose entry smear did not include an endocervical component but whose exit smear did (group B), in those whose entry smear did include an endocervical component but whose exit smear did not (group C), and in those in whom neither smear contained an endocervical component (group D). Incidences of CIN in the latter 3 groups were adjusted for age against the incidences in group A.

Results.—An endocervical component was included in 55% of entry smears and 52% of exit smears. The prevalence of CIN on exit smears that included an endocervical component was 4%, compared with 1.4% of exit smears with no endocervical component. The incidence of definite or equivocal CIN was highest in group A, and standardized incidence ratios were .86 for group B, .41 for group C, and .31 for group D. Women whose first smear did not include an endocervical component had a significantly lower incidence of definite cytologic evidence of CIN.

Conclusions.—Women with negative smears that lack an endocervical component need not be rescreened any earlier than those whose negative smears do include an endocervical component. Early repeat testing involves a large cost and engenders a high level of patient anxiety. In addition, samples from some women will not yield endocervical cells, even if they are taken with special instruments.

▶ Despite the format of the Bethesda classification system, the previous expert cytopathologist consensus was that an endocervical or metaplastic cell sample was not an absolute requirement for an adequate Pap smear specimen (1). Absence of an endocervical component is a particularly prevalent finding in postmenopausal women (2), and it is unfortunate that this analysis did not segregate out this important group. Many laboratories now report specimens in premenopausal women lacking an endocervical component as "less than optimal" rather than as unsatisfactory, and this study lends support to practitioners who either bring these women back for retesting in 6 months or redouble their efforts to ensure annual retesting. Ambiguities are likely to remain in the practice of cytology despite the proliferation of consensus groups.—R.M. Austin, M.D., Ph.D.

References

1. Gilbert FE, et al: *Gynecol Oncol* 1:271, 1973.
2. Kline TS, Solomon D: *Diagn Cytopathol* 7:1, 1991.

Cytologic Identification of Clinically Occult Proliferative Breast Disease in Women With a Family History of Breast Cancer

Marshall CJ, Schumann GB, Ward JH, Riding JM, Cannon-Albright L, Skolnick M (Univ of Utah)

Am J Clin Pathol 95:157–165, 1991 1–48

Objective.—There is reason to believe that in many women proliferative breast disease (PBD) may be present for some time in a diffuse, clinically inapparent form from which masses later arise. Whether 4-quadrant sampling of breast tissue by fine-needle aspiration (FNA) can detect PBD in the absence of an identifiable mass was investigated.

Subjects.—Fifty-one first-degree relatives of women with breast cancer were enrolled in the study. None had a breast lesion on physical examination or mammography at the time of entry into the study. The mean age was 44 years.

Findings.—All 8 breast quadrants were sampled in 45 of the 51 subjects. Benign hyperplastic ductal epithelium was found in 50 quadrants from 21 women. Atypical hyperplastic epithelium was found in 8 samples from 4 women. One of these women later had microcalcification and malignant cells in the same quadrant where atypical hyperplasia had been found. Computerized image analysis demonstrated significant differences in nuclear area, perimeter, and diameter between samples of atypical hyperplasia and those of benign hyperplasia.

Conclusions.—Proliferative breast disease can be detected by 4-quadrant FNA biopsy in clinically normal breasts. Nuclear enlargement is a major feature of atypical hyperplasia.

▶ The authors used FNA to identify background changes in palpably and mammographically normal breasts of first-degree relatives of women with breast cancer. A potential practical application could be the use of random-quadrant FNA to ascertain the type of fibrocystic disease in a woman's breast, determine her risk for subsequent carcinoma in conjunction with other factors, and thereby perhaps change the type of follow-up for these women, depending on the findings.

The authors conclude that FNA quadrant sampling is useful in the detection and characterization of clinically inapparent fibrocystic disease and identifies both proliferative changes and atypical proliferative changes. Their study, however, is limited by relatively sparse data on the cytopathologic definition of atypical ductal hyperplasia as it relates to the histopathologic definition in wide use today (1).—G.F. Worsham, M.D.

Reference

1. Dupont WD, Page DL: *N Engl J Med* 312:146, 1985.

Touch Preparation Cytology of Breast Lumpectomy Margins With Histologic Correlation

Cox CE, Ku NN, Reintgen DS, Greenberg HM, Nicosia SV, Wangensteen S (Univ of South Florida)

Arch Surg 126:490–493, 1991 1–49

Introduction.—Local recurrences after lumpectomy and radiotherapy might reflect the presence of residual microscopic disease at the time of resection. Present methods of evaluating the margins assess little more

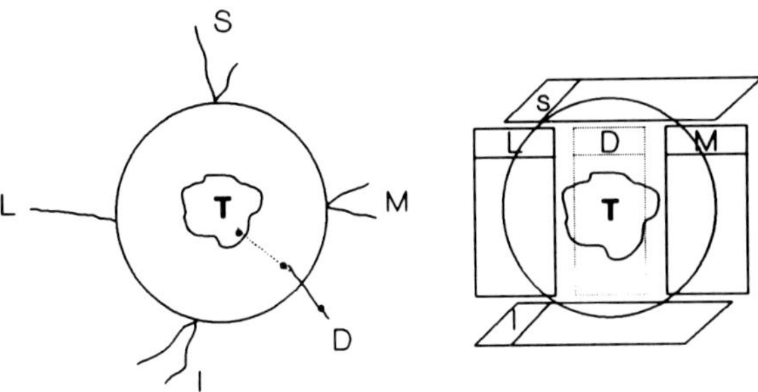

Fig 1–9.—Schematic diagram of touch preparation cytology of lumpectomy specimens. Lumpectomy margins were first oriented by various sutures *(left)* and then sampled by touch preparation cytology *(right)*. *S* indicates superior; *M*, medial; *D*, deep; *I*, inferior; *L*, lateral; and *T*, tumor. (Courtesy of Cox CE, Ku NN, Reintgen DS, et al: *Arch Surg* 126:490–493, 1991.)

than 10% to 15% of the surface area of a given specimen. Touch preparation cytology now has been evaluated as a rapid means of detecting microscopic disease in breast lumpectomy margins (Fig 1–9).

Methods.—Data were reviewed on 162 patients who had breast conservation surgery in 1984–1990; 114 of them were evaluated prospectively. About 4–6 slides were acquired for a specimen 5 cm in diameter, and cell samples were obtained by touch preparation cytology. A specimen from the tumor itself served as a positive cytologic control.

Results.—Tumor extended to the gross margin in 10 of the 111 patients. Frozen-section study demonstrated malignancy in 17 patients (table). Malignant cells were found by touch preparation cytology in 25 lumpectomy margins. Study of permanent histologic sections showed positive margins in 22 lumpectomy specimens. The overall accuracy of touch preparation cytology was 97%.

Conclusion.—Touch preparation cytology is an accurate way of topographically assessing lumpectomy margins. It complements frozen-section study of the lumpectomy margins and reduces the need for repeated resection of the margins as a separate procedure. It is hoped

Correlation Between Gross, Frozen Section, Permanent Histologic, and Touch Preparation Cytologic Examinations of Lumpectomy Margins

	Type of Examination			
Margins	**Gross**	**Cytologic**	**Frozen Section**	**Permanent**
True-positive	10	22	17	22
True-negative	86	86	89	89
False-positive	3	3	0	. . .
False-negative	12	0	5	. . .

(Courtesy of Cox CE, Ku NN, Reintgen DS, et al: *Arch Surg* 126:490–493, 1991.)

that this method will help to reduce local recurrences of cancer after breast conservation treatment.

▶ As conservative procedures become more prevalent for breast cancer, pathologists have become more creative in their approach to the evaluation of specimen margins at the time of surgery. One of the most widely used protocols for evaluation is based on a recommendation from the National Surgical Adjuvant Breast Project (1). A practical problem with this method, which is well described and illustrated, is the large number of blocks required to perform a relatively complete evaluation of the margins. If the surgeon believes that this is necessary at the time of the initial surgery, the cryostat time may exceed what is reasonable for the surgical procedure.

Using a cytologic method that reduced specimen processing time to 15 minutes, the authors were able to achieve good correlation with the final examination by permanent section. Despite meticulous attention to the margins of resection, however, many other factors appear to be involved in local recurrence. One study (2) showed residual tumor in 14 of 47 patients with clear or close margins and no residual tumor in 19 of 40 patients with positive margins. Specific subsets of breast carcinoma and particular characteristics (e.g., lymphatic permeation, extent of intraductal carcinoma, and the presence of comedocarcinoma) have all been suggested as predictors of local recurrence. Further, the role of radiation therapy in "cleaning up" potential residual cardinoma in all of the above groups remains a debated issue among surgeons, radiation therapists, and pathologists (3,4).

Until further consensus develops on these other issues, the authors of the present paper are to be commended for developing a technique that manages the time required yet provides topographical information regarding specific areas of margin involvement at the time of conservative breast cancer surgery.— G.F. Worsham, M.D.

References

1. Fisher ER, et al: *Cancer* 57:1717, 1986.
2. Frazier TG, et al: *Arch Surg* 124:37, 1989.
3. Vicini F, et al: *Ann Surg* 214:200, 1991.
4. Haffty BG, et al: *J Clin Oncol* 9:997, 1991.

Cytopathologic Diagnosis of Benign Lesions Simulating Choroidal Melanomas

Char DH, Miller TR, Crawford JB (Univ of California, San Francisco)
Am J Ophthalmol 112:70–75, 1991 1–50

Background.—Fine-needle aspiration (FNA) biopsy is accurate for the diagnosis of uveal melanoma, but its role in atypical nonmelanomatous pigmented lesions is uncertain. Three patients referred for evaluation of suspected uveal melanomas were found to have benign pigmented proliferations on FNA biopsy.

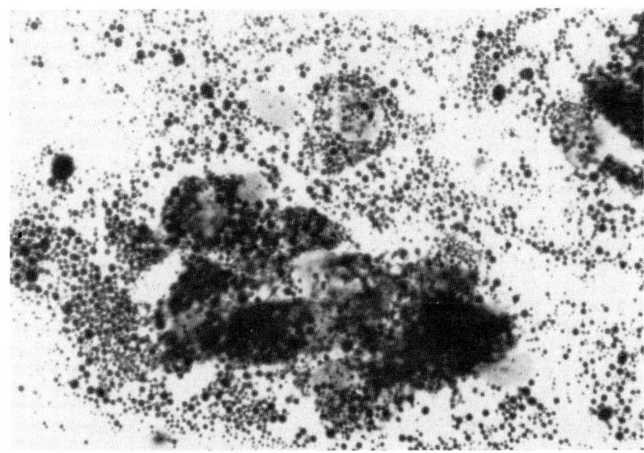

Fig 1–10.—Cytopathology of a pigmented epithelial adenoma. Note the large pigment granules. Uveal melanomas are not associated with pigment granules of this size. (May-Giemsa-Grunewald; original magnification, ×40.) (Courtesy of Char DH, Miller TR, Crawford JB: *Am J Ophthalmol* 112:70–75, 1991.)

Findings.—All 3 patients had a ciliochoroidal tumor. Ultrasound appearances were consistent with a uveal melanoma in 2 patients. Fine-needle aspiration biopsy specimens were identified correctly in the operating room as benign tumors. Two patients had pigment epithelial adenomas and 1 had a melanocytoma. Large, uniformly spherical pigment granules and benign-appearing cells were noted (Fig 1–10), and the granules displayed a refractile quality in low illumination. Microscopic examination of the resected tumors, using Papanicolaou and May-Giemsa-Grunewald stains, confirmed the findings on FNA biopsy. The tumor consisted of well-differentiated pigment epithelial cells with large pigment granules and no significant cellular atypia. The pigment granules were much larger than those observed in uveal melanomas. The tumors were resected successfully in 2 patients with good visual outcome. The third patient had the eye removed.

Conclusion.—Fine-needle aspiration biopsy can often differentiate a benign-simulating pigmented intraocular lesion from uveal melanoma.

▶ These 3 cases indicate an important potential for FNA in evaluation of pigmented tumors of the eye. In 2 cases, ciliary body tumors were judged to represent malignant melanoma on the basis of noninvasive evaluation. In each case, intraoperative FNA with rapid stain yielded a benign diagnosis, and in each case the lesion was removed and a useful eye was preserved. In the third case, aspiration of a suspicious choroidal lesion yielded a benign diagnosis, and the patient was followed by observation alone with no further surgery despite some further enlargement of the lesion. Five years later, the eye was removed because of pain from other causes, and histologic examination confirmed the benign nature of the lesion. In addition to the usual nuclear criteria, the authors emphasize the importance of large pigment granules in the cells of these benign lesions.—J.A. Tucker, M.D.

A Quantitative Comparison of Light and Electron Microscopic Diagnoses in Specimens Obtained by Fine-Needle Aspiration Biopsy

Dardick I, Yazdi HM, Brosko C, Rippstein P, Hickey NM (Toronto Gen Hosp; Ottawa Civic Hosp)

Ultrastruct Pathol 15:105–129, 1991 1–51

Objective.—Fine-needle aspiration (FNA) biopsy is used increasingly as a primary diagnostic tool. The relevance of ultrastructural examination of FNA biopsy specimens as an adjunctive procedure in establishing a diagnosis was studied.

Methods.—Initial diagnoses based on light microscopy were compared to those established by electron microscopy on 279 FNA biopsy specimens obtained under radiologic control during a 3-year period. Electron microscopy of needle rinse material was performed to clarify undifferentiated or poorly differentiated tumors, to distinguish primary and secondary tumors, to examine small cell tumors in children, to make a "sarcoma versus carcinoma" diagnosis, or to confirm the findings of light microscopy (Table 1).

Results.—Fifty-seven FNA biopsy specimens (20.4%) were considered inadequate for diagnostic studies. In the remaining 222 specimens, electron microscopy provided a specific or unsuspected diagnosis not possible by light microscopy in 7.7%. It provided a diagnosis consistent with light microscopic findings, a specific diagnosis from a set of differential diagnoses, or additional information that was clinically relevant in 19.4%. Electron microscopy contributed additional information that was not rel-

Table 1.—Indications for Electron Microscopy of FNA Biopsy Specimens

Clarification of undifferentiated or poorly differentiated (look-alike) neoplasms
Carcinoma
Malignant melanoma
Malignant lymphoma
Sarcoma
Small cell tumors in children
Neuroendocrine neoplasms (primary or metastatic)
Differential diagnosis of
Sarcomas
Mediastinal and retroperitoneal tumors
Renal and adrenal tumors
Malignant mesothelioma and carcinoma
Hepatocellular carcinoma and adenocarcinoma
Determination of primary site of certain metastatic tumors
Confirmation of light microscopic diagnosis

(Courtesy of Dardick I, Yazdi HM, Brosko C, et al: *Ultrastruct Pathol* 15:105–129, 1991.)

Table 2.—Contribution of Electron Microscopy to FNA Biopsy Diagnoses

Group	Role	Number of specimens	Percentage of total specimens
1	Major contribution	17	7.7
2	Confirmatory, clinical value	43	19.4
3	Confirmatory, limited value	45	20.3
4	No contribution	117	52.6
		222	100.0
5	Inadequate specimen	57/279	20.4

(Courtesy of Dardick I Yazdi HM, Brosko C, et al: *Ultrastruct Pathol* 15:105–129, 1991.)

evant clinically in 20.3%, and it made no contribution in 56.2% because the light and electron microscopic diagnoses were the same (Table 2). Overall, electron microscopy made a major contribution to the final cytologic diagnosis in 27.1% of specimens. The lung and the liver accounted for 75% of the specimens examined by electron microscopy that resulted in final cytopathologic diagnoses, with significant differences from light microscopic findings.

Conclusion.—Most FNA biopsy specimens, particularly from the lung and liver, are well suited to ultrastructural examination. Electron microscopy improves both the cytologic diagnostic criteria and the reliability of FNA diagnoses. It also reveals crucial aspects of architectural organization and cytologic details.

▶ Electron microscopy is often overlooked as an adjunctive technique in cytologic diagnosis. The authors demonstrate that electron microscopy can often provide clinically relevant information in the evaluation of fine-needle aspirates. Significantly, material for ultrastructural examination was obtained not by an additional pass of the aspiration needle, but from needle rinses after preparation of smears. This technique yielded adequate material for ultrastructural study in about 80% of cases. Further, rapid processing of the material enabled routine reporting of the ultrastructural findings within 48 hours of collection. Although histochemical or immunoperoxidase stains may sometimes obviate the need for ultrastructural examination of difficult cases, this report emphasizes the useful role electron microscopy can play in selected fine-needle aspirates.—J.A. Tucker, M.D.

Diagnostic Value of Brush Cytology in the Diagnosis of Bile Duct Carcinoma: A Study in 65 Patients With Bile Duct Strictures

Rabinovitz M, Zajko AB, Hassanein T, Shetty B, Bron KM, Schade RR, Gavaler JS, Block G, Van Thiel DH, Dekker A (Univ of Pittsburgh)

Hepatology 12:747–752, 1990 1–52

Background.—It is difficult to differentiate malignant strictures of the extrahepatic bile ducts from benign strictures, especially in patients who have primary sclerosing cholangitis. Brush cytology may provide a specific diagnosis in these cases, but there are few data on this application. A large series of patients with bile duct carcinoma (BDC) was investigated to determine the diagnostic accuracy of brush cytology.

Methods.—In a 5-year period, 65 patients with intrahepatic or extrahepatic biliary strictures who underwent brush cytology were available for subsequent analysis. Each patient had at least 1 brushing after undergoing percutaneous transhepatic biliary drainage. Twenty-eight patients had benign intrahepatic or extrahepatic biliary strictures (Fig 1–11), and 37 had BDC (Fig 1–12). Diagnoses were confirmed subsequently at operation or autopsy. The 14 patients still alive after 4 years were considered to have benign lesions.

Results.—The first brushing was positive in 40% of patients with BDC; an additional 11% had suspicious but not diagnostic cells. Second brushings were done in 13 patients whose initial brushings were negative; 38% of these specimens were malignant and 24% were suspicious. Malignant cells were found in all 3 patients who underwent a third brushing.

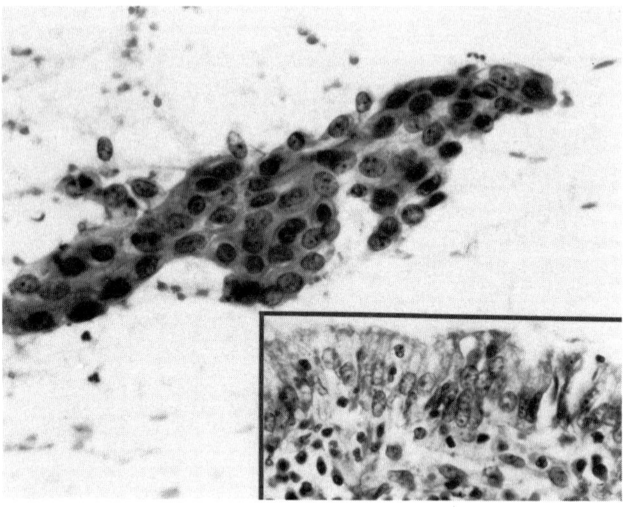

Fig 1–11.—Atypical (benign) epithelial cells in patient with primary sclerosing cholangitis. Note disparity in nuclear size and loss of honeycomb pattern. Papanicolaou stain; original magnification, ×500. **Inset,** histologic section from liver transplant showing slightly irregular bile duct epithelial lining cells with proper orientation to the basement membrane. Note also the mild, chronic submucosal inflammatory infiltrate. Hematoxylin-eosin; original magnification, ×500. (Courtesy of Rabinovitz M, Zajko AB, Hassanein T, et al: *Hepatology* 12:747–752, 1990.)

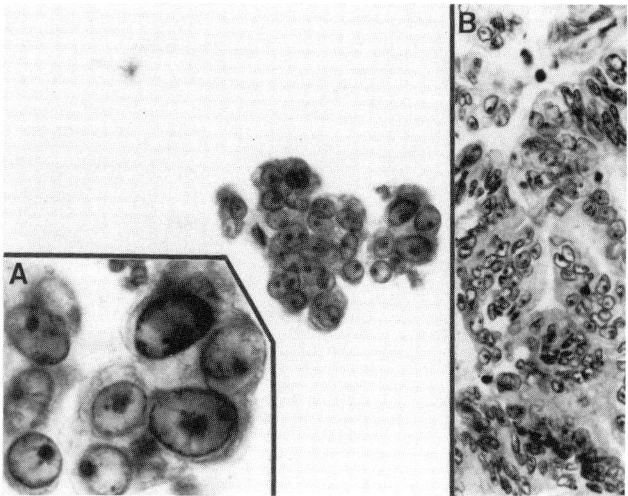

Fig 1–12.—Loosely cohesive group of malignant epithelial cells with molding and overlapping of nuclei, which contain jagged nucleoli and prominent parachromatin clearing. Papanicolaou stain; original magnification, ×500. **Inset A,** Papanicolaou stain; original magnification, ×1250. **Inset B,** hematoxylin-eosin; original magnification ×500. (Courtesy of Rabinovitz M, Zajko AB, Hassanein T, et al: *Hepatology* 12:747–752, 1990.)

In the group with benign strictures, 2 patients had suspicious findings on the first but not the second brushing. The probability of BDC was reduced to 43% after a single negative or suspicious brushing, to 32% after 2 negative tests, and to 0% after 3 negative tests. These probabilities fell to 41%, 20%, and 0%, respectively, when suspicious findings were excluded.

Conclusions.—Brush cytology for detection of BDC has a low yield on the first test, but its sensitivity increases with repeated attempts. Patients with 3 negative results have less than a 5% probability of having BDC. Percutaneous transhepatic cholangiography and bile duct cytologic studies are useful in establishing the diagnosis.

▶ The differential diagnosis of well-differentiated adenocarcinoma from inflammatory processes involving the bile ducts has always been a challenging activity both in surgical pathology and cytopathology. Despite the success of fine-needle aspiration (FNA) cytology in diagnosing mass lesions in the pancreas, our experience is that tumors of the extrahepatic bile ducts frequently do not present with distinct masses, are difficult to visualize by imaging studies, and therefore are diagnosed either by brush or exfoliative cytology or, more commonly, at the time of surgery. This study is the largest reported series of patients in whom BDC was diagnosed by this technique.

In only a minority of patients who subsequently were proved to have carcinoma was the diagnosis made on the initial procedure. In these authors' hands, however, negative brushings on 3 repeat procedures excluded a malignant diagnosis. Because the brushings were obtained attendant to the drainage procedure, complications, including transient hemobilia (3 patients), bile leakage around the catheter tract (2 patients), and infection (5 patients), were thought to be related to the drainage procedure itself. The authors provide useful illustrations of the cases they considered atypical but likely to be benign, suspicious, and malignant.

Our experience with exfoliative cytology from this anatomical site has, like the authors' impression of the literature, been hampered by poor cellular preservation and low sensitivity. This paper provides useful quantitative and qualitative information in the application of brush cytology to the types of cases encountered in any large hospital practice.—G.F. Worsham, M.D.

Cytologic Criteria to Distinguish Hepatocellular Carcinoma From Nonneoplastic Liver

Cohen MB, Haber MM, Holly EA, Ahn DK, Bottles K, Stoloff AC (Univ of California, San Francisco; Columbia Univ; Stanford Univ, Palo Alto)
Am J Clin Pathol 95:125–130, 1991 1–53

Objective.—Fine-needle aspiration biopsy smears of liver aspirates from 52 patients with hepatocellular carcinoma (HCC) and 30 with various nonneoplastic conditions, including cirrhosis and fatty change, were

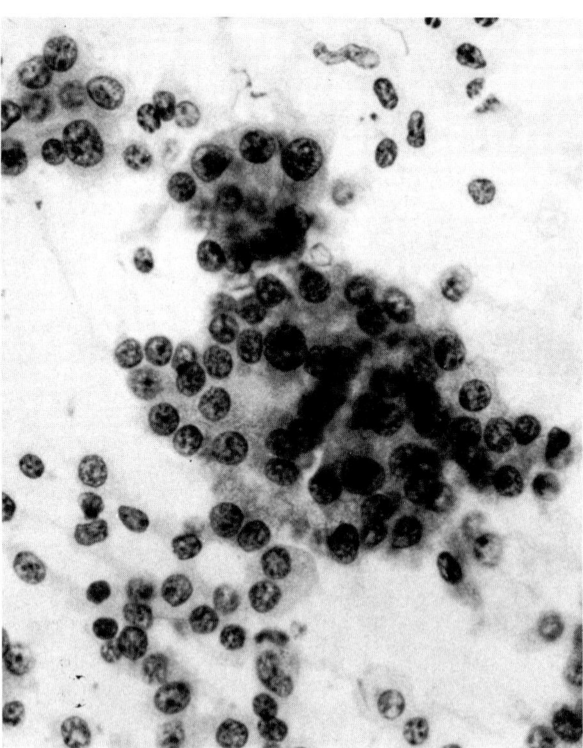

Fig 1–13.—Acinar pattern. (Courtesy of Cohen MB, Haber MM, Holly EA, et al: *Am J Clin Pathol* 95:125–130, 1991.)

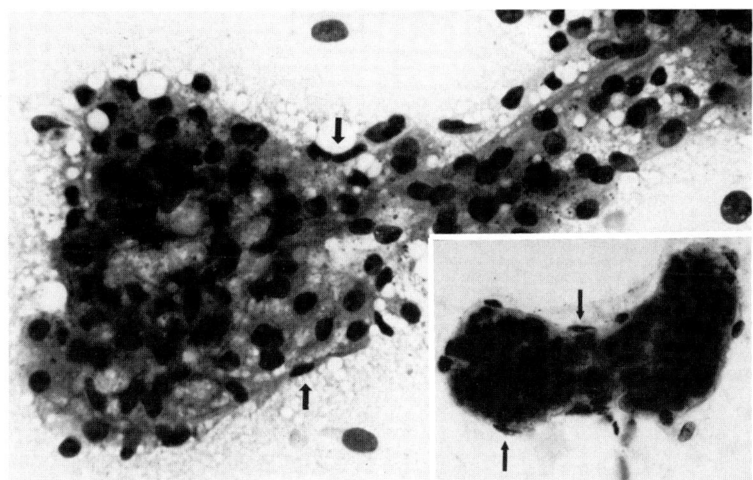

Fig 1–14.—Trabecular pattern. *Arrows* point to endothelial cells. May-Grünwald-Giemsa; original magnification, ×250. **Inset,** Papanicolaou-stained smear; original magnification, ×250. (Courtesy of Cohen MB, Haber MM, Holly EA, et al: *Am J Clin Pathol* 95:125–130, 1991.)

reviewed. Stepwise logistic regression analysis was undertaken to identify cytologic features that distinguish HCC from nonneoplastic liver.

Findings.–No single cytologic feature adequately identified HCC. An acinar or pseudoglandular pattern (Fig 1–13) was found in 38% of HCC smears and in 7% of control specimens. A trabecular pattern (Fig 1–14) was present in two thirds of HCC samples and in 10% of nonneoplastic liver smears. Hyperchromasia was seen in one third of HCC and 10% of control specimens. Pleomorphism, found in 71% of HCC smears, also was present in 30% of nonneoplastic samples. More than half of the HCC smears and only 7% of control smears had multiple nucleoli of varying sizes and shapes. Atypical naked hepatocytic nuclei were present in nearly three fourths of HCC samples and in only 3% of samples from nonneoplastic liver.

Diagnostic Usefulness.—When a trabecular pattern, an increased nuclear/cytoplasmic ratio, and atypical naked hepatocytic nuclei all were present, the method was 100% sensitive and 87% specific for HCC. The positive and negative predictive values were 93% and 100%, respectively.

Conclusion.—The use of key cytologic criteria can make fine-needle aspiration biopsy a more accurate way of diagnosing HCC.

▶ Small biopsy specimens, either surgical or cytologic, represent challenging material for the differential diagnosis noted above. The authors provide excellent illustrations of common and discriminatory features as well as the 3 features they refer to as key criteria: trabecular pattern, increased nuclear to cytoplasmic ratio, and atypical naked nuclei. Using these 3 key criteria, the authors note that they would have misclassified 4 of 30 cirrhotic livers (13%) as HCC. They (and we) conclude that there will be "continued difficulty [in] distinguishing nonneoplastic liver conditions from very well-differentiated HCCs."—G.F. Worsham, M.D.

Immunocytochemical Profile of Benign and Carcinomatous Effusions: A Practical Approach to Difficult Diagnosis

Esteban JM, Yokota S, Husain S, Battifora H (City of Hope Natl Med Ctr, Duarte, Calif)

Am J Clin Pathol 94:698–705, 1990 1–54

Background.—In cytodiagnosis of effusions, it may be difficult to distinguish between reactive mesothelium or histiocytes and cancer cells, especially in patients who have undergone radiation therapy or chemotherapy. An attempt was made to determine which monoclonal antibodies (MoAbs) are most useful for the routine study of serous effusions by a conventional immunostaining method.

Methods.—Sixty effusions diagnosed by standard cytologic criteria from 1986 to 1989 were reviewed in a blinded fashion. There were 18 malignant, 18 benign, and 24 equivocal effusions from the pleural, peritoneal, and pericardial cavities. The specimens were investigated with a panel of 7 available MoAbs (cytokeratins, vimentin, EMA, B72.3, α-CEA, HMFG-2, and Leu-M1) and with the lectin *Ulex europaeus* I. A slightly modified avidin-biotin complex was used as the immunocytochemical method.

Results.—All of the malignant specimens reacted with EMA and HMFG, 94% with B72.3, and 61% with α-CEA. The following combinations were also positive in malignant cases: EMA plus B72.3 in 94%, EMA plus α-CEA in 61%, and EMA plus α-CEA plus B72.3 in 55%. Seven of the benign specimens reacted with HMFG, 2 each with EMA and B72.3, and 1 with EMA plus B72.3. These findings were used to classify the equivocal effusions as malignant (14) or benign (10). The diagnoses were confirmed by follow-up effusions obtained within 3 months in all but 5 patients. The EMA plus B72.3 combination showed malignant cells in 94% of cases. There was a 3.5% incidence of false positive findings.

Conclusions.—The MoAbs EMA, B72.3, and α-CEA are highly sensitive and specific in detecting malignant cells in effusions. A panel of these MoAbs can be used to make a precise diagnosis in questionable cases, without adapting available immunocytochemical techniques. No neoplasm should be diagnosed as malignant on the basis of reactivity with a single MoAb.

▶ A reflection of the interest this common problem generates is that 6 of 34 of the abstracts (18%) in the cytopathology sections at the International Academy of Pathology meeting in 1991 were studies involving this differential diagnosis. An additional article earlier in the same journal (1) used a similar immunocytochemical panel approach with MoAbs to EMA, CEA, B72.3, and Leu-M1, and found positivity in 96%, 77%, 58%, and 42% of adenocarcinomas, respectively. These determinants were not found in mesotheliomas and reactive fusions. Two studies reported in abstract form (2,3) found BER-EP4, a MoAb directed against 2 glycoproteins in most epithelial cells, but not in mesothelial cells, useful in this differential diagnosis.

Another approach reported in abstract form (4) suggested the usefulness of chromosome analysis in effusions that yielded equivocal results on more routine examinations. These authors identify specific chromosome aberrations previously reported in malignant mesotheliomas, and their presence was able to confirm the diagnosis of malignant mesothelioma. This last study did not compare less costly approaches.—G.F. Worsham, M.D.

References

1. Nance KV, Silverman JS: *J Clin Pathol* 95:867, 1991.
2. Diaz Arias A, et al: *Mod Pathol* 24-A:4(suppl), 1991.
3. Frisman DM, et al: *Mod Pathol* 25-A:4(suppl), 1991.
4. Granadaos, et al: *Mod Pathol* 25-A:4(suppl), 1991.

Distinction Between Carcinoma Cells and Mesothelial Cells in Serous Effusions: Usefulness of Immunohistochemistry

Tickman RJ, Cohen C, Varma VA, Fekete PS, DeRose PB (Emory Univ)

Acta Cytol 34:491–496, 1990 1–55

Introduction.—It can be difficult to distinguish between reactive and malignant mesothelial cells in serous effusions. The ability of a battery of immunoperoxidase tests to distinguish between carcinomatous and benign effusions was studied in 90 lesions—69 carcinomatous effusions, 2 malignant mesotheliomas, and 19 lesions with reactive cells only.

Methods.—The 2-step immunoperoxidase detection system used Brigati's capillary gap immunocytochemical staining method and the Code-On Immunochemistry System. Samples were stained with antibodies to Leu-M1, B72.3, epithelial membrane antigen (EMA), carcinoembryonic antigen (CEA), and vimentin.

Findings.—The most useful markers were EMA and vimentin. Epithelial membrane antigen reacted with 86% of carcinomas, and vimentin reacted with 90% of samples from patients with reactive mesothelial cells only. Staining with antibodies to Leu-M1, B72.3, and CEA also was helpful (table).

Frequency of Immunopositivity in Benign and Malignant Serous Effusions

	No. of	Frequency of immunopositivity (%)				
Diagnosis	**cases**	**EMA**	**Vimentin**	**CEA**	**B72.3**	**Leu-M1**
Carcinomas						
Breast	23	91.3	4.3	8.6	52.2	34.4
Ovary	16	100.0	12.5	6.3	81.2	43.8
Lung	10	100.0	0.0	20.0	80.0	70.0
GI tract	7	71.4	0.0	100.0	57.1	28.6
Miscellaneous	13	76.9	0.0	46.2	53.8	15.4
Reactive mesothelial cells	19	5.3	94.7	5.3	0.0	5.3

(Courtesy of Tickman RJ, Cohen C, Varma VA, et al: *Acta Cytol* 34:491–496, 1990.)

Conclusion.—The routine use of a panel of immunoperoxidase tests to assess cell blocks from serous effusions appears justified when cells suspicious for carcinoma are present. Most lesions can be diagnosed with a combination of anti-EMA and antivimentin antibodies.

Forensic Pathology

Firearm Fatalities in Victoria, Australia, 1988

Selway R (Corpus Christi College, Cambridge, England)
Med Sci Law 31:167–174, 1991 1–56

Objective.—A survey was made of gunshot deaths occurring in Victoria, Australia, in 1988. The 138 deaths yielded an incidence of 3.2/100,000. Whereas 71% of the deaths were suicides, 24% were homicides.

Analysis.—Twice as many males as females were homicide victims. Female homicide victims chiefly were shot by their husbands. Nearly half of all homicides were of a domestic nature. Another 15% represented criminals shot by the police. Only 3 women shot themselves, whereas 11 were homicide victims. Gunshot deaths were most prevalent in the summer months. There was evidence of illicit drug use in 5 instances. Alcohol intake was evident in one third of the cases.

Summary.—Gunshot deaths are a major part of all homicides in Victoria and also account for a significant number of suicides. Considering how many individuals own guns, the number of accidental firearm deaths is reassuringly low (2% of the present series).

Gunshot Suicides in Victoria, Australia, 1988

Selway R (Corpus Christi College, Cambridge, England)
Med Sci Law 31:76–80, 1991 1–57

Objective.—Ninety-six gunshot suicides occurring in Victoria, Australia, in 1988 were analyzed. The incidence was 2.25/100,000 population. The median age was 40 years; only 3 victims were females.

Associations.—The most frequent concomitants of suicide in this series were psychiatric disorder and poor physical health. Alcohol problems, an argument or loss of a friend, and contact with the police also were not infrequent correlates of suicide. Nearly one third of the victims exhibited evidence of drinking before the event.

Circumstances.—Only 10% of suicides were witnessed. About 75% took place at home—frequently in the bedroom. Handguns were used less often than in other countries; 63 cases involved use of a rifle. The weapon was found in the victim's hands in only one fifth of evaluable cases.

Conclusions.—Access to a gun provides an effective means of committing suicide, lessening the need for planning. Alcohol use not infrequently has a role in prompting a gunshot suicide. More restrictive gun ownership laws might lessen the frequency of these suicides.

An Investigation of the Pattern of Firearms Fatalities Before and After the Introduction of New Legislation in Denmark

Thomsen JL, Albrektsen SB (Univ Inst of Forensic Medicine, Copenhagen)
Med Sci Law 31:162–166, 1991 1–58

Background.—On January 1, 1986, a new and rigorous Firearms Act was implemented in Denmark. Firearms fatalities before and after 1986 were compared to assess the effects of this new legislation and the patterns of firearm fatalities.

Data Analysis.—From 1984 through 1987, 276 firearm fatalities occurred—an incidence of 3/100,000 living inhabitants. Most were suicides (86%), and only 4 were accidental deaths, 2 resulting from "Russian roulette." There were no hunting accidents. Most fatalities involved men and occurred in private homes. Suicides were usually by shots in the head, most often into the mouth. The location was more sporadic in homicides, with no shots fired into the mouth. Those in the suicide group were more often married than those in the homicide group. Among suicides, 31% occurred in persons with chronic alcohol and/or drug abuse problems.

Results.—The numbers of suicides and homicides decreased after the introduction of the new Firearms Act. This reduction, however, could not be attributed to the new law, because there was no specific decrease in the number of shotgunt fatalities, but a general preventive effect was possible. Compared with previous Danish investigations covering the 10-year period between 1957 and 1966 and between 1970 and 1979, there was an increase in the total number of suicides with firearms and the total and relative numbers of homicides.

Implications.—There is a need for more information and more restrictive legislation to limit the number of firearms in the population.

▶ The above reports (Abstracts 1–56, 1–57, and 1–58) from these foreign countries serve to underscore the extreme paucity of such information in the United States. This despite the fact that firearms are a major source of death and injury in this country.

There is a virtual absence of basic data from the United States, e.g., where the shootings occur, what the characteristics are of the victims or shooters, the relationship to alcohol and drugs, and so on. In this information vacuum, national debate continues regarding handgun legislation. The National Academy of Science on Trauma Research has recommended the formation of an injury control center as part of the Centers for Disease Control. Nonetheless, the question raised by Jagger and Deitz remains largely unanswered (1).—W.A. Gardner, Jr., M.D.

Reference

1. Jagger J, Dietz PE: Death and injury by firearms: Who cares? *JAMA* 255:3143, 1986.

Inadequacy of Death Certification: Proposal for Change
Ashworth TG (Walsgrave Hosp, Coventry, England)
J Clin Pathol 44:265–268, 1991 1–59

Introduction.—The death certificate is a vital source of demographic information. The cause of death as listed on the death certificate is used by those who collect and publish morbidity and mortality data. This information serves as a basis for designing government policies and is used in support of funding new research projects. It is generally agreed that the listed cause of death is often inaccurate, and that autopsy is the only means of validating the actual cause.

Problem.—In England and Wales, the overall 1987 necropsy rate was 26%, considered high by any standard. Yet, the morbidity and mortality statistics based on this body of data are seriously flawed, mainly because of omission of important information on the death certificate. This problem arises from the fact that only those conditions thought to have contributed directly to the death are listed, whereas conditions that did not contribute directly to the death but might be important to public health are not included on the death certificate in its current format. Additional information on conditions that do not specifically contribute to the cause of death but may be important for future studies should be included in an addendum to the existing death certificate.

Examples.—Examples of conditions not directly related to the cause of death and thus would not be included on the death certificate are the following: incidentally detected carcinomas and tumors; malignancies treated successfully years earlier; gallstones; peptic ulcers; the severity of cerebral, coronary, and aortic atheroma; normally functioning prosthetic heart valves inserted years earlier; functioning kidney transplants; and diabetes mellitus. Many of these conditions could be listed by family physicians who complete the death certificate even if no autopsy was performed. The extra time it takes to list the additional information on the death certificate would have important ramifications for future studies and government policies.

Conclusion.—Expanding the information on the death certificate to include conditions and factors that did not contribute directly to the cause of death would limit errors and provide an important research source for future studies.

▶ This is a worthwhile proposal. The suggested check-list format should be considered as having the additional advantage of being easly computerized.—W.A. Gardner, Jr., M.D.

2 Cardiovascular System

Morphologic Comparison of Patients With Mitral Valve Prolapse Who Died Suddenly With Patients Who Died From Severe Valvular Dysfunction or Other Conditions

Dollar AL, Roberts WC (Natl Heart, Lung, and Blood Inst, Bethesda, Md)

J Am Coll Cardiol 17:921–931, 1991 2–1

Introduction.—Mitral valve prolapse commonly affects about 5% of the American population. The morphological findings from patients with mitral valve prolapse not associated with any other possibly fatal condition were compared with the mitral valve prolapse associated with a potentially fatal disorder determined at necropsy.

Methods.—Between January 1956 and February 1990, the hearts of 101 patients were diagnosed as having had mitral valve prolapse by the Pathology Branch of the National Heart, Lung, and Blood Institute. Of these 101 cases, 81 were available for restudy. After all exclusions, 56 patients aged 16–70 years were included in the study.

Results.—The table presents the morphological and clinical findings in 49 patients without congenital heart disease. Of the 56 total patients, 22 died suddenly of cardiac disease; 4 had significant coronary artery disease, 2 had mitral valve replacement, and 1 had cyanotic congenital disease; 15 had no explanation for their death except for mitral valve prolapse. Of these last 15 patients, 10 were women. The hearts of the 15 patients had a mean weight of 398 g, and the mitral valve anulus was dilated in 12. Also, the anterior mitral leaflet appeared elongated in 12 patients. When compared with other patients with mitral valve prolapse, the 15 who died suddenly were significantly younger at death (mean, 39 years vs. 52 years), had a reduced frequency of mitral regurgitation, and had a lower amount of ruptured chordae tendineae previously; also, the group included more women. In 7 patients congenital heart disease was present, and 8 had Marfan's syndrome.

Implications.—Relatively young women with mitral valve prolapse, but without mitral regurgitation or any other recognized condition, may be at greater risk of dying suddenly.

▶ The clinical and morphological substrates for the rare complication of sudden death in patients with mitral valve prolapse remain enigmatic, but they have included a family history of sudden death, abnormal resting ECG, and redundant valve leaflets or extensive endocardial fibrous plaques. Based on the findings described in this paper, clinicians may need to maintain a heightened level of aware-

Clinical and Morphological Features of Mitral Valve Prolapse at Necropsy Unassociated With Other Congenital Cardiovascular Anomalies (49 Patients, Aged 16–70 years)

Patient Category	+SCD −MR −CAD	+SCD +MR −CAD	+SCD −MR +CAD	−SCD +MR −CAD	−SCD −MR −CAD	Total (%)
No. of patients	14	3	3	10	19	49
Mean age (yr)	38 ± 17	50 ± 17	65 ± 3	55 ± 13	49 ± 17	48 ± 17
Women/men	10/4	0/3	0/3	3/7	6/13	19/30
Heart weight (g)	379 ± 96	770 ± 105	462 ± 103	577 ± 180	397 ± 131	458 ± 167
MV anulus >10 cm	11/14	1/1	2/3	8/8	6/10	29/36 (81)
TV anulus >14 cm	1/13	1/2	0/3	2/9	1/10	5/37 (14)
AML length >2.0 cm	11/13	1/1	2/3	2/4	3/6	19/27 (70)
PML length >1.5 cm	10/13	1/1	3/3	4/4	3/6	21/27 (78)
Absent chordae	4/12	0/1	2/2	6/8	2/6	14/29 (48)
LV cavity dilated (grade 3/4 or 4/4)	0/14	1/3	0/3	3/9	1/19	5/48 (10)
CA narrowed >75% in CSA	0/14	0/3	3/3	3/9	1/15	7/44 (16)
LV necrosis	0/14	0/3	1/3	0/10	0/18	1/48 (2)
LV fibrosis	0/14	1/3	1/3	2/10	1/18	5/48 (10)
Grade of MVP						
Mild	3/14	0/1	0/3	0/5	2/11	5/34 (15)
Moderate	4/14	0/1	2/3	2/5	7/11	15/34 (44)
Severe	7/14	1/1	1/3	3/5	2/11	14/34 (41)
Endocardial fibrous plaque under PML	10/14	1/1	1/3	6/7	5/9	23/34 (68)
Mitral annular calcium						
Grade 1–2/4	3/14	0/2	1/3	1/7	2/17	7/43 (16)
Grade 3–4/4	1/14	0/2	0/3	2/7	2/17	5/43 (12)
Valvular competent PFO	3/11	1/3	1/3	1/5	1/8	7/31 (23)
Redundant FO membrane	3/11	0/3	1/3	2/5	0/7	6/30 (20)
SCD due to MVP	14/14	1/3	0/3	0/10	0/19	15/49 (31)
The Marfan syndrome	2/14	0/3	0/3	2/10	4/19	8/49 (16)
Mitral valve replacement	0/14	2/3	0/3	1/10	0/19	3/49 (6)

Abbreviations: *AML*, anterior mitral leaflet; *CA*, coronary artery; *CAD*, fatal coronary artery disease; *CSA*, cross-sectional area; *FO*, fossa ovale; *LV*, left ventricular; *MR*, severe mitral regurgitation; *MV*, mitral valve; *MVP*, mitral valve prolapse; *PFO*, patent foramen ovale; *PML*, posterior mitral leaflet; *SCD*, sudden cardiac death; *TV*, tricuspid valve; −, absent; +, present.

(Courtesy of Dollar AL, Roberts WC: *J Am Coll Cardiol* 17:921–931, 1991.)

ness when systolic clicks are discovered in young patients (particular women) who have no evidence of mitral regurgitation.—J.B. Atkinson, M.D., Ph.D.

Isolated Noncompaction of Left Ventricular Myocardium: A Study of Eight Cases

Chin TK, Perloff JK, Williams RG, Jue K, Mohrmann R (Univ of California, Los Angeles)

Circulation 82:507–513, 1990) 2–2

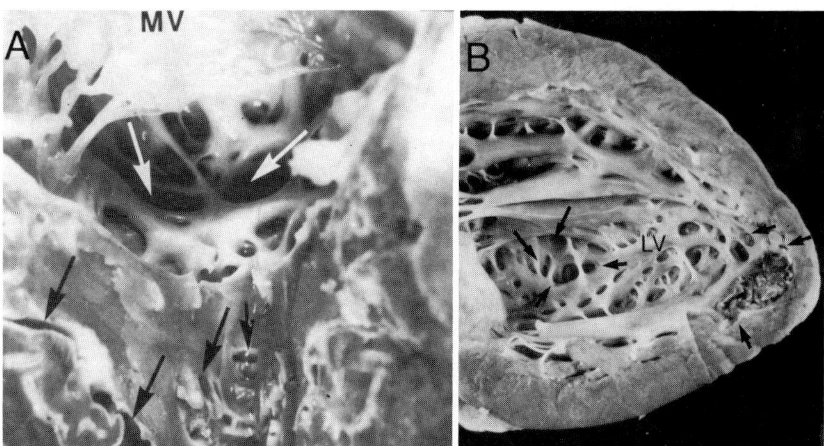

Fig 2–1.—**A,** photograph of necropsy specimen from boy aged 2.3 years showing gross morphological features of noncompaction. Abnormally numerous, excessively prominent trabeculations and deep intertrabecular recesses *(arrows)* shown from 2 perspectives in perpendicular, cross-section *(black arrows)* and endocardial surface *(white arrows).* **B,** photograph of necropsy specimen from woman aged 22.5 years showing thrombi *(black arrows)* in cross-section within intertrabecular recesses at apex of left ventricle (LV). *White arrows* identify excessively numerous, deep intertrabecular recesses that penetrate endocardial surface. (Courtesy of Chin TK, Perloff JK, Williams RG, et al: *Circulation* 82:507–513, 1990.)

Introduction.—Isolated noncompaction of left ventricular myocardium (INVM) is a rare disorder caused by an arrest in endomyocardial morphogenesis. Eight patients with INVM were studied, 3 at necropsy.

Findings.—The 5 male and 3 female patients were aged 11 months to 22.5 years at presentation (mean, 8.9 years). Two-dimensional echocardiograms showed numerous, excessively prominent trabeculations and deep intertrabecular recesses in all 8 patients. When assessed by a quantitative echocardiographic X-to-Y ratio, the depths of the intertrabecular recesses were significantly greater than in normal controls. The X-to-Y ratio decreased progressively from the level of the papillary muscles to the apex. At necropsy the left ventricular endomyocardial morphology corresponded to the echocardiographic images in 3 patients (Fig 2–1). Clinically, 5 patients had ventricular arrhythmias and 5 had depressed left ventricular systolic function. Systemic embolization occurred in 3 patients. Noncardiac malformations included a distinctive facial dysmorphism in 3 patients, together with motor and speech defects. Four patients exhibited familial recurrence of INVM.

Conclusions.—These 8 patients represent the largest study population of INVM to date. Isolated noncompaction of left ventricular myocardium is a rare if not unique disorder that affects both sexes from infancy through young adulthood. Two-dimensional echocardiography is diagnostic of INVM. This disorder is associated with a high risk of cardiovascular complications, including depressed left ventricular function, ventricular arrhythmias, and endocardial clot with systemic embolization. Furthermore, INVM may be associated with facial dysmorphism and familial recurrence.

▶ The clinical and morphological description of noncompliance of the ventricular myocardium has implications above and beyond the characterization of a relatively rare cardiac disorder. In a broader sense, it gives pathologists a conceptual framework when analyzing ventricular architecture in complex congenital heart disease of various types, particularly in univentricular hearts with "indeterminate" ventricular morphology.—J.B. Atkinson, M.D., Ph.D.

Human Abdominal Aortic Aneurysms: Immunophenotypic Analysis Suggesting an Immune-Mediated Response

Koch AE, Haines GK, Rizzo RJ, Radosevich JA, Pope RM, Robinson PG, Pearce WH (Northwestern Univ)

Am J Pathol 137:1199–1213, 1990 2–3

Introduction.—Inflammatory cells appear to be important in the immunopathogenesis of atherosclerosis. Because atherosclerosis is the most common cause of abdominal aortic aneurysm (AAA), inflammatory cells may also be involved in the immunopathogenesis of AAA. The potential role of inflammatory cells in the development of AAA was investigated.

Methods.—Tissue samples were obtained from the infrarenal abdominal aortas of 32 patients. Four normal aortas were obtained at autopsy, 6 aortas were obtained during surgery for occlusive aortic disease, and 23 aortas were obtained from patients operated on for aneurysmal disease, 5 having inflammatory aneurysms and 17 having typical AAA. Five monoclonal antibodies were used for the study (anti-CD3, anti-CD19, anti-CD11c, anti-CD4, and anti-CD8).

Findings.—Tissue samples from normal aortas contained little inflammation. In contrast, tissue from diseased aortas showed significant numbers of inflammatory cells, 67% to 80% of which were CD3-positive T lymphocytes. The locations of the T lymphocytes varied by disease. In occlusive disease, 25% of the CD3-positive T lymphocytes were found in the adventitia with the remainder in the media. In AAA and inflammatory aneurysm tissue, CD3-positive T lymphocytes were found predominantly in the adventitia. In all 3 pathologic groups, CD19-positive B lymphocytes were found mainly in the adventitia. The adventitial CD4-positive:CD8-positive ratio was greater in AAAs than in the other groups. Further, CD11c-positive macrophages were found throughout the diseased tissues.

Conclusion.—Aneurysmal disease may progress from occlusive disease, and it is characterized by an increase in and redistribution of chronic inflammatory cells. Although it is possible that the inflammation seen in aneurysmal tissue may be an epiphenomenon, these changes suggest that aneurysmal disease represents an immune-mediated response. The antigen(s) stimulating the process have not yet been identified. Suggested candidates include components of the vessel wall, modified lipoproteins, phospholipids, and the like.

Low Density Lipoprotein-Containing Circulating Immune Complexes and Coronary Atherosclerosis

Tertov VV, Orekhov AN, Kacharava AG, Sobenin IA, Perova NV, Smirnov VN
(USSR Cardiology Research Ctr, Moscow)

Exp Molec Pathol 52:300–308, 1990 2–4

Background.—Sera from most patients with coronary heart disease has been shown to induce lipid accumulation by cultured smooth muscle cells from aortic intima uninvolved by atherosclerosis. Additional experimental evidence suggested that factors interacting with low-density lipoprotein (LDL) might induce this abnormality. A study was undertaken to evaluate the role of LDL-containing circulating immune complexes in initiation of intracellular lipid accumulation.

Study.—Blood levels of LDL-containing immune complexes were determined in 122 healthy donors and in 108 patients with coronary heart disease. Immune complexes were isolated and added to cultures of smooth muscle cells from unaffected human aortic intima. Apolipoprotein B– immunoglobulin complexes were determined in microtiter plate studies.

Observations.—Sera from most patients with coronary heart disease led to a twofold to fivefold rise in the lipid content of smooth muscle cells from uninvolved intima. Incubating smooth muscle cells with circulating immune complexes isolated from atherogenic serum produced a 1.5- to threefold increase in intracellular cholesterol. The complexes contained apolipoprotein B at a level correlating closely with the total cholesterol content. The ratio of cholesterol to apolipoprotein B was characteristic of LDL. The ability of sera to induce lipid accumulation in cultured cells correlated directly with the cholesterol and apolipoprotein B levels in circulating immune complexes.

Discussion.—It appears that LDL-containing immune complexes are responsible for the atherogenic potential of sera from patients with coronary heart disease.

▶ Koch et al. (Abstract 2–3) have shown a change in the number and distribution of inflammatory cells in the wall of the aorta with progression of atherosclerotic disease and speculate that this change supports a role of the immune response in development of atherosclerotic lesions. They suggest several possible inciting agents for this process, including modified lipoproteins. Tertov et al. (Abstract 2–4) have demonstrated that circulating immune complexes containing apolipoprotein B and cholesterol can be isolated from the serum of patients with coronary heart disease, and that these complexes can induce accumulation of cholesterol in cultured smooth muscle cells.

An understanding of the pathogenesis of atherosclerosis has eluded us to date. Numerous theories have been proposed, all of which have some merit but none of which provides a total explanation. It is possible, indeed probable, that like many other processes, atherosclerosis is the end product of multiple pathways of cell damage. The idea that one of these involves immune complex formation and/or immune-mediated damage to vessel walls raises the possibility of new avenues of prevention and therapy for at least some patients with atherosclerosis. For example, LDL apheresis, described as a therapeutic tool in familial hypercholesterolemia, makes even more sense if viewed in the context of therapy for immune complex disease (1). These studies require confirmation, of course, and additional investigation to insure that the formation of immune complexes and the like is not a secondary rather than a primary event.

Other potential mechanisms for stimulation of atherogenesis by LDL have been reviewed recently (2).—B.D. Bennett, M.D., Ph.D.

References

1. Keller C: *Atherosclerosis* 86:1, 1991.
2. Steinberg D, et al: *JAMA* 264:3047, 1990.

Illustrated Histopathologic Classification Criteria for Selected Vasculitis Syndromes

Lie JT, for the American College of Rheumatology Subcommittee on Classification of Vasculitis (Mayo Clinic and Found, Rochester, Minn)
Arthritis Rheum 33:1074–1087, 1990 2–5

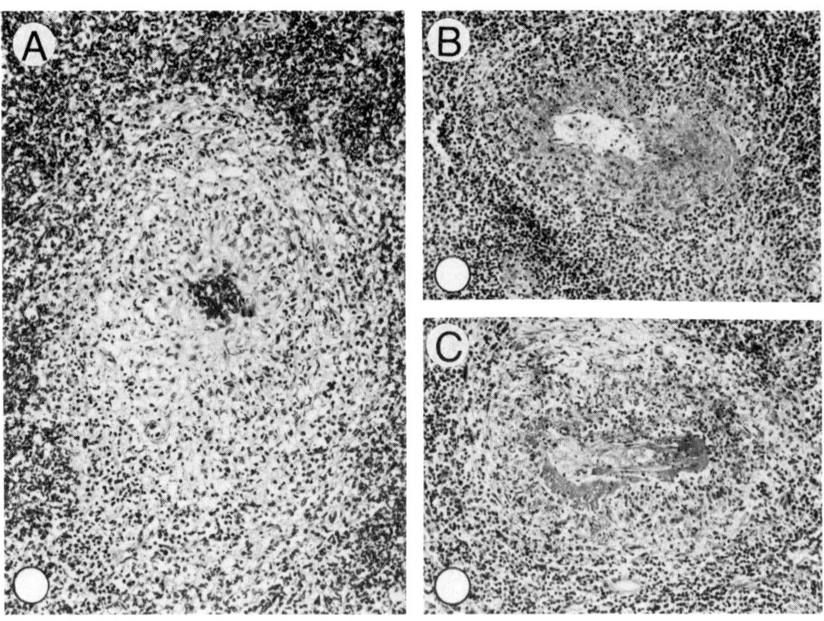

Fig 2–2.—Vascular and extravascular lesions of spleen in Churg-Strauss syndrome. **A,** typical extravascular eosinophilic granuloma with a central zone of necrosis, surrounded by a mixed cell infiltrate with prominent epithelioid cells. **B** and **C,** necrotizing vasculitis with fibrinoid necrosis and eosinophil-rich inflammatory infiltrate (hematoxylin-eosin; original magnification, ×160.) (Courtesy of Lie JT, American College of Rheumatology Subcommittee on Classification of Vasculitis: *Arthritis Rheum* 33:1074–1087, 1990.)

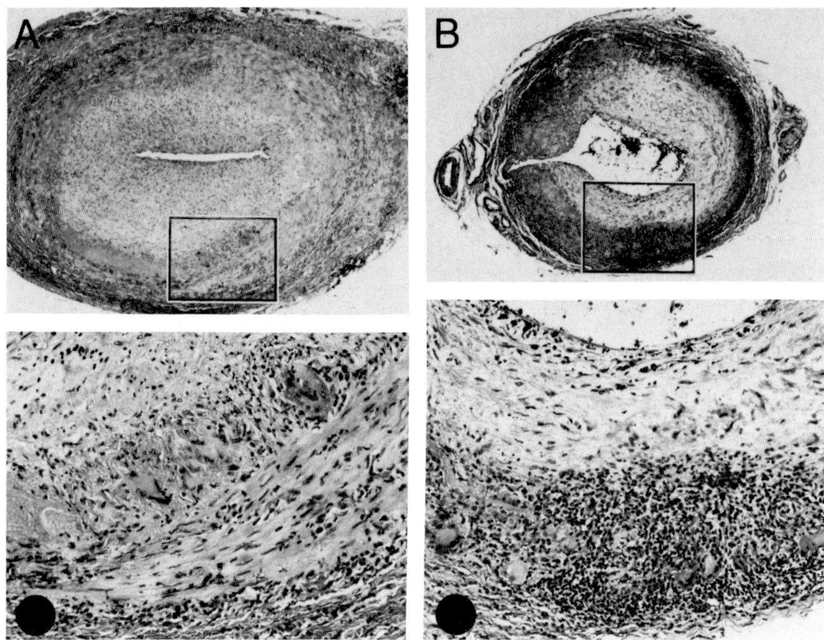

Fig 2–3.—Variations of the histopathology of active temporal (giant cell) arteritis. **Top,** 2 positive biopsies with near occlusion of the arterial lumens. **Bottom,** higher magnification of boxed areas from top views showing the usual location of giant cells in granulomatous inflammation at the intima-media junction (**A**) and the less common location of intense granulomatous inflammation in the media and extending into the adventitia (**B**) (hematoxylin-eosin; original magnifications: top, ×40; bottom, ×160.) (Courtesy of Lie JT, American College of Rheumatology Subcommittee on Classification of Vasculitis: *Arthritis Rheum* 33:1074–1087, 1990.)

Introduction.—The vasculitides are difficult to classify as they often have overlapping clinical and pathologic features. A definitive diagnosis of vasculitis almost always requires histologic documentation. The success of a biopsy diagnosis of vasculitis depends on the pathologist's experience, selection and preparation of tissues, sample size, chronologic age of the disease, and the patient's previous treatment. A standardized histopathologic classification for diagnosing the vasculitides was developed.

Methods.—Seven major vasculitis syndromes that have been generally accepted as distinct clinical entities were selected for the study, including polyarteritis nodosa, Churg-Strauss syndrome (Fig 2–2), Wegener's granulomatosis, hypersensitivity vasculitis, Henoch-Schönlein purpura, giant cell arteritis (Fig 2–3), and Takayasu arteritis. The biopsy material submitted from 278 patients was reviewed to formulate criteria that would apply to the stereotypical cases in each of the 7 categories. The pathology data from another 1,079 patients also were used in the classification.

Conclusion.—Although each of the 7 major vasculitis syndromes selected for inclusion in the classification has its own unique histopathologic features, overlap is common. A biopsy diagnosis of vasculitis does not stand alone, and a definitive diagnosis usually requires consideration of the patient's clinical history, physical findings, and angiographic data.

▶ This article is an excellent summary of criteria for the histopathologic diagnosis of several of the vasculitis syndromes. Although it is recognized that many of these criteria are overlapping and distinction between these cases may not always be possible using histopathology alone, the definition of these criteria is quite useful and the lesions are extremely well illustrated. This article is part of a series on the American College of Rheumatology 1990 criteria for classification of the various vasculitides (1–9).—B.D. Bennett, M.D., Ph.D.

References

1. Bloch DA, et al: *Arthritis Rheum.* 33:1068, 1990.
2. Lightfoot RW, et al: *Arthritis Rheum* 33:1088, 1990.
3. Masi AT et al: *Arthritis Rheum* 33:1094, 1990.
4. Laevitt RV, et al: *Arthritis Rheum* 33:1101, 1990.
5. Calabrese LH: *Arthritis Rheum* 33:1108, 1990.
6. Mills JA, et al: *Arthritis Rheum* 33:1114, 1990.
7. Hunder GG, et al: *Arthritis Rheum* 33:1122, 1990.
8. Arend WP, et al: *Arthritis Rheum* 33:1129, 1990.
9. Fries JF, et al: *Arthritis Rheum* 33:1135, 1990.

Bacillary Epithelioid Angiomatosis Occurring in an Immunocompetent Individual

Cockerell CJ, Bergstresser PR, Myrie-Williams C, Tierno PM (Univ of Texas, Dallas; George Washington Univ; New York Univ)
Arch Dermatol 126:787–790, 1990 2–6

Background.—Patients with AIDS may have an unusual subcutaneous vascular proliferative condition in which clusters of bacilli are found within the vascular lesion. Oral erythromycin resolves this condition. This type of infectious disorder developed in a patient without HIV infection who had no risk factors for the development of AIDS.

Case Report.—Man, 37, had a recurrent, red papular rash on the right forearm for 18 months (Fig 2–4). The rash consisted of lesions that ranged in diameter from 5 mm to 1 cm. Some lesions had disappeared spontaneously but, as lesions cleared, others formed. No risk factors for HIV exposure were found after rigorous questioning by at least 4 physicians. Two separate serologic HIV tests using the Western blot technique did not find any circulating antibody to the HIV. The patient observed that this condition appeared to start after his pet parakeet walked on the affected arm. The bird had a history of respiratory allergy that responded to corticosteroid therapy but had no active infectious disease. Partial resolution of the condition occurred after treatment with oral trimethoprim-sulfamethoxazole for 14 days. During the next 3 months of erythromycin therapy (2–3 g/day), scattered new lesions continued to appear. Local cryosurgery successfully cured these new lesions.

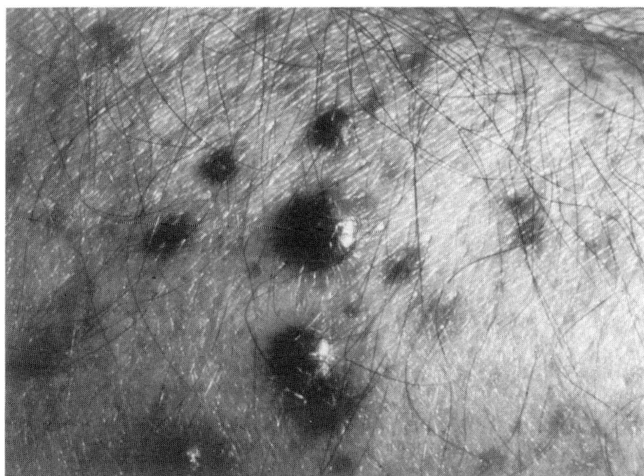

Fig 2–4.—Close-up reveals the purplish vascular nature of individual papules. (Courtesy of Cockerell CJ, Bergstresser PR, Myrie-Williams C, et al: *Arch Dermatol* 126:787–790, 1990.)

Methods and Findings.—Hematoxylin-eosin stain and Warthin-Starry silver stains (pH 3.8) were used to detect the presence of bacteria in biopsied tissue from the lesion site. The hematoxylin-eosin–stained sections of 3 skin lesions demonstrated lobular proliferations of small round blood vessels composed of closely adherent cuboidal endothelial cells with abundant cytoplasm. Microbiological tests were positive for coccobacillus, and electron microscopic analysis demonstrated the usual characteristics of bacilli.

Implications.—This condition was described as bacillary epithelioid angiomatosis (BEA) in a patient who did not have an HIV infection or any risk factors for such an infection. This is the first known report of such an event. Once physicians begin to recognize this condition and use the Warthin-Starry silver and hematoxylin-eosin stains to detect bacteria, more cases of this vascular proliferative disorder probably will be reported.

▶ Bacillary epithelioid angiomatosis, described in 1983, is thought to be a new disease. The vast majority of cases have been identified in patients with AIDS. In this study, the authors describe a patient who had no evidence of HIV infection or other immunodeficiency in whom cutaneous lesions were clinically and histologically identical to those seen in immunocompromised patients with bacillary angiomatosis. Although the bacteria recovered from this patient were similar ultrastructurally to the bacteria recovered from immunocompromised patients with the disease, several differences were noted in culture characteristics and in response to therapy. These differences suggest that this patient's infection may have been caused by a more virulent strain of the organism.—J.S. Metcalf, M.D.

Acute Rheumatic Fever in New York City (1969 to 1988): A Comparative Study of Two Decades

Griffiths SP, Gersony WM (Columbia Univ; Babies Hosp of the Columbia-Presbyterian Med Ctr, New York)

J Pediatr 116:882–887, 1990 2–7

Background.—In the early 1980s, the seeming disappearance of acute rheumatic fever (ARF) was reported in the United States. Between 1984 and 1988, scattered resurgences of ARF occurred in several areas. The annual incidence and presentation of rheumatic fever in the past 20 years were examined.

Methods.—The records of all patients with ARF admitted to a New York City hospital between 1969 and 1988 were reviewed. Patients were classified by major manifestations in the acute attack based on the revised Jones criteria.

Results.—There were 115 reported attacks of ARF between 1969 and 1988; 104 were first attacks and 11 were recurrences. The maximum number of cases in a year, 18, occurred in 1969. Thereafter, the annual incidence was greatly reduced until a resurgence occurred in 1985 and 1986, when ARF was diagnosed in 25 patients. The frequency of major manifestations and the severity of carditis in the 1980s did not differ from these findings in the 1970s. Fifty-one patients had polyarthritis alone; 31, carditis alone; and 28, both carditis and polyarthritis. Five had chorea. Congestive heart failure occurred in 17 carditis attacks. One of these patients died of fulminant disease in 1982. Most of the affected population was urban and low income, and lived in crowded communities. More than half of the patients were Hispanic, predominantly from the Dominican Republic.

Conclusions.—This prevalence of ARF emphasizes the need for early detection and treatment of streptococcal pharyngitis. The fact that 9.5% of the attacks were recurrent indicates failure to comply with antimicrobial prophylaxis, which reaffirms the need for better secondary prevention programs.

▶ This paper emphasizes the necessity for continuing to educate health care personnel regarding classic examples of disease, even though under ideal circumstances the disease should no longer occur. The relationship between streptococcal pharyngitis and ARF is well known, and with proper therapy both initial and recurrent attacks are almost entirely preventable. This study should heighten physician awareness of the necessity for appropriate evaluation of all cases of pharyngitis, and also for the extension of such simple health care benefits to low-income urban areas.—B.D. Bennett, M.D., Ph.D.

A Distinctive Cardiovascular Lesion Resembling Histiocytoid (Epithelioid) Hemangioma: Evidence Suggesting Mesothelial Participation

Luthringer DJ, Virmani R, Weiss SW, Rosai J (Yale Univ; Armed Forces Inst of Pathology, Washington, DC)

Am J Surg Pathol 14:993–1000, 1990 2–8

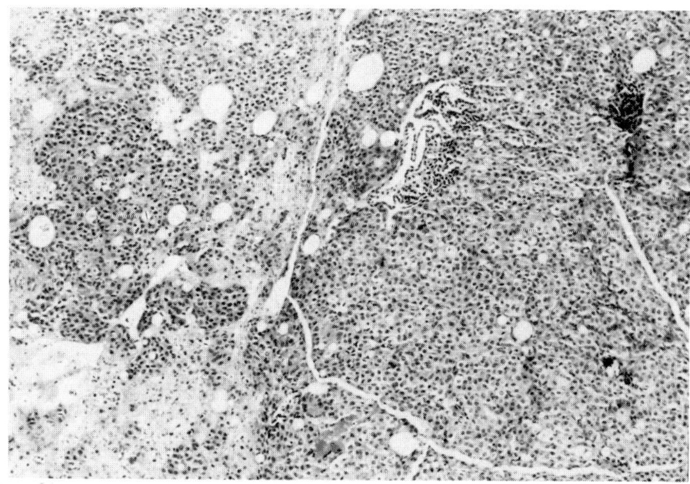

Fig 2–5.—Solid cell clusters are surrounded by fibrin and occasionally separated by large round empty spaces. (Courtesy of Luthringer DJ, Virmani R, Weiss SW, et al: *Am J Surg Pathol* 14:993–1000, 1990.)

Introduction.—In 1979, Rosai et al. suggested the term "histiocytoid hemangioma" for a condition of endothelial proliferation having a distinctive histiocytoid appearance. Some of these lesions have clear neoplastic features and can metastasize; they are called "epithelioid hemangioendotheliomas." A cardiovascular lesion resembling histiocytoid (epithelioid) hemangioma occurred in 14 patients.

Clinical Picture.—The 7 men and 7 women had an average age of 51 years. Several lesions were attached to the endocardium of the left atrial wall or to valve tissue, whereas 3 were floating freely within the pericardial sac. Eight patients were operated on because of severe mitral valve disease. None of the 9 patients followed had evidence of a recurrent lesion.

Pathology.—The lesions, all solitary, ranged from 1 cm to 3 cm in size and usually were seen as a small fleshy mass adhering loosely to the endocardial wall. Solid clusters of cells were seen within a network of fibrin and red blood cells, resembling a thrombus or blood clot (Fig 2–5). Most cells were round to polygonal in shape (Fig 2–6) and had a histiocytoid or epithelioid appearance. Mitotic figures were very infrequent. Myocardium was not identified in any case. The cytoplasm of smaller cells consistently stained strongly for keratin.

Conclusion.—A reactive mesothelial origin is the most likely explanation of this lesion.

▶ The recognition of benign mesothelial proliferation involving the heart and pericardium and its distinction from true neoplasms (hemangiomas, mesotheliomas) may have implications at the time of frozen-section diagnosis. The authors speculate that the pathogenesis of these lesions may relate to previous cardiac invasive procedures (e.g., catheterization), but other conditions that elicit a reac-

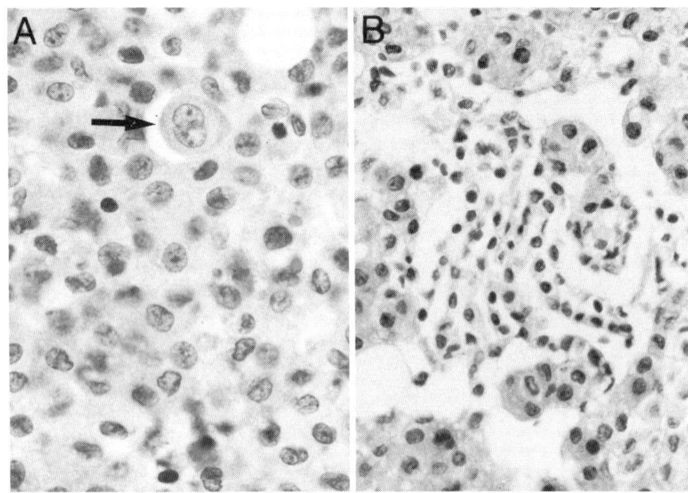

Fig 2–6.—High-power view of the proliferating cells. **A**, large cell with acidophilic cytoplasm and bilobed nucleus (*arrow*) is seen amid smaller, uniform cells with a bland nuclear appearance. **B**, small cells arranged in tubule-like formations can be seen among the larger cuboidal cells. (Courtesy of Luthringer DJ, Virmani R, Weiss SW, et al: *Am J Surg Pathol* 14:993–1000, 1990.)

tive mesothelial response (e.g., mediastinal irradiation for malignancy) may alsounderlie this condition in some patients.—J.B. Atkinson, M.D., Ph.D.

Spindle Cell Haemangioendothelioma: A Clinicopathological and Immunohistochemical Study Indicative of a Non-Neoplastic Lesion

Fletcher CDM, Beham A, Schmid C (St Thomas' Hosp, London; Univ of Graz, Austria)

Histopathology 18:291–301, 1991 2–9

Introduction.—Thirty-five spindle cell hemangioendotheliomas have been reported. They occur in patients of widely varying age but often begin in childhood or early adult life. Up to half of the patients have had multiple lesions. Only one previously reported tumor has metastasized, and this was after 19 recurrences. Twenty further patients with these tumors have been identified.

Patients.—Twelve patients had multiple lesions, whereas 8 had a solitary nodule. The lower extremity was the most common tumor site. Most lesions occurred distally on the extremities. Among the 10 patients followed over the long term, in those with multiple lesions new tumors tended to develop over many years in areas adjacent to previous lesion sites. One patient had lesions resembling epithelioid hemangioendothelioma; subsequently, a well-differentiated angiosarcoma developed in the same part of the body.

Pathology.—Circumscribed nodules, present in the dermis or superficial subcutis, consisted mainly of thin-walled, variably dilated vascular spaces and solid spindle cell areas. The dilated spaces often contained thrombi. The cells lacked nuclear hyperchromasia and, with one exception, did not exhibit mitotic activity. Bundles of eosinophilic smooth muscle cells were identified, as were large malformed vessels resembling those of an arteriovenous malformation.

Interpretation.—Spindle cell hemangioendothelioma appears to be a nonneoplastic vascular lesion, possibly a reactive one, arising in conjunction with locally abnormal blood flow.

▶ These authors hypothesize that the rare tumor, spindle cell hemangioendothelioma, is a form of vascular malformation. Additional cases are necessary to test this hypothesis.—A.J. Garvin, M.D.

The Immunophenotype of Hemangiopericytomas and Glomus Tumors, With Special Reference to Muscle Protein Expression: An Immunohistochemical Study and Review of the Literature

Porter PL, Bigler SA, McNutt M, Gown AM (Univ of Washington)

Mod Pathol 4:46–52, 1991 2–10

Introduction.—Traditionally, both hemangiopericytomas and glomus tumors have been thought to arise from proliferation of the pericytes. However, ultrastructural studies indicate the presence of well-developed smooth muscle myofibrils and dense bodies in the cells of glomus tumors, whereas hemangiopericytomas more closely resemble normal pericytes. Immunocytochemical studies were conducted to define the immunophenotype of these 2 tumors, particularly with regard to expression of muscle-specific actin and desmin.

Methods.—Antibodies to vimentin, low–molecular-weight cytokeratins (35βH11), muscle actins (HHF35), desmin (clone 33), S100 protein, nerve growth factor receptor (NGFR5), myelin-associated glycoprotein (CD57), factor VIII-related antigen, and *Ulex* lectin were localized using the avidin-biotin immunoperoxidase method in formalin-fixed, paraffin-embedded tissue from 16 glomus tumors and 11 hemangiopericytomas.

Results.—Muscle-specific actin was present in 88% of glomus tumors and desmin was found in 19%. In contrast, desmin and muscle actins were absent in all hemangiopericytomas. Three different "nerve sheath"–associated marker proteins, including CD57, S100 protein, and nerve growth factor receptor, were present in a subset of both tumors. Vimentin expression was consistently present in both hemangiopericytomas and glomus tumors.

Conclusion.—This study demonstrates the immunohistochemical expression of smooth-muscle actin in most glomus tumors. In contrast, although muscle-specific actin has been identified in normal pericytes, there is no evidence of an analogous expression in hemangiopericytomas.

▶ In 1956, Arthur Purdy Stout postulated that the glomus tumor and the hemangiopericytoma, which he had named, originated from the pericyte (1). Subsequent studies have failed to demonstrate all of the cellular features of the pericyte in hemangiopericytomas, most notably the lack of smooth muscle expression. In this series, a few hemangiopericytomas expressed some nonspecific markers of peripheral nerve. Additional monoclonal antibodies will be necessary to identify the cell of origin of the hemangiopericytoma.—A.J. Garvin, M.D., Ph.D.

Reference

1. Stout AP: *Lab Invest* 5:217, 1956.

Incidental Glomus Coccygeum: When a Normal Structure Looks Like a Tumor

Albrecht S, Zbieranowski I (Univ of Toronto)

Am J Surg Pathol 14:922–924, 1990 2–11

Background.—Tumors of the glomus, a specialized arteriovenous anastomosis in the distal extremities, are easily diagnosed. Two reports

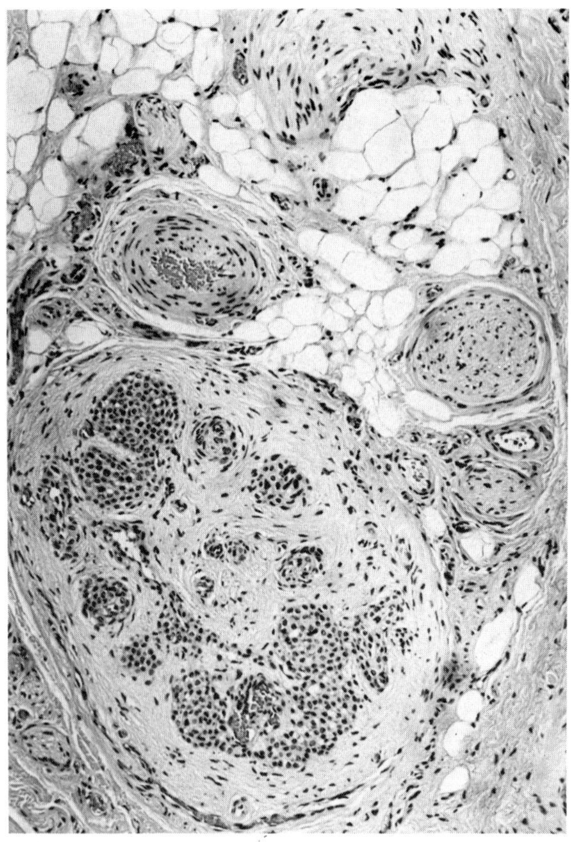

Fig 2–7.—Numerous nerve twigs surround 1 of the individual glomus nodules. (Courtesy of Albrecht S, Zbieranowski I: *Am J Surg Pathol* 14:922–924, 1990.)

of the removal of glomera coccygea during pilonidal sinus excision appear similar to earlier descriptions of tumors of the coccygeal glomus.

Methods.—Two patients, aged 30 years and 40 years, each had a pilonidal sinus in the usual location and underwent deep excision of the sinuses.

Pathology.—Microscopic analysis revealed that both pilonidal sinus specimens had a typical appearance, with related dermal inflammation and fibrosis. The glomus bodies, found in the deep subcutaneous tissue, consisted of clustered nodules .28–2.1 mm in diameter. Each of these nodules was encapsulated and contained a loose, fibroblastic stroma (Fig 2–7). The stroma contained nests of rounded epithelioid cells that surrounded small blood vessels in the same way as the glomus. Many nerve twigs also were noted.

Conclusions.—These findings suggest that pathologists should be familiar with the appearance of normal glomus in the distal extremities, because they may be found unexpectedly in a specimen taken from the coccygeal region.

▶ Normal anatomical structures posing as neoplasms are part of the every day pitfalls of surgical pathology practice. These authors add yet another structure, the glomus coccygeum, to a growing list that includes such diverse entities as the juxta oral organ of Chievitz (1), urachal remnants at the dome of the bladder, and the pineal gland. The authors point to a number of case reports in which this normal finding has been reported erroneously as a glomus tumor and has been said to be the cause of coccydynia. In addition to tumors of the glomus apparatus, the epithelioid cells resemble ependymal cells and presumably could be mistaken initially for an extraspinal sacrococcygeal ependymoma.—G.F. Worsham, M.D.

Reference

1. Tshen TA, Fechner RE: *Am J Surg Pathol* 3:147, 1979.

QBEnd/10: A New Immunostain for the Routine Diagnosis of Kaposi's Sarcoma

Sankey EA, More L, Dhillon AP (Royal Free Hosp, London)
J Pathol 161:267–271, 1990 2–12

Introduction.—Kaposi's sarcoma is seen increasingly often in AIDS patients, but it is not always easy to diagnose. Several endothelial markers have been described for this tumor, but immunocytochemical methods have so far not been helpful.

Methods.—A new IgG1 murine monoclonal antibody, QBEnd/10, was raised against CD34 in human placental endothelial cells. The antibody can be applied to formalin-fixed, paraffin-embedded tissue and stains the spindle cells of Kaposi's sarcoma. Twenty-two cutaneous lesions from 9 patients with Kaposi's sarcoma were examined.

Findings.—QBEnd/10 clearly immunostained spindle cells in patch,

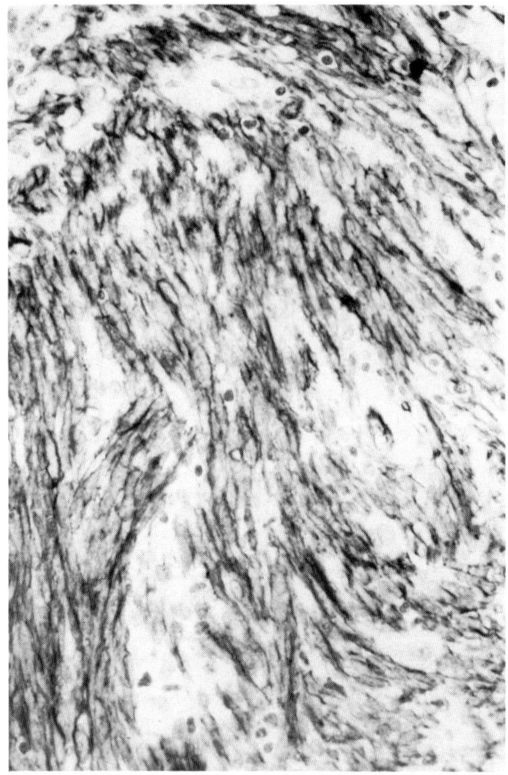

Fig 2–8.—QBEnd/10 immunostaining of a nodular Kaposi's sarcoma showing intense cytoplasmic staining of the spindle cells. (Courtesy of Sankey EA, More L, Dhillon AP: *J Pathol* 161:267–271, 1990.)

plaque, and nodular lesions of the tumor (Fig 2–8), but not those in vascular or spindle cell tumors. Spindle cells of Kaposi's sarcoma stained only weakly and irregularly for factor VIII-related antigen and not at all for *Ulex europaeus* agglutinin 1 (UEA-1).

Conclusion.—Kaposi's sarcoma can be reliably diagnosed by immunostaining routinely prepared tissue with QBEnd/10.

▶ The diagnosis of Kaposi's sarcoma is often difficult to discern from other spindle cell neoplasms. Unfortunately, the factor VIII-related antigen and reactivity with the lectin *U. europaeus* is too often destroyed by routine processing in paraffin-embedded material. The development of a specific monoclonal antibody similar to the one described here would be an excellent aid in the diagnosis of Kaposi's sarcoma.—A.J. Garvin, M.D., Ph.D.

3 Hematopoietic System

Composite Lymphoma: A Clinicopathologic Analysis of Nine Patients With Hodgkin's Disease and B-Cell Non-Hodgkin's Lymphoma

Gonzalez CL, Medeiros LJ, Jaffe ES (Natl Cancer Inst, Bethesda, Md)

Am J Clin Pathol 96:81–89, 1991 3–1

Background.—Composite lymphomas involving the same lymph node or extranodal site are usually 2 separate types of non-Hodgkin's lymphoma (NHL), reflecting 2 expressions of the same progenitor cell population. On occasion, however, subtypes of Hodgkin's disease (HD) and NHL coexist.

Results.—Eleven samples of composite lymphoma involving HD and NHL from 9 patients were reviewed. Two patients had recurrent tumors. The initial specimen from 1 recurrence showed follicular and diffuse large-cell NHL with unclassifiable HD; a specimen obtained during relapse showed diffuse large-cell NHL with nodular sclerosis HD. In the other recurrence the NHL component was follicular mixed in both specimens, whereas the HD component was nodular sclerosis in the initial specimen and interfollicular in that obtained during relapse. Of the remaining patients, the HD component was nodular sclerosis or of mixed cellularity in 3 cases each and unclassifiable in 1. The NHL component was diffuse large cell and diffuse large cell immunoblastic in 2 cases each and follicular and diffuse large cell, diffuse mixed small and large cell, or lymphocytic lymphoma of intermediate differentiation in 1 case each (table). Of 9 specimens tested, the NHL component was positive for leukocyte common antigen (LCA) and negative for Leu-M1. A B cell phenotype was suggested by the finding of L26-positive and UCHL-1 negative neoplastic cells. Reed-Sternberg and Hodgkin's cells from the HD component were Leu-M1 positive and LCA negative in 5 of 7 cases, suggesting an immunophenotype typical of non–lymphocyte-predominant HD. Two specimens contained malignant cells negative for Leu-M1 and LCA.

Conclusions.—Cases of composite HD and NHL are uncommon, and even less common is NHL and coexistent non–lymphocyte-predominant HD. When such lymphomas occur, they usually involve a B cell NHL coexisting with HD. There may therefore be a close relationship between malignant HD cells and B lymphocytes.

▶ Our concepts about HD are undergoing dramatic changes. The nodular variant of lymphocyte-predominant HD has many clinical, immunophenotypic, and morphological features that suggest a B cell origin for this neoplasm. Although there is a growing body of evidence that Reed-Sternberg (RS) cells are lymphoid, conflicting information is presented in the literature as to the B or T cell nature of these cells. The current study supports a B cell origin for the RS cells

Summary of Pathologic and Immunophenotypic Data

Case No.	*Biopsy Site*	*NHL Diagnosis (%)**	*NHL Cell Phenotype*	*HD Diagnosis (%)**	*RS/H Cell Phenotype*
1	Cervical lymph node	Large-cell immunoblastic (75%)	LCA+, L26+, LeuMl−, UCHL−1−	Nodular sclerosis (25%)	LeuMl+, LCA−, L26+, UCHL−1−
2A	Inguinal lymph node	Follicular and diffuse large-cell (NA)	LCA+, L26+, LeuMl−, UCHL−1−	Unclassified (NA)	LeuMl+, LCA−, L26+, UCHL−1−
2B	Supraclavicular lymph node	Diffuse large-cell (90%)	LCA+, L26+, LeuMl−, UCHL−1−	Nodular sclerosis (10%)	LeuMl+, LCA−, L26−, UCHL−1−
3	Stomach	Diffuse large-cell (90%)	LCA+, L26+, LeuMl−, UCHL−1−	Mixed cellularity (10%)	LeuMl−, LCA−, L26−, UCHL−1−
4	Inguinal lymph node	Follicular and diffuse large-cell (50%)	Not done	Nodular sclerosis (50%)	Not done
5	Cervical lymph node	Large-cell immunoblastic (75%)	LCA+, L26+, LeuMl−, UCHL−1−	Mixed cellularity (25%)	Not technically satisfactory
6	Cervical lymph node	Diffuse mixed small and large-cell (95%)	LCA+, L26+, LeuMl−, UCHL−1−	Unclassified (5%)	LeuMl+, LCA−, L26−, UCHL−1−
7	Mediastinum	Diffuse large-cell (50%)	LCA+, L26+, LeuMl−, UCHL−1−	Nodular sclerosis (50%)	Not technically satisfactory
8A	Cervical and inguinal lymph nodes	Follicular mixed small cleaved and large-cell (75%)	Monoclonal IgMk LCA+, L26+, LeuMl−, UCHL−1−	Nodular sclerosis (25%)	LeuMl+, LCA−, L26−, UCHL−1−
8B	Submandibular lymph node	Follicular mixed small cleaved and large-cell (90%)	Not done	Interfollicular (10%)	Not done
9	Inguinal lymph node	Lymphocytic lymphoma of intermediate differentiation (90%)	Monoclonal IgMλ LCA+, L26+, LeuMl−, UCHL−1−	Mixed cellularity (10%)	LeuMl−, LCA−, L26−, UCHL−1−

*Percentage of biopsy specimen involved by either NHL or HD.
NA, not applicable. In case 2A the NHL and HD components were intimately admixed.
(Courtesy of Gonzalez CL, Medeiros LJ, Jaffe ES: *Am J Clin Pathol* 96:81–89, 1991.)

in some cases of non–lymphocyte-predominant HD. It is likely that HD is more than one entity and includes both T and B cell neoplasms.—J.B. Cousar, M.D.

Monocytoid B-Cell Lymphoma: A Study of 36 Cases

Ngan B-Y, Warnke RA, Wilson M, Takagi K, Cleary ML, Dorfman RF (Stanford Univ; Little Company of Mary Hosp, Torrance, Calif; Jikei Univ, Tokyo)

Hum Pathol 22:409–421, 1991 3–2

Background.—Monocytoid B cell lymphoma (MBCL) is an unusual lymphoma in which the neoplastic cells closely resemble reactive monocytoid B lymphocytes. Clinicopathologic study of 36 patients with MBCL included immunohistochemical and immunogenetic studies.

Patients.—The patients were 30 women and 6 men, confirming the reported predilection for females (table). The mean age was 59.8 years. Thirty patients initially had lymphadenopathy, localized in most cases. There was a propensity for the paraparotid or intraparotid glands to be affected; the salivary glands were affected in 5 cases. Patients had the symptom complex of autoimmune disease, with 8 having Sjögren's syndrome; 1, systemic lupus erythematosus; 1, Raynaud's phenomenon; and 2, monoclonal gammopathy. Twenty-three patients were followed for up to 20 years; 15 were alive and well at last follow-up.

Findings.—Seven patients had "composite lymphomas" and 7 had association with or progression to a higher grade lymphoma, usually large cell. The latter finding was associated with more aggressive behavior by the lymphoma. The B cell nature of the lymphoma was apparent on immunohistochemical study of 20 patients. Nine of 15 frozen or paraffin biopsy specimens showed immunoglobulin light chain restriction. In all frozen biopsy specimens, monocytoid B cells were stained with at least 1 monoclonal B cell antibody. One specimen stained with LeuM5 and 1 with LeuM3. Monocytoid B cells had an average reactivity of less than 10% with the proliferation marker Ki-67, in keeping with the indolent behavior of MBCL. The t(14;18) chromosomal translocation did not seem to play a causative role.

Conclusions.—Monocytoid B cell lymphoma appears to have morphological and clinical features distinct from other subclasses of low-grade lymphomas. It may be associated with other autoimmune disorders or may represent a true composite lymphoma. There may be an overlap between MBCL and lymphomas arising from mucosa-associated lymphoid tissue.

▶ Monocytoid B cell lymphoma is a recently described entity that is being recognized with increasing frequency. Other authors have also suggested a relationship with Sjögren's syndrome (1) and low-grade B cell lymphomas of mucosa-associated lymphoid tissue (2).—J.B. Cousar, M.D.

References

1. Shin SS, et al: *Hum Pathol* 22:422, 1991
2. Weiss LM: *Hum Pathol* 22:407, 1991.

Clinicopathologic Information on the 36 Patients With Monocytoid B Cell Lymphomas

Patient No.	Age (yr)/Sex	Biopsy Site	Clinicopathologic Features	Treatment	Patient Status/Years
1	60/F	P/LN	Sjögren's syndrome, LA, BLEL	None	AL/4
2	61/M	C/LN	Composite lymphoma (MBCL with SLL), LA	None	AL/1
3	78/F	CH	Discordant lymphoma (SLL, MBCL), CH; no LA	Chemotherapy	LR/3
4	67/M	P/LN	Sjögren's syndrome, LA	Parotidectomy	LR/12
5	74/F	C/I/LN	LA	NA	NA
6	75/F	Breast	No LA	Resection	AL/4
7	67/F	C/LN/T	Cervical-mediastinal mass, LA, T; composite lymphoma (MBCL with FLCL)	Chemotherapy	AL/4
8	58/F	I/LN	Sjögren's syndrome, SLE, gammopathy, splenomegaly, evolved to DLCL, LA	Radiation/chemotherapy	Dead/1
9	52/F	A/LN/BM	Sjögren's syndrome evolved to DLCL, LA	Chemotherapy	Dead/2
10	29/F	C/LN	Polyclonal gammopathy, LA	Chemotherapy	AL/4
11	31/M	C/LN	LA	Radiation	LR/3
12	70/M	A/LN	Splenomegaly, abdominal/thoracic adenopathy	Chemotherapy	AL/3
13	35/F	P/LN	Hodgkin's, nodular sclerosing, 13 yr previously, LA	Parotidectomy	AL/3
14	69/F	P/LN	Sjögren's syndrome, LA	Parotidectomy	AL/1
15	51/F	Stomach	ST; composite lymphoma (MBCL with follicular and diffuse LCL)	Resection	NA
16	79/M	MTM	Composite lymphoma (MBCL with FSCL), LA	Resection	NA
17	48/F	S/LN	Composite lymphoma (MBCL with FLCL), LA evolved to DLCL	Chemotherapy	Dead/1

18	68/F	ST/LN	LA, intra-abdominal mass	Resection/chemotherapy	AL/5
19	58/F	C/LN	Local recurrence, LA	Radiation/chemotherapy	AL/4
20	66/M	A/Med/LN	LA	NA	NA
21	53/F	P/LN	Hodgkin's, nodular sclerosis, 9 yr previously, evolved to DLCL, LA	Parotidectomy	AL/7
22	65/F	I/A/LN	Adenocarcinoma of ovary, LA	Chemotherapy for ovarian carcinoma	AL/1
23	80/F	S/LN	LA, evolved to mixed small and large cell	Radiation	LR/4
24	80/F	S/LN	LA	Chemotherapy	AL/1
25	66/F	SM/LN	LA	NA	NA
26	75/F	P/LN	Sjögren's syndrome	Parotidectomy	AL/1
27	54/F	C/LN/T	Composite lymphoma (MBCL with FSCL), evolution to LCL in thyroid, LA	None	AL/20
28	35/F	P,P/LN	LA, recurrent parotiditis	Resection	NA
29	32/F	C/LN	LA, Sjögren's syndrome; composite lymphoma (MBCL with mixed small and large cell) with plasmacytoid changes	None	NA
30	54/F	P,S/LN	Sialadenitis, 8 yr, BLEL	None	NA
31	66/F	S/LN	LA	None	NA
32	44/M	P,P/LN	BLEL	None	NA
33	36/F	P	BLEL	None	NA
34	67/F	C/LN	LA	None	NA
35	85/F	C/LN	LA	None	NA
36	64/F	Breast, P/LN	Sjögren's syndrome, focal evolution to DLCL	None	AL/1

Abbreviations: A, axillary; *AL,* alive and well; *BLEL,* "benign" lymphoepithelial lesion; *BM,* bone marrow; *C,* cervical; *CH,* chest wall; *DLCL,* diffuse large cell lymphoma; *FLCL,* follicular large cell lymphoma; *FSCL,* follicular small cleaved cell lymphoma; *I,* inguinal; *LA,* lymphadenopathy; *LN,* lymph node; *LR,* local recurrence; *MED,* mediastinum; *MTM,* mesenteric mass; *NA,* not available; *P,* parotid; *S,* scalene; *SLE,* systemic lupus erythematosus; *SM,* submandibular; *ST,* stomach; *T,* thyroid; *SLL,* small lymphocytic lymphoma. (Courtesy of Ngan B-Y, Warnke RA, Wilson M, et al: *Hum Pathol* 22:409–421, 1991.)

Mantle Zone Lymphoma: A Clinicopathologic Study of 22 Cases

Duggan MJ, Weisenburger DD, Ye YL, Bast MA, Pierson JL, Linder J, Armitage JO (Univ of Nebraska; Sun Yat-Sen Univ of Med Sciences, Guangzhou, China)

Cancer 66:522–529, 1990 3–3

Background.—Mantle zone lymphoma (MZL) is a type of follicular non-Hodgkin's lymphoma characterized by proliferating small lymphoid cells in wide mantles around benign germinal centers (Fig 3–1). Past studies have suggested that MZL is the follicular variant of diffuse intermediate lymphocytic lymphoma.

Findings.—Twenty-two MZLs were evaluated. In addition to follicular growth, focal areas of diffuse involvement occurred in nearly 40% of the cases. Usually, the tumor cells were predominantly the small lymphoid type or the intermediate lymphocytic type (Fig 3–2). Immunoperoxidase staining showed the phenotype of MZL to be identical to that of the mantle zones of benign reactive follicles apart from staining with LN5.

Patients.—The median patient age was 63 years; only 3 patients were younger than age 50 years. More than half of the patients had B symptoms at the time of diagnosis. Most of the patients (73%) received multidrug chemotherapy at the outset. Eleven patients experienced complete remission, but 5 later died of lymphoma. Seven of the 9 nonresponsive patients died. The overall median survival time was 88 months at last follow-up. A lymphocyte count of more than 4,000/μL predicted survival, as did fewer than 10 mitoses and fewer than 40 large lymphoid cells per 10 high-power fields.

Conclusions.—Mantle zone lymphoma is a distinctive form of low-grade non-Hodgkin's lymphoma.

▶ The relationship between various morphological categories of neoplasms composed of small B lymphocytes is incompletely understood (see Abstract 3–4). It is hoped that, with new techniques (e.g., molecular genetic analysis)

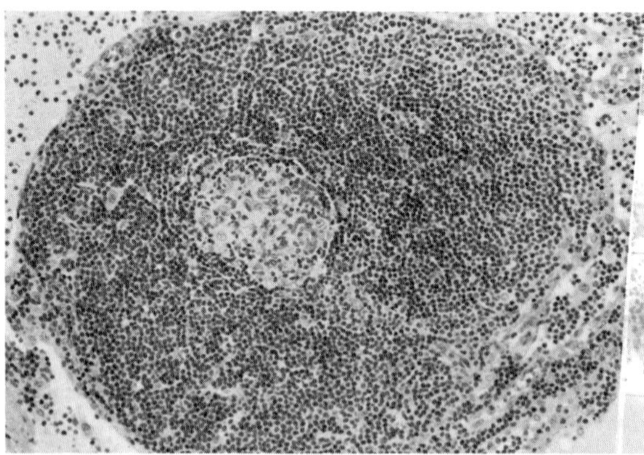

Fig 3–1.—Lymph node showing a follicle with a small germinal center that is surrounded by a wide mantle of neoplastic lymphoid cells. Hematoxylin-eosin; original magnification, ×20. (Courtesy of Duggan MJ, Weisenburger DD, Ye YL, et al: *Cancer* 66:522–529, 1990.)

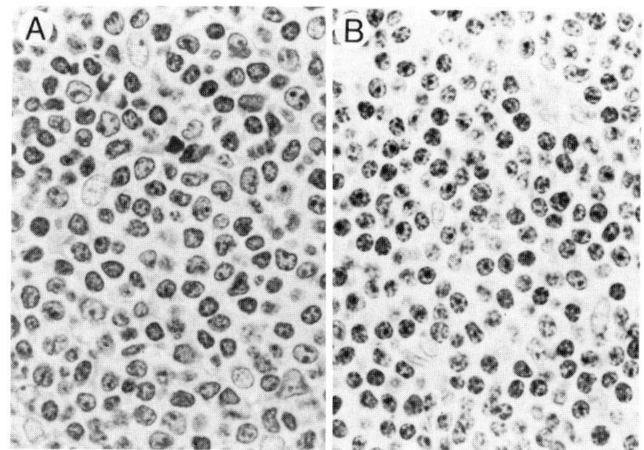

Fig 3–2.—**A,** lymph node showing intermediate lymphocytic lymphoma composed of small to medium-sized cells with irregular nuclear contours. **B,** lymph node showing small lymphocytic lymphoma composed of small cells with uniformly round nuclei. Hematoxylin-eosin; original magnification, ×200. (Courtesy of Duggan MJ, Weisenburger DD, Ye YL, et al: *Cancer* 66:522–529, 1990.)

these neoplasms will become better defined. This study provides some insight into the clinical behavior of MZLs.—J.B. Cousar, M.D.

Lymphocytic Lymphoma of Intermediate Differentiation: Morphologic and Immunophenotypic Spectrum and Clinical Correlations

Lardelli P, Bookman MA, Sundeen J, Longo DL, Jaffe ES (Natl Cancer Inst, Bethesda, Md)

Am J Surg Pathol 14:752–763, 1990 3–4

Background.—There is controversy regarding strict diagnostic criteria for lymphocytic lymphoma of intermediate differentiation (IDL). In addition, the distinction among small lymphocytic lymphomas, chronic lymphocytic leukemia, IDL, and follicular center cell lymphomas is not always evident. Thirty-three patients with IDL were reviewed to define the histopathologic spectrum of the disease and to study morphological and immunophenotypic features that may have prognostic relevance.

Methods.—Twenty-seven samples were analyzed immunophenotypically, and the clinical records of 22 patients were reviewed. There was a male-to-female ratio of 3.4:1, and the median age was 58 years.

Results.—At presentation, all patients had stage III or stage IV disease and 5 had primary extranodal disease. Only 3 patients survived relapse free for longer than 2 years. The median survival was 56.3 months. There were 14 specimens with a morphologically diffuse or only vaguely nodular growth pattern and 18 with a mantle zone pattern (Fig 3–3) and naked germinal centers. For patients with the mantle zone pattern the median survival was 77.4 months. Irregular or cleaved small lymphoid cells (Fig 3–4) with a mitotic rate ranging from 5 to 62 per 20 high-power fields made up the neoplastic population. Seven samples showed a histologically distinctive variant with blastic cytologic features. This was associated with a higher mitotic index and an average survival of 24.9

months. No transformation from a large cell or small noncleaved lymphoma was observed, in contrast to the histologic progression often seen in follicular lymphomas. A mature B cell phenotype with monoclonal Ig and B cell surface antigens was found in all cases, and CD5 positivity was seen in 78% of specimens. Of 6 CD5-negative samples, 3 were from mucosa-associated extranodal sites. Although CD10 was expressed in 52% of tumors and CD25 in 44%, they were not correlated clinically. There was a positive correlation between the proliferative rate measured by Ki-67 and the mitotic index, but neither had a significant effect on survival.

Conclusions.—Lymphocytic lymphoma of intermediate differentiation is a distinct subtype of non-Hodgkin's lymphoma. It may be considered a low-grade lymphoma, although blastic cytologic findings are associated with a more aggressive clinical course. Long-term remissions are rare, even in aggressively treated patients.

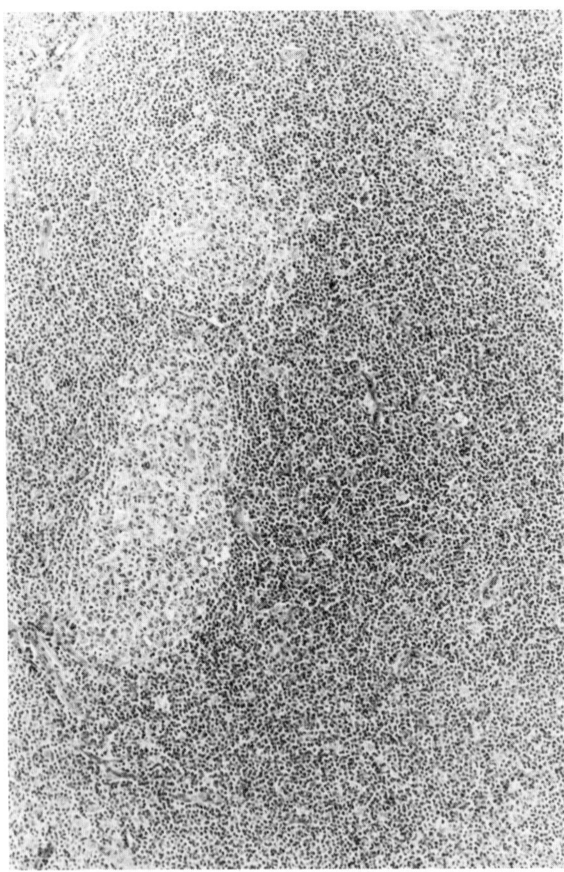

Fig 3–3.—Mantle zone lymphoma of growth with naked germinal centers lacking lymphoid cuffs. It is surrounded by expansive mantles, producing a vaguely nodular growth pattern. (Courtesy of Lardelli P, Bookman MA, Sundeen J, et al: *Am J Surg Pathol* 14:752–763, 1990.)

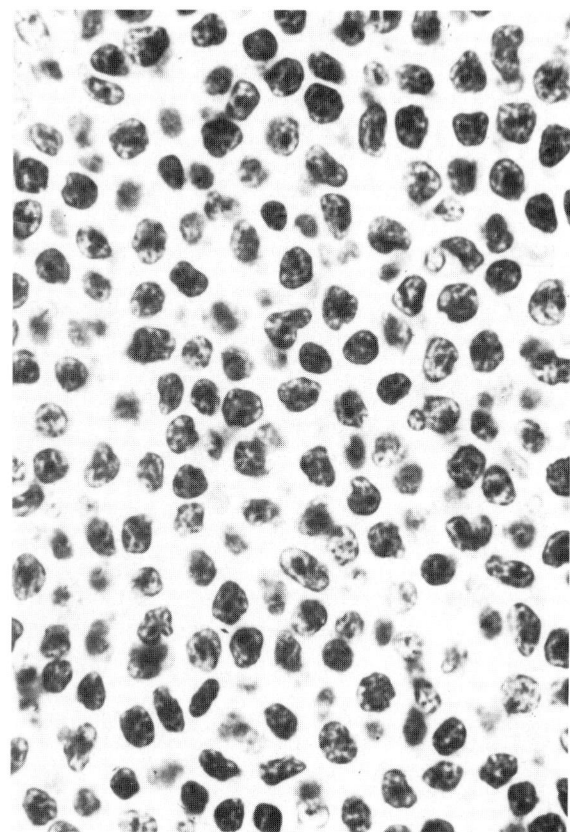

Fig 3–4.—Neoplastic cell population of IDL showing small lymphocytes with slightly indented nuclei and coarse chromatin; original magnification, ×1,000. (Courtesy of Lardelli P, Bookman MA, Sundeen J, et al: *Am J Surg Pathol* 14:752–763, 1990.)

▶ A recent study has suggested that molecular genetic analysis of a centrocytic lymphoma, which is similar if not identical to most IDLs, may be useful in the recognition of these neoplasms. Specifically, rearrangement of the chromosome 11 *bcl*-1 was shown in many patients with centrocytic lymphomas (1).—J.B. Cousar, M.D.

Reference

1. Williams ME, et al: *Blood* 78:493, 1991.

The Value of Immunophenotyping on Paraffin Sections in the Identification of T-Cell Rich B-Cell Large-Cell Lymphomas: Lineage Confirmed by J_H Rearrangement

Osborne BM, Butler JJ, Pugh WC (Univ of Texas, Houston)

Am J Surg Pathol 14:933–938, 1990 3–5

Introduction.—The T-cell-rich B cell lymphoma (TCRBCL), is a difficult clinical entity to diagnose because of the small number of malignant B cells that are present. Immunophenotyping of paraffin-embedded lymphoid tissue can be useful in identifying the minority population of large neoplastic B cells. The utility of this diagnostic approach was validated in 7 cases.

Pathology.—These 7 cases were identified initially as diffuse mixed cell lymphoma of possible peripheral T cell lineage. However, the large cells proved to be immunoreactive with L-26 (pan B cell marker). The smaller lymphocytes reacted with UCHL-1 and Leu-22 (pan T cell markers). The diagnosis of TCRBCL was confirmed by detection of immunoglobulin heavy and light chain gene rearrangements, with germ line configuration of the T cell receptor β-chain gene in all cases.

Conclusions.—These studies confirm the usefulness of immunophenotyping of paraffin sections in the diagnosis of TCRBCL. Further studies of more patients with TCRBCLs are required to understand its clinical significance.

▶ This unusual type of B cell lymphoma can best be recognized with paraffin section immunoperoxidase studies utilizing L26 (CD20). One wonders how many cases reported as peripheral T cell lymphomas before the availability of the newer phenotypic and genotypic markers were really TCRBCL!—J.B. Cousar, M.D.

Primary Large-Cell Lymphoma of the Thymus: A Diffuse B-Cell Neoplasm Presenting as Primary Mediastinal Lymphoma

Davis RE, Dorfman RF, Warnke RA (Stanford Univ)

Hum Pathol 21:1262–1268, 1990 3–6

Background.—It has been thought that large cell non-Hodgkin's lymphomas arising primarily in the thymus are of B lymphocyte origin, even though the thymus is normally the organ of T lymphocyte differentiation. Apart from their predominantly B cell lineage, primary mediastinal non-lymphoblastic non-Hodgkin's lymphomas usually are immunoglobulin negative and have a distinctive large cell morphology, often with sclerosis and clear cytoplasm.

Patients.—Fifteen nonlymphoblastic non-Hodgkin's lymphomas involving the thymus, diagnosed between 1980 and 1989, were studied. A total of 118 tumors involving the mediastinum occurred during this period. All of the patients had an anterior mediastinal mass without apparent involvement of other sites. The mean age at presentation was 29 years.

Histopathology.—The morphological features closely resembled those described in several series of primary nonlymphoblastic non-Hodgkin's lymphoma. Sclerosis was a consistent finding (Fig 3–5) but was quite variable in extent. Mitotic figures also were variable, as was necrosis. Thirteen cases were classified as diffuse large cell non-Hodgkin's lym-

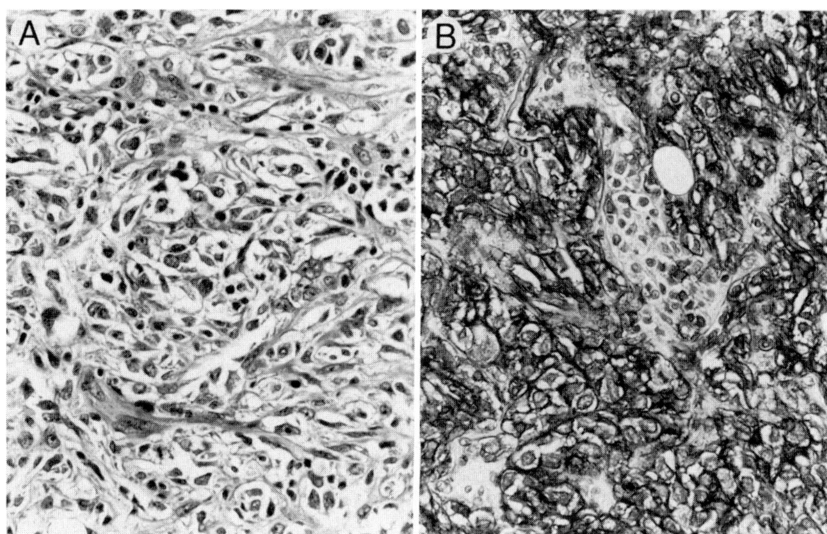

Fig 3–5.—**A,** a representative area from the thymic lymphoma in the case shows tumor cells with pale cytoplasm and angular nuclei, surrounded by small lymphocytes and bands of sclerosis. Hematoxoylin-eosin; original magification , ×400. **B,** immunohistochemical stain using L26 antibody on lymphoma in the case shows strong cell membrane staining of large neoplastic cells; a group of small lymphocytes is unstained. Hematoxylin-eosin stain; original magnification, ×400. (Courtesy of Davis RE, Dorfman RF, Warnke RA: *Hum Pathol* 21:1262–1268, 1990.)

phoma and 2 were classified as immunoblastic lymphoma. Multinucleated cells were not present consistently. Reactive cells were predominantly lymphocytes, but histiocytes also were seen. In all cases but 1, the large atypical neoplastic cells exhibited specific membrane staining with L26.

Conclusion.—Nonlymphoblastic non-Hodgkin's lymphomas primary in the thymus and the mediastinum are similar B lineage neoplasms. Both may well have a thymic B cell origin because the thymus contains substantial numbers of resident B cells in the medulla and extraparenchymal septa.

▶ This study illustrates, among other things, that the complexity and number of different B cell neoplasms have been greatly underestimated.—J.B. Cousar, M.D.

Immunophenotyping of Non-Hodgkin's Lymphomas in Paraffin-Embedded Tissue Sections: A Comparison With Genotypic Analysis

Elghetany MT, Kurec AS, Schuehler K, Forbes BA, Duggan DB, Davey FR
(State Univ of New York, Syracuse)
Am J Clin Pathol 95:517–525, 1991 3–7

Background.—Immunophenotyping of non-Hodgkin's lymphomas (NHLs) in paraffin-embedded tissue sections can be done with several

TABLE 1.—Immunophenotyping 33 Genotypic B Cell Lymphomas

Case	*Dx*	*UCHL-1*	*MT-1*	*MT-2*	*4KB5*	*MB-1*	*MB-2*	*L-26*	*LN-2*	*Mac 387*	*LCA*	*IP:PT*	J_H	J_κ	*TCR-β*	*FC/FS*
1	SL	−	+	+	+	+	+	+	−	−	+	B-cell	R	(−)	G	B-cell
2	SL	−	+	−	+	+	+	+	−	−	+	B-cell	R	(−)	G	B-cell
3	SL	−	−	+	+	+	+	+	−	−	+	B-cell	R	(−)	G	(−)
4	FSC	−	−	+	+	+	+	+	+	−	+	B-cell	R	(−)	G	B-cell
5	FSC	−	−	−	+	+	+	+	+	−	+	B-cell	R	(−)	G	B-cell
6	FSC	−	−	−	+	+	+	+	+	−	+	B-cell	R	R	G	B-cell
7	FSC	−	−	−	+	+	+	+	+	−	+	B-cell	R	(−)	G	(−)
8	FSC	−	−	−	+	+	+	+	+	−	+	B-cell	R	(−)	G	(−)
9	FSC	−	+	+	+	+	+	+	+	−	+	B-cell	R	(−)	G	B-cell
10	FMC	−	−	+	+	−	+	+	−	−	+	B-cell	G	R	G	(−)
11	FMC	−	−	−	−	−	+	+	+	−	+	B-cell	R	(−)	G	(−)
12	FMC	−	−	+	+	+	+	+	+	−	+	B-cell	R	(−)	G	(−)
13	FMC	−	−	−	+	+	+	+	−	−	+	B-cell	R	(−)	G	B-cell
14	FMC	−	−	+	+	+	+	+	−	−	+	B-cell	R	(−)	G	B-cell
15	FMC	−	−	+	+	+	+	+	+	−	+	B-cell	R	R	G	(−)
16	DSC	−	−	+	+	+	+	+	−	−	+	B-cell	R	(−)	G	B-cell

17	DMC	−	−	−	+	+	+	+	+	−	+	B-cell	R	(−)	G	B-cell
18	DMC	−	−	−	+	−	+	+	−	−	+	B-cell	R	(−)	G	B-cell
19	DLC	−	+	−	−	−	−	+	+	−	+	B-cell	R	(−)	G	B-cell
20	DLC	−	−	+	−	+	−	+	+	−	+	B-cell	R	(−)	G	B-cell
21	DLC	−	−	+	+	+	+	+	+	−	+	B-cell	R	R	G	B-cell
22	DLC	−	−	+	+	+	+	+	−	−	+	B-cell	R	R	G	B-cell
23	DLC	−	−	−	+	+	+	+	−	−	+	B-cell	R	(−)	G	(−)
24	DLC	−	−	+	+	+	−	+	−	−	+	B-cell	R	R	G	B-cell
25	DLC	−	−	−	−	−	+	+	+	−	+	B-cell	R	(−)	G	(−)
26	DLC	−	−	−	+	+	+	+	+	−	+	B-cell	R	(−)	G	B-cell
27	LIB	+	−	−	+	+	+	+	+	−	+	B-cell	G	R	G	(−)
28	LIB	−	−	+	+	+	+	−	−	−	+	B-cell	R	(−)	G	(−)
29	LIB	−	−	−	+	+	+	+	−	−	+	B-cell	R	(−)	G	(−)
30	LIB	−	−	−	+	+	−	+	+	−	+	B-cell	R	(−)	G	(−)
31	LIB	−	−	+	+	+	+	+	+	−	+	B-cell	R	R	G	B-cell
32	MZL	−	−	+	+	+	+	+	+	−	+	B-cell	R	(−)	G	(−)
33	MZL	−	−	+	+	+	+	+	+	−	+	B-cell	R	(−)	G	B-cell

Abbreviations: SL, malignant lymphoma small lymphocytic; *FLC*, follicular large cell; *DLC*, diffuse large cell; *LBL*, lymphoblastic lymphoma; *IP:PT*, immunophenotype: paraffin-embedded tissues; *FC/FS*, flow cytometry or frozen section immunophenotyping; *FSC*, follicular small cleaved cell; *DSC*, diffuse small cleaved cell; *LIB*, large cell immunoblastic; *FMC*, follicular mixed cell; *DMC*, diffuse mixed cell; *MZL*, mantle zone lymphoma; *LCA*, leukocyte common antigen; (−), not performed; *R*, rearranged; *G*, germline.

(Courtesy of Elghetany MT, Kurec AS, Schueler K, et al: *Am J Clin Pathol* 95:517–525, 1991.)

TABLE 2.—Immunophenotyping 6 Genotypic T-Cell Lymphomas

Case	*Dx*	*UCHL-1*	*MT-1*	*MT-2*	*4KB5*	*MB-1*	*MB-2*	*L-26*	*LN-2*	*Mac 387*	*LCA*	*IP:PT*	J_H	J_κ	*TCR-β*	*FC/FS*
34	DMC	−	+	−	+	+	−	+	−	−	+	B-cell	G	(−)	R	T-cell
35	DLC	−	−	−	−	−	−	−	+	−	+	?	G	(−)	R	T-cell
36	DLC	+	+	−	−	−	−	−	−	−	−	T-cell	G	(−)	R	T-cell
37	LIB	−	+	−	−	−	−	−	−	−	+	T-cell	G	(−)	R	T-cell
38	LIB	−	+	+	−	−	−	−	−	−	+	T-cell	G	(−)	R	T-cell
39	LBL	+	+	−	−	−	+w	−	−	−	+	T-cell	G	(−)	R	T-cell

Abbreviations: w, weak staining of 20% of cells. Other abbreviations as in Table 1.
(Courtesy of Elghetany MT, Kurec AS, Schuehler K, et al: *Am J Clin Pathol* 95:517–525, 1991.)

currently available monoclonal antibodies (MoAbs). A comparative study was done to determine the reliability of these agents in predicting genotypes.

Methods.—An alkaline phosphatase-antialkaline phosphatase technique was used to study 44 surgical specimens obtained from patients with NHL. The MoAbs used were leukocyte common antigen (CD45), Mac 387, L26, 4KB5, MB1, MB2, LN2, UCHL1, MT1, and MT2. Gene rearrangement studies for the immunoglobulin heavy chain and for the T cell receptor β chain were done to determine the lineages of the neoplastic cells.

Results.—A B cell lineage was determined in 75% of specimens (Table 1), T cell lineage in 14% (Table 2), and mixed or undetermined lineage in 11%. Lineage assignments by paraffin section immunophenotyping and those by gene rearrangement studies were concordant in 95% of lymphomas with an unequivocally defined genotype. The most sensitive MoAb for detecting the B cell genotype was L26. For detecting the T cell genotype, MT1 was the most sensitive and UCHL1 was the most specific.

Conclusions.—Lineage assignment of NHLs in paraffin sections appears to reflect the corresponding genotype when an appropriate MoAb panel is used. The MoAbs accurately reflect the genotypic expression determined by DNA analysis in most B cell lymphomas and in fewer T cell lymphomas. There is a continuing need for more specific MoAbs, especially for those against T cells.

▶ One "take home" message from this study is that L26 appears to be a very good marker of B cell lineage in paraffin-embedded tissue—something to keep in mind if you are planning to set up a diagnostic immunoperoxidase service in your laboratory.—J.B. Cousar, M.D.

Peripheral T-Cell Lymphomas: A Clinicopathologic Study of 75 Cases

Chott A, Augustin I, Wrba F, Hanak H, Öhlinger W, Radaszkiewicz T (Univ of Vienna; Inst of Pathology, Vienna and Linz, Austria)

Hum Pathol 21:1117–1125, 1990 3–8

Background.—A classification system for peripheral T cell lymphomas (PTL) was developed, i.e., the "Updated Kiel Classification of Non-Hodgkin's Lymphomas." To assess the utility of this low- and high-grade classification system, 75 PTLs, excluding mycosis fungoides and Sezary's syndrome, were classified and then examined morphologically, immunologically, and by patient survival.

Findings.—Of the 75 lymphomas, 37 were classified as low grade (table). These included T cell chronic lymphocytic leukemia, 3; lymphoepithelioid, 4; angioimmunoblastic, 22; T zone, 6; and pleomorphic small cell PTL, 2. The other 38 lymphomas were classified as high grade and included 24 pleomorphic medium and large cell types; immunoblastic, 1;

Distribution of 75 Peripheral T Cell Lymphomas Classified According to the "Updated Kiel Classification of Non-Hodgkin's Lymphomas"

Classification	No.
Low-grade	
Lymphocytic-chronic lymphocytic leukemia	3
Lymphoepithelioid (Lennert's lymphoma)	4
Angioimmunoblastic (AILD, LGR-X)	22
T zone	6
Pleomorphic small cell	2
High-grade	
Pleomorphic, medium and large cell	24
Immunoblastic	1
Large-cell anaplastic (Ki-1-positive)	13

Abbreviations: AILD, angioimmunoblastic lymphoma with dysproteinemia; *LGR-X,* lymphogranulomatosis X.

(From Chott A, Augustin I, Wrba F, et al: *Hum Pathol* 21:1117–1125, 1990. Courtesy of Radaszkiewicz T, Lennert K: *Dtsch Med Wochenschr* 100:1157—1163, 1975.)

and large cell anaplastic Ki-1-positive PTL, 13. Only high-grade PTLs had loss of pan-T antigens.

Patients.—Of the 75 patients, 60 had lymphadenopathy and 15 had extranodal disease. Symptoms of B cell lymphoma occurred in 43 cases. Bone marrow involvement was detected in 12 patients with non–T-cell chronic lymphocytic leukemia. Most patients cases assessed were in stage III or IV. Of the 60 intensively treated patients, 37% experienced complete remission, and 15 continued in complete remission at a median of 24 months. The overall median survival rate was 23 months. Pleomorphic medium and large cell PTL was the most aggressive, with a median survival of 8 months. Correlated with a significantly decreased survival were B cell lymphoma symptoms, bone marrow involvement, and a Ki-67-positive response. Age, stage, and grade were not correlated with survival.

Conclusions.—Classification of PTLs into low- and high-grade malignancies was not useful for prognosis in this series of 75 patients. However, because Ki-67 reactivity was associated with poor survival, it may be a useful prognostic tool.

▶ Peripheral T cell lymphomas exhibit considerable morphological and clinical heterogeneity. In another study of low-grade node-based peripheral T cell lymphomas, the clinicopathologic features of 110 angioimmunoblastic, T-zone, and lymphoepithelial lymphomas were described (1). An overlapping spectrum of histologic appearances was noted, and immunologic studies revealed that the neoplastic cells were usually of the T helper phenotype.—J.B. Cousar, M.D.

Reference

1. Nakamura S, et al: *Cancer* 67:2565, 1991.

Comparison of Anaplastic Large Cell Ki-1 Lymphomas and Microvillous Lymphomas in Their Immunologic and Ultrastructural Features

Kinney MC, Glick AD, Stein H, Collins RD (Vanderbilt Univ; Freie Universität, Berlin)

Am J Surg Pathol 14:1047–1060, 1990 3–9

Background.—Anaplastic large cell Ki-1 malignant lymphomas (MLs) have a pleomorphic infiltrate with a sinus growth pattern. Microvillous ML is also a large cell malignant lymphoma with a sinus growth pattern. These 2 MLs were compared immunologically and ultrastructurally to determine whether ultrastructural features are sufficient to distinguish between them.

Pathology.—Immunologic studies were carried out on 23 lymphomas and ultrastructural studies were done on 14 anaplastic large cell Ki-1 MLs. Findings were compared to those in 7 microvillous MLs. Thirteen of the 23 anaplastic large cell Ki-1 MLs were predominantly of T cell type, 3 were B cell, and in 7 cases the type was not well defined. Six of the 7 microvillous MLs expressed monotypic immunoglobulin and 1 appeared to be a B cell type (Fig 3–6). All microvillous MLs were Ki-1 negative and epithelial membrane antigen (EMA) negative, whereas most Ki-1 MLs were positive, with the exception of the B cell type (Fig 3–7). Ultrastructural studies indicated that Ki-1 ML was more variable and

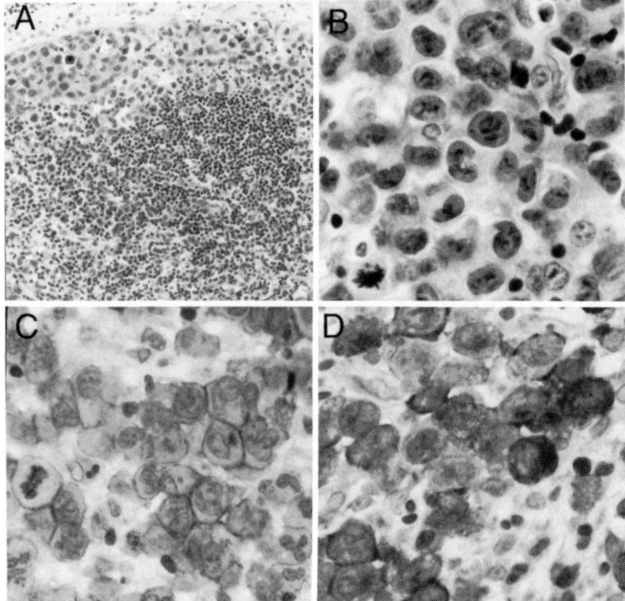

Fig 3–6.—**A**, anaplastic large cell Ki-1 lymphoma showing typical sinus growth pattern. **B**, tumor is composed of pleomorphic large cells with irregular, often indented nuclei and abundant cytoplasm. **C**, immunoperoxidase staining for Ber-H2, demonstrating both membrane and Golgi zone reactivity. **D**, immunoperoxidase stain for EMA, showing strong positivity. (Courtesy of Kinney MC, Glick AD, Stein H, et al: *Am J Surg Pathol* 14:1047–1060, 1990.)

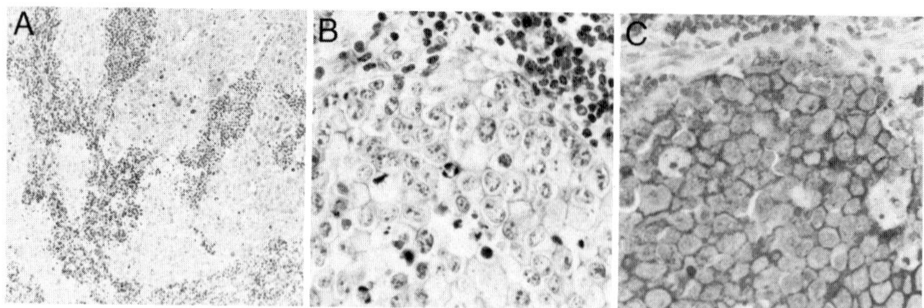

Fig 3–7.—A, microvillous lymphoma showing sinus infiltrate. B, tumor cells with large round to slightly irregular nuclei and abundant cytoplasm. C, immunoperoxidase stain for L26, with tumor cells having distinct membrane reactivity. (Courtesy of Kinney MC, Glick AD, Stein H, et al: *Am J Surg Pathol* 14:1047–1060, 1990.)

had more nuclear irregularity than microvillous ML. Many cytoplasmic processes were present in microvillous MLs, as well as in some of the Ki-1 MLs.

Conclusions.—Both anaplastic large cell Ki-1 ML and microvillous ML have a sinus growth pattern and can have cytoplasmic projections. These 2 types of ML cannot be differentiated on the basis of morphology alone. Both immunologic and ultrastructural studies are necessary to distinguish between these 2 types of ML.

▶ Malignant lymphomas of large cells that demonstrate a sinusoidal growth pattern in lymph nodes are difficult to distinguish from metastatic carcinoma, melanoma, and malignant histiocytosis (see Abstract 3–10). Now that monoclonal antibodies functional in paraffin-embedded material are available, distinction of these neoplasms is greatly facilitated.—J.B. Cousar, M.D.

Malignant Histiocytosis: A Reassessment of Cases Previously Reported in 1975 Based on Paraffin Section Immunophenotyping Studies

Wilson MS, Weiss LM, Gatter KC, Mason DY, Dorfman RF, Warnke RA (Stanford Univ; Univ of Oxford, England)

Cancer 66:530–536, 1990 3–10

Background.—The term malignant histiocytosis is sometimes applied to a syndrome with systemic proliferation of cells with the cytologic appearance of atypical histiocytes. Understanding of the malignant histiocytoses has been improved by the availability of immunologic markers for T and B lymphocytes and the application of molecular biology techniques. With these current concepts, biopsy specimens from a series of 15 patients reported to have malignant histiocytosis in 1975 were reclassified.

Methods.—Histologic materials were available for 15 of the 29 original patients. The antibodies used were the anti-B-cell L-26; the anti-T-cell UCHL1, Leu 22, and T3; and various others, including Ber-H2, PD7, and KP1, which detect a formalin-resistant epitope of Ki-1, leukocyte common antigen, and monocyte/macrophage-derived cells, respectively.

Immunophenotypic Findings in Patients With "Malignant Histiocytosis"

Patient	Histologic pattern	Age (yr)/sex	L-26	Leu 22	UCHL1	CD3	KP1	BerH2	PD7	Conclusion
1	LC, sinusoidal/diffuse	14/M	−	+	+	+	−	+(f)	+	T lineage, Ki-1 lymphoma
2	LC, polymorphous, sinusoidal	52/F	−	+	+	+	−	+	−	T lineage, Ki-1 lymphoma
3	LCNC, red pulp	51/M	−	+	+	−	−	+(f)	+	T lineage, Ki-1 lymphoma
4	LC, histiocytic, diffuse	25/M	−	+	+	−	−	+	+	T lineage, Ki-1 lymphoma
5	LC, polymorphous, paracortical	2/F	−	+	−	−	−	+	−	T lineage, Ki-1 lymphoma
6	LC, sinusoidal	3/M	−	+	−	−	−	+	+	T lineage, Ki-1 lymphoma
7	LC, polymorphous, sinusoidal/diffuse	65/M	−	+	+	+	−	−	+	T lineage lymphoma
8	LC, red pulp	31/F	−	+	+	+	−	−	+	T lineage lymphoma
9	LC, sinusoidal/diffuse	5/M	−	+	+	+	−	−	+	T lineage lymphoma
10	LCNC, sinusoidal	53/M	+	+	−	−	−	−	+	B lineage lymphoma
11	LC, sinusoidal	37/F	+	−	−	−	−	−	+	B lineage lymphoma
12	LC, pleomorphic, sinusoidal	9/M	−	−	−	−	−	+	−	Ki-1 lymphoma, uncertain lineage
13	LC, histiocytic, sinusoidal	3/M	−	−	−	−	−	+	−	Ki-1 lymphoma, uncertain lineage
14	LC, pleomorphic, red pulp	41/M	−	−	−	−	−	−	−	Uncertain lineage
15	Histiocytic, sinusoidal	11/M	−	−	+	+	−	−	−	IAHS

Abbreviations: IAHS, infection-associated hemophagocytic syndrome; *LC,* large cell; *LCNC,* large cell, noncleaved; *f,* focal staining; *L-26,* B-cell marker; *UCHL1, Leu 22, CD3,* primarily T-cell markers; *KP1,* macrophage marker; *BerH2,* formalin-resistant epitope of Ki-1; *PD7,* leukocyte common antigen.

(Courtesy of Wilson MS, Weiss LM, Gatter KC, et al: *Cancer* 66:530–536, 1990.)

Results.—Nine lymphomas, 6 of which coexpressed Ki-1, had a profile consistent with T lineage (table). Two lymphomas had a B lineage. No specific lineage characteristics were expressed by 3 lymphomas, although 2 were positive for Ki-1. No lymphoma expressed KP1. A variety of patterns was seen in the 12 lymph node biopsy specimens. In the spleen, mostly red pulp involvement was seen. One patient seemed to have a virus-associated hemophagocytic syndrome.

Conclusions.—Most malignant histiocytoses appear to be T-lineage-associated hematolymphoid neoplasms, with only rare monocyte-macrophage origins. It is recommended that the term malignant histiocytosis be abandoned for a more descriptive one, e.g., sinusoidal large cell lymphoma. The former term may be used if there is compelling immunohistochemical evidence of a histiocytic origin.

▶ Malignant histiocytosis is an extraordinarily rare neoplasm. Now that better methods are available to evaluate the lineage of hematopoietic-lymphoid cells, we recognize that many cases previously reported as malignant histiocytosis are likely to be unusual types of T or B cell neoplasms. It is interesting that at least 8 of the 15 cases in the present series were reclassified as Ki-1 positive lymphomas. A broader review of Ki-1-positive lymphomas and their differentiation from malignant histiocytosis, metastatic carcinoma, Hodgkin's disease, and other lymphomas involving lymphoid sinuses is available (1).—J.B. Cousar, M.D.

Reference

1. Kinney MC, et al: *Pathol Annu* 26:1, 1990.

4 Respiratory System and Thorax

Crack Lung: An Acute Pulmonary Syndrome With a Spectrum of Clinical and Histopathologic Findings

Forrester JM, Steele AW, Waldron JA, Parsons PE (Univ of Colorado)

Am Rev Respir Dis 142:462–467, 1990 4–1

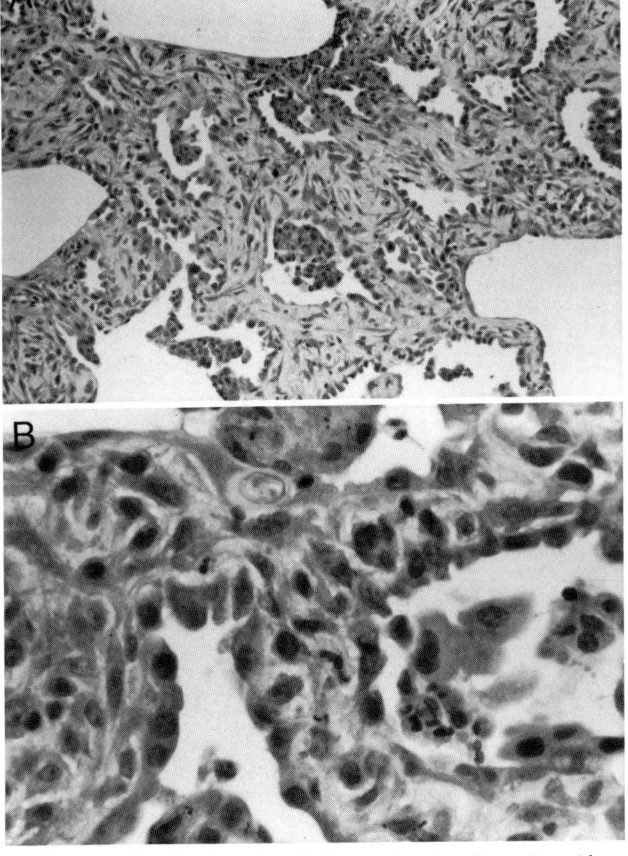

Fig 4–1.—**A,** open lung biopsy demonstrating edematous, broadened interstices with reactive mesenchymal cells and prominent alveolar lining cell reaction. Aggregates of hemosiderin-laden macrophages are present in many alveolar lumens (hematozylin-eosin; original magnification, ×40). **B,** eosinophils with bilobed nuclei are present in the interstitium and intermingled with macrophages in the alveolar lumens. Note the hyperplastic alveolar lining cells and the reactive interstitial mesenchymal cells (hematoxylin-eosin; original magnification, ×160). (Courtesy of Forrester JM, Steele AW, Waldron JA, et al: *Am Rev Respir Dis* 142:462–467, 1990.)

Background.—The manifestations of acute pulmonary injury complicating inhalation of freebase cocaine are variable. Four patients had an acute pulmonary syndrome after inhaling at least 1 g of freebase cocaine.

Patients.—Two patients had a prolonged hospital course characterized by fever, dyspnea, hypoxemia, hemoptysis, and respiratory failure. Chest radiographs showed diffuse alveolar infiltrates. Lung biopsy specimens (Fig 4–1) revealed diffuse alveolar damage, alveolar hemorrhage, and marked inflammatory cell infiltration, particularly of eosinophils. There was striking deposition of immunoglobulin E in lymphocytes and in alveolar macrophages. Clinical and radiographic improvement was noted during corticosteroid therapy. The other 2 patients had a self-limited pulmonary injury associated with acute dyspnea and diffuse alveolar infiltrates but without respiratory failure and fever.

Summary.—These cases provide evidence that inhalation of freebase cocaine can cause an acute pulmonary syndrome. The crack-associated lung injury may resolve rapidly without specific therapy, or it may persist with worsening hypoxemia, fever, diffuse pulmonary infiltrates, and respiratory failure. The persistent form may respond to systemic corticosteroid therapy.

▶ It is becoming clear that there is a spectrum of histopathologic changes seen in "crack lung." Mild to severe hemorrhage with hemosiderin formation is common, and fibrosis suggestive of diffuse damage can sometimes be found. The presence of a heavy deposition of IgE in one of the patients examined is intriguing and, at the risk of making too much of a single case, suggests that some cases of "crack lung" may represent an acute hypersensitivity reaction rather than a direct toxic injury.—R.A. Harley, M.D.

A Clinicopathologic Study of 34 Cases of Diffuse Pulmonary Hemorrhage With Lung Biopsy Confirmation

Travis WD, Colby TV, Lombard C, Carpenter HA (Natl Cancer Inst, Bethesda, Md; Mayo Clinic and Found, Rochester, Minn; El Camino Hosp, Mountainview, Calif)

Am J Surg Pathol 14:1112–1125, 1990 4–2

Objective.—It often is difficult to interpret lung biopsy specimens obtained from patients who have diffuse pulmonary hemorrhage (DPH). An approach to the differential diagnosis of DPH was developed from experience with 31 patients having open lung biopsy and 3 others undergoing transbronchial biopsy. All had a primary histologic finding of DPH.

Clinical Findings.—Most of the patients had hemoptysis, dyspnea, and diffuse pulmonary infiltrates on chest radiography. Some, however, had a more chronic and less specific presentation. Most patients had clearly defined associated disorders, predominantly vasculitis (14 patients, 41%). Eleven patients had syndromes that proved difficult to classify.

Histopathologic Findings.—Acute bleeding with intra-alveolar red blood cells was a constant finding. Capillaritis was present in 88% of cases. Three of the 5 patients with Wegener's granulomatosis had granulomas in their biopsy specimens, and 2 of these had arteritis. Pleuritis was seen in 6 cases. Positive immunofluorescence findings were observed in patients with Wegener's disease and antibasement membrane antibody (ABMA)-mediated DPH.

Outcome.—Most patients received steroids, and some received cyclophosphamide as well. All 4 patients with idiopathic pulmonary hemorrhage recovered. One of 4 patients with ABMA-mediated DPH and 2 of those with Wegener's granulomatosis died. Two of 3 patients with systemic necrotizing vasculitis recovered. Two patients with unclassified pulmonary-renal syndromes died, 2 recovered but had renal failure, and 1 did well.

Recomendations.—If DPH is suspected clinically or on frozen-section study, a small piece of unfixed lung tissue should be snap frozen and another sample saved for electron microscopy.

▶ In addition to detailed information on DPH syndromes, this relatively large collection of cases describes immunofluorescence and electron microscopic findings not readily available in textbooks.—R.A. Harley, M.D.

Pulmonary Alveolar Proteinosis Associated With *Pneumocystis carinii:* Ultrastructural Identification in Bronchoalveolar Lavage in AIDS and Immunocompromised Non-AIDS Patients

Tran Van Nhieu J, Vojtek A-M, Bernaudin J-F, Escudier E, Fleury-Feith J (Hôpital Henri-Mondor, Créteil, France; Centre Hospitalier Intercommunal de Créteil)

Chest 98:801–805, 1990 4–3

Background.—In pneumonitis caused by *Pneumocystis carinii,* bronchoalveolar lavage fluid contains foamy honeycombed material representing *P. carinii* cysts. In addition, another extracellular material more suggestive of alveolar proteinosis has also been observed.

Patients.—An ultrastructural study of lavage fluid was undertaken in 37 patients, 26 of whom had *P. carinii* pneumonitis (PCP). Nineteen of these patients had AIDS and 7 were immunodeficient secondary to heart or kidney transplantation. Eleven immunocompromised patients without PCP also were studied.

Findings.—Samples of fluid from patients with PCP contained, in addition to honeycombed material, an accumulation of extracellular material that resembled phospholipid surfactant, sometimes mixed with *P. carinii* cysts. In 9 cases the finding of abundant phospholipid material with myelin tubular laminated structures suggested associated pulmonary alveolar proteinosis. This type of material was not found abundantly in lavage samples from immunocompromised patients without PCP.

Discussion.—Lipoproteinaceous material accumulates in the alveoli in some patients with PCP, but its pathophysiologic significance is uncertain. It appears that the association of PCP and pulmonary alveolar proteinosis is not rare.

▶ This is an intriguing observation, but the presence of excessive surfactant-derived material in alveolar spaces may not necessarily justify the designation "pulmonary alveolar proteinosis." Proteinosis reactions in varying degrees occur in a number of conditions (e.g., adjacent to foci of tuberculosis, in response to fine silica and aluminum dust). If the dose of the causative agent is reduced, the resulting accumulation of phospholipid debris does not have the light microscopic appearance of alveolar proteinosis. Perhaps the term should be reserved for those cases in which the light microscopic appearance is similar to that seen in idiopathic alveolar proteinosis. (This is a matter of semantics and does not detract from the observation that this reaction occurs at the ultrastructural level in patients with PCP.)—R.A. Harley, M.D.

Typical and Atypical Bronchopulmonary Carcinoids: A Clinicopathologic and Flow Cytometric Study

El-Naggar AK, Ballance W, Abdul Karim FW, Ordóñez NG, McLemore D, Giacco GG, Batsakis JG (Univ of Texas, Houston; Roche BioMed Lab, Greenville, NC: Case Western Reserve Univ)

Am J Clin Pathol 95:828–834, 1991 4–4

Background.—Bronchopulmonary carcinoids have a variable, unpredictable clinical course. Recent studies have shown that DNA content is correlated with the biological behavior of some tumors. The clinical rele-

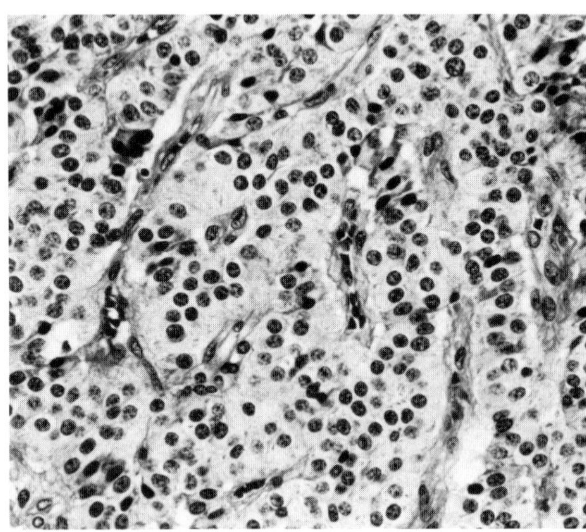

Fig 4–2.—Typical carcinoid *(upper, left)* displaying organoid pattern and uniform cells. Hematoxylin-eosin; original magnification, ×250. (Courtesy of El-Naggar AK, Ballance W, Abdul Karim FW, et al: *Am J Clin Pathol* 95:828–834, 1991.)

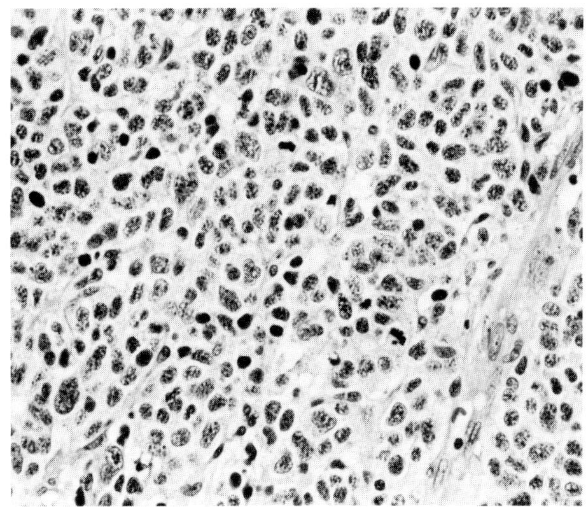

Fig 4–3.—Atypical carcinoid *(upper, right)* presenting cellular pleomorphism and mitotic figures. Hematoxylin-eosin; original magnification, ×250. (Courtesy of El-Naggar AK, Ballance W, Abdul Karim FW, et al: *Am J Clin Pathol* 95:828–834, 1991.)

vance of measuring the DNA content and proliferative cellular fraction in typical and atypical bronchopulmonary carcinoids was examined.

Methods and Findings.—The clinicopathologic and flow cytometric features of 47 bronchopulmonary carcinoids were compared with patient survival. Aneuploidy was more frequently associated with tumor size and lymph node or vascular involvement. An aneuploid DNA content occurred significantly more often in histologically atypical than in typical

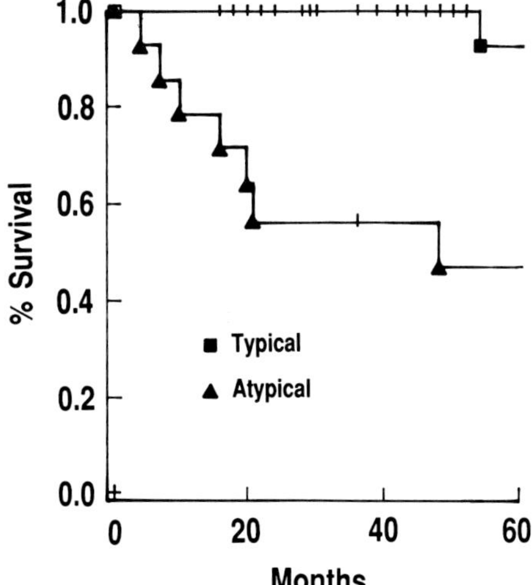

Fig 4–4.—Survival distribution of histologically typical and atypical bronchopulmonary carcinoids by Kaplan-Meier method. (Courtesy of El-Naggar AK, Ballance W, Abdul Karim FW, et al: *Am J Clin Pathol* 95:828–834, 1991.)

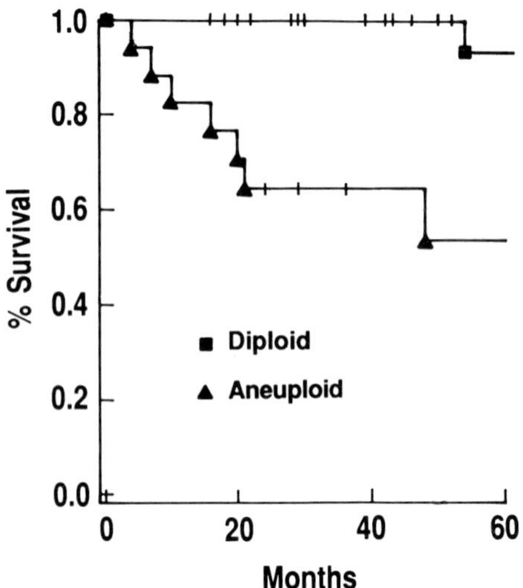

Fig 4–5.—Survival distribution by Kaplan-Meier method for diploid and aneuploid bronchopulmonary carcinoids. (Courtesy of El-Naggar AK, Ballace W, Abdul Karim FW, et al: *Am J Clin Pathol* 95:828–834, 1991.)

carcinoid neoplasms. According to Cox proportional hazard model analysis, the histologic category and ploidy patterns were important predictors. Primary tumor size and the presence of vascular involvement also significantly predicted outcome. Histologically atypical carcinoids with diploid DNA content were less aggressive than their aneuploid counterparts (Figs 4–2 to 4–5).

Conclusions.—In this study, DNA analysis by flow cytometry was a valuable predictor of the clinical course of bronchopulmonary carcinoids. Determination of DNA content can complement the microscopic assessment of bronchopulmonary carcinoids and may possibly assist in identifying histologically atypical neoplasms that have a variable biological course. Tumor size and the presence of vascular invasion are also important prognostic indicators.

▶ The ancillary technique of flow cytometry was valuable in assessment of bronchopulmonary carcinoids by identifying those with an aggressive clinical course. The presence of vascular invasion and tumor size were also important in the clinical outcome.—A.J.Garvin, M.D., Ph.D.

Fine Needle Aspiration Cytology of Pulmonary Carcinoid Tumors

Anderson C, Ludwig ME, O'Donnell M, Garcia N (Hartford Hosp, Hartford, Conn)

Acta Cytol 34:505–510, 1990 4–5

Background.—Carcinoid lung tumors account for only 1% to 2% of primary pulmonary neoplasms. Reports of the cytologic diagnosis of these neoplasms have rarely included references to plexiform vascularity, which may be of primary diagnostic importance. A fine-needle aspiration (FNA) cytologic study of pulmonary carcinoid tumors was carried out.

Methods.—Twenty-four pulmonary carcinoid tumors initially sampled by FNA were reviewed. The diagnosis of carcinoid tumor was confirmed in 23 cases. The exception, which closely resembled a carcinoid tumor in the FNA specimen, proved to be a sclerosing hemangioma.

Findings.—All typical spindle cell carcinoids and atypical carcinoids were diagnosed and classified correctly. The original cytologic diagnosis of the 15 typical round cell carcinoids was lymphoma in 2 cases and benign bronchial lining cells in another 2. Diagnostic errors were therefore more likely in "typical" carcinoids. Frequently stripped cytoplasm, coupled with the almost universal plexiform vascularity, would have permitted an accurate cytologic diagnosis in virtually all cases.

Conclusions.—Familiarity with the spectrum of cytologic features in FNA specimens allows a reproducible diagnosis and classification of pulmonary carcinoid tumors. Diagnostic errors seem to be more likely in "typical" carcinoids, whose cells can be confused with bronchial lining cells or lymphocytes.

Long-Term Follow-Up of Classical Bronchial Carcinoid Tumors: Clinicopathologic Observations

Warren WH, Gould VE (Rush Med College, Chicago)

Scand J Thorac Cardiovasc Surg 24:125–130, 1990 4–6

Background.—A clinicopathologic classification of the neuroendocrine tumors found in the bronchopulmonary tract was developed to reduce confusion in nomenclature and taxonomy. The bronchial carcinoids are those cancers that express eutopic neuropeptides and serotonin. More aggressive tumors more often express ectopic neuropeptides, e.g., adrenocorticotropic hormone (ACTH).

Patients.—Long-term follow-up was made of 36 patients with suspected bronchial carcinoids who underwent resection; in 27 of them, bronchial carcinoid was confirmed according to the classification of Gould et al. The remaining 9 patients did not have tumors that conformed histologically with the strictly defined carcinoid and were excluded.

Methods.—The original histologic sections were reviewed. When possible, paraffin sections of tumors were analyzed by immunohistochemistry with antibodies to several neuropeptides and serotonin, neuron-specific enolase (NSE), chromogranin, and the recently isolated neuroendocrine glycoprotein, synaptophysin.

Findings.—The patients ranged in age from 14 to 73 years. Of the 27 patients followed for at least 10 years, 15 had conservative surgery, with distant metastases occurring in only 2 patients. Radiotherapy relieved bone pain in the latter 2 patients and chemotherapy stopped the disease in 1. All tumors expressed NSE, and most showed immunoreactivity for chromogranin A and/or synaptophysin. Serotonin was the most frequently produced neuroendocrine product, whereas α-MSH was present in 8 samples, ACTH in 1, and β-endorphin in 1. Immunohistochemical profiles did not differentiate between patients with nodal metastases or those in whom distant metastases would eventually develop.

Conclusion.—Although bronchial carcinoids do not demonstrate any malignant tendency after resection, long-term follow-up is recommended. The alteration of the neuropeptide and ACTH profiles of these tumors does not appear to affect long-term survival.

So-Called Minute Chemodectoma of the Lung: An Electron Microscopic and Immunohistochemical Study

Torikata C, Mukai M (Keio Univ, Tokyo)

Virchows Archiv A Pathol Anat 417:113–118, 1990 4–7

Background.—The so-called minute pulmonary chemodectoma is a curious, small, lung tumor that occurs primarily in women. The nature and origin of the proliferation cells are not understood. The first report of this tumor described the component cells as resembling chemoreceptor cells. Electron microscopic studies, however, have found no evidence of neuronal characteristics. Rather, they have found a close resemblance to meningothelial cells. An electron microscopic and immunohistochemical assessment was made of minute chemodectoma of the lung.

Methods.—All lung tissues were fixed and processed for routine histologic study. Serial sections of minute chemodectomas were immunostained for actin, muscle actin, vimentin, desmin, cytokeratin, EMA, S-100 protein, neuron-specific enolase, myosin, and myoglobin. Formalin-fixed, paraffin-embedded tissues from 2 patients were used for electron microscopy.

Findings.—The results of electron microscopic study were similar to those previously described. In 1 of the 2 cases, however, tumor cells were filled with abundant cytofilaments, which gave them an occasional dense, patchlike appearance. Immunostaining for myosin and vimentin was positive in all tumor cells. Epithelial membrane antigen staining did not occur.

Conclusions.—Minute pulmonary chemodectomas exhibit smooth muscle cell differentiation when closely associated with the small pulmonary veins. There appears to be no evidence of meningothelial cell differentiation. Notably, myosin-like molecules have been found in human nonmuscle cells.

▶ Although meningiomas have been reported in a number of odd locations, it is a relief that the present study suggests that minute chemodectomas, which are relatively common, are not of meningothelial origin, a suggestion that has always strained the imagination. The authors' classification of these as neoplasms is not necessarily accurate. They may also be considered simply a hyperplastic phenomenon. In any case, they point to the presence of a cell in the lung of which we know nothing, except that it can form minute chemodectomas. Our ideas concerning the nature of this cell continue to form under the influence of studies such as this.—R.A. Harley, M.D.

Pulmonary Blastomas

Koss MN, Hochholzer L, O'Leary T (Univ of Southern California; Armed Forces Inst of Pathology, Washington, DC)

Cancer 67:2368–2381, 1991 4–8

Background.—Pulmonary blastoma is a rare tumor of the lung. It is made up of immature mesenchyme and/or epithelium that morphologically mimics the embryonal pulmonary structure. The prognosis is poor, and the histologic appearance does not readily predict the clinical course. The clinical, gross, microscopic, and immunohistochemical features of 52 tumors were correlated with their prognostic significance.

Methods.—Gross pathologic parameters were determined from surgical pathology reports. One to 25 microscopic glass slides were studied for each tumor, and the peroxidase-antiperoxidase technique was used to stain paraffin sections from 38 tumors.

Results.—The tumors were found in 28 women and 24 men; the mean and median age was 35, with a unimodal age peak in the fourth decade. There were only 2 patients younger than age 10 years, both of whom had biphasic blastomas. There were no symptoms in 41% of the patients. A peripheral or midlung mass with no predilection for any lobe was the typical chest radiographic finding. Twenty-eight tumors were well-differentiated fetal adenocarcinomas (WDFAs), composed solely of malignant glands of embryonal appearance, 24 tumors had a biphasic appearance. Cytokeratin, carcinoembryonic antigen, milk fat globulin, and, often, chromogranin were found in the malignant epithelium. In the malignant stromal cells, vimentin, actin, and, less commonly, desmin and myoglobin, were found. The WDFA tumors tended to be smaller than the biphasic tumors, were less likely to show pleural effusion on chest radiography, and were more likely to be asymptomatic. They were less likely to contain giant or bizarre tumor cells, or 30 or more mitoses per 10 high-power fields. Fourteen percent of patients with WDFAs died within a mean follow-up of 97 months, and 52% of patients with biphasic tumors died within a mean of 49 months. Factors most highly correlated with poor prognosis in the patients with WDFAs were the presence of thoracic adenopathy on chest radiographs and of metastasis at presentation, followed by tumor recurrence. The most significant indicator in those with biphasic tumors was recurrence, followed by metastasis at presentation and by tumor size of 5 cm or larger.

Conclusions.—Histologic classifications and gross and clinical findings can be useful indicators of prognosis. Although the distinction between WDFAs and biphasic tumors is prognostically valid, the 2 should not be considered histogenetically distinct.

▶ Few pathologists have the opportunity to see more than 1 or 2 pulmonary blastomas. This series of 52 cases may be viewed as the "definitive study" of blastoma of the lung.—R.A. Harley, M.D.

Alveolar Epithelial Hyperplasia and Adenocarcinoma of the Lung
Nakanishi K (Natl Defense Med College, Tokorozawa, Saitama, Japan)
Arch Pathol Lab Med 114:363–368, 1990 4–9

Background.—Peripheral adenocarcinoma of the lung is often observed in an area of pulmonary fibrosis or scar. Alveolar epithelial hyperplasia (AEH) is consistently found in diffuse interstitial pulmonary fibrosis. Atypical AEH in such settings is thought to be precancerous. However, AEH changes also sometimes occur in regions without pulmonary fibrosis. The pathogenesis of peripherally occurring, well-differentiated adenocarcinoma of the lung was examined in relation to AEH.

Methods.—Lung cancer specimens were obtained for pathologic study and assessed immunohistochemically, morphometrically, and electron microscopically. Specimens of interstitial pulmonary fibrosis were excluded, eliminating the effects of diffuse lung scarring on the development of neoplasia. Overall, 70 specimens with various types of pulmonary carcinomas were examined.

Findings.—Fifteen specimens had coexistent typical or atypical AEH lesions. No transition areas from AEH to neoplasm were found. Immunohistochemical assessment revealed significant differences in the reactions of carcinoembryonic and blood group antigens between typical and atypical AEH. However, there were no significant differences between atypical AEH lesions and adenocarcinoma. The morphometry of the mean nuclear regions showed highly significant differences between atypical AEH lesions and adenocarcinoma. Many Clara granules in atypical AEH cells were found on electron microscopy.

Conclusions.—These findings do not prove that AEH lesions are precancerous. However, the existence of Clara granules in atypical AEH cells should raise speculation on the histogenetic relationship of AEH and pulmonary adenocarcinoma.

▶ This study is intriguing to those interested in peripheral lung cancers and atypical hyperplasias. One wonders how many of us might categorize some of these grossly visible lesions with bizarre nuclear forms as early alveolar cell carcinomas.—R.A. Harley, M.D.

Clear Cell Tumor of the Lung: Immunohistochemical and Ultrastructural Evidence of Melanogenesis
Gaffey MJ, Mills SE, Zarbo RJ, Weiss LM, Gown AM (Univ of Virginia; Henry Ford Hosp, Detroit; City of Hope Natl Med Ctr, Duarte, Calif; Univ of Washington)
Am J Surg Pathol 15:644–653, 1991 4–10

Background.—Clear cell tumors of the lung (CCTLs) are rare tumors of uncertain differentiation. Prompted by earlier evidence of melanocytic differentiation in CCTL and the availability of additional melanocytic markers, a study was undertaken to find evidence of melanocytic differentiation in CCTL.

Methods.—Ultrastructural and immunohistochemical studies with preliminary enzymatic digestion were performed on 9 CCTLs.

Findings.—The tumors appeared as well-circumscribed, unencapsulated, peripheral nodules unassociated with bronchi or major blood vessels. Microscopically, the cells were polygonal with clear-to-eosinophilic cytoplasm and ovoid, centrally placed nuclei. The immunohistochemical staining patterns showed strong reactivity with the antimelanocytic markers HMB-45 (7 tumors) and HMP-50 (6 tumors) and focal positivity for S-100 (9 tumors), neuron-specific enolase (3 tumors), synaptophysin (1 tumor), and Leu-7 (1 tumor). Furthermore, the expression of vimentin and NK1-BETEB, an antibody directed against a glycoprotein located on the inner melanosomal membrane, was observed in 1 CCTL for which snap-frozen tissue was available. Ultrastructural studies of 3 CCTLs fixed in glutaraldehyde showed the full morphological spectrum of melanosomes in 2 and aberrant melanosomal forms in the third. Neurosecretory granules also were evident in 1 CCTL with melanosomes. In contrast, none of the remaining 5 CCTLs studied, either from formalin-fixed or paraffin-retrieved specimens, demonstrated melanosomes.

Conclusions.—There was evidence of melanocytic differentiation in CCTL. This feature may be used to distinguish CCTL from other clear cell tumors.

▶ Clear cell tumors of the lung are composed of periodic-acid Schiff-positive, diastase-sensitive cells, hence the designation "sugar tumor." Although these rare tumors remain enigmatic, the findings reported in this article represent a significant step forward in the understanding of these lesions. The unexpected, convincing evidence of melanogenesis may be useful for the identification of these lesions and for further thought regarding their origin.—J.A. Tucker, M.D.

Elevated Serum Levels of Soluble Interleukin-2 Receptors in Small Cell Lung Carcinoma

Yamaguchi I, Nishimura Y, Kiyokawa T, Matsuzaki H, Ishii T, Kubota K, Kawahara M, Furuse K, Yoshinaga T, Kinuwaki E, Takatsuki K (Kumamoto Univ; Natl Kinki Central Hosp for Chest Diseases, Sakai; Kumamoto Chuo Hosp, Japan)

J Lab Clin Med 116:457–461, 1990 4–11

Background.—Small cell lung carcinoma (SCLC) is an aggressive malignancy with a poor prognosis. Soluble interleukin-2 receptor (sIL-2R) is detectable at low levels in healthy individuals, at higher levels in those with lymphocyte activation, and at particularly elevated levels in patients with certain hematologic malignancies. The level of sIL-2R was examined in the serum of 47 healthy controls, 21 patients with SCLC, and 37 patients with non-SCLC.

Methods.—An enzyme-linked immunoassay was used to measure the concentration of sIL-2R in serum samples. In patients with SCLC the level of sIL-2R was measured serially throughout therapy.

Results.—The mean serum level of sIL-2R in patients with SCLC was 3.8 times higher than in healthy controls and 1.9 times higher than in patients with non-SCLC. Six of the 21 patients with SCLC had levels of sIL-2R that ranged from 5 to 52 times the mean level observed in healthy controls. In the patient with the highest levels of sIL-2R, tumor cells in the pleural fluid reacted to anti–IL-2R antibodies. In this patient there was a good correlation between tumor activity and detectable levels of sIL-2R over time. In patients with SCLC who responded to therapy, there was a corresponding decrease in levels of sIL-2R.

Conclusion.—Some SCLCs appear to secrete sIL-2R. Serial measurement of serum levels of sIL-2R in these patients can be used as a noninvasive marker of the progress of the disease and its response to therapy.

Neoplasms Associated With Pulmonary Eosinophilic Granuloma

Tomashefski JF Jr, Khiyami A, Kleinerman J (Case Western Reserve Univ)
Arch Pathol Lab Med 115:499–506, 1991 4–12

Objective.—Lung tissue was sampled from 21 patients in whom primary pulmonary eosinophilic granuloma (PEG) was diagnosed. Ten patients had a neoplasm as well, which in 9 instances was malignant.

Findings.—The patients with tumors were older than the others, and all were heavy smokers. All of those without tumors who could be evaluated also smoked. Four patients had either primary carcinoma or carcinoid tumor of the lung, whereas 2 had lymphoproliferative malignancies and 3, extrapulmonary carcinomas. The most common symptoms associated with PEG in patients with tumors were dyspnea and cough; 2 patients were asymptomatic. Seven patients had pulmonary infiltrates.

Outcome.—One patient died of metastatic cancer and another survived with widespread metastatic disease. During follow-up, PEG progressed in 3 patients, and in 3 others it either resolved or remained stable. Six patients received prednisone in treatment of PEG.

Conclusions.—There may be more than a random association between PEG and neoplasia. Cigarette smoking is an important risk factor for both PEG and lung carcinoma. In patients with an underlying malignant tumor, PEG can stimulate pulmonary metastases. Open lung biopsy may be necessary to rule out these lesions.

Hematologic Neoplasia Associated With Primary Mediastinal Germ-Cell Tumors

Nichols CR, Roth BJ, Heerema N, Griep J, Tricot G (Indiana Univ, Indianapolis; St Catherine's Hosp, East Chicago, Ind)
N Engl J Med 322:1425–1429, 1990 4–13

Characteristics of the 16 Patients With Mediastinal Germ Cell Tumors

Characteristic	Value
Median age (range) — yr	22 (16–33)
Histologic diagnosis	
Teratocarcinoma	11
Endodermal sinus tumor	2
Unclassified germ-cell tumor	1
Benign teratoma	1
Serologic diagnosis only	1
Serum markers	
Alpha-fetoprotein*	
No. with elevated levels/no. of patients (%)	15/16 (94)
Median (range) — ng/ml	1420 (<5–13,690)
Human chorionic gonadotropin†	
No. with elevated levels/no. of patients (%)	6/16 (38)
Median (range) — mIU/ml	9 (<1.56–596)
Chemotherapy for germ-cell tumor	
Cisplatin + vinblastine +/− bleomycin	5
Cisplatin + etoposide + bleomycin	9
None	2
Response	
Complete	7
Partial	3
Could not be evaluated	6
Time to diagnosis of hematologic tumor	
Simultaneous diagnosis	5
Within 12 mo	8
Median (range) — mo	6 (0–122)

*Normal level <25 ng/mL.
†Normal level <1.56 mIU/mL.
(Courtesy of Nichols CR, Roth BJ, Heerema N, et al: *N Engl J Med* 322:1425–1429, 1990.)

Background.—In 1985, several patients with primary mediastinal germ cell tumors and hematologic neoplasia were reported. It was thought that the cisplatin-based induction therapy of the primary mediastinal germ cell tumor was not the cause of the hematologic neoplasia. A series of 16 patients with hematologic neoplasia associated wtih mediastinal germ cell tumors were seen between 1983 and 1988. Twenty-eight similar cases have been reported previously.

Findings.—The clinical and cytogenetic characteristics of these patients are presented in the table. The findings suggested that the hematologic neoplasia did not result from cisplatin-based chemotherapy. Only patients with nonseminomatous mediastinal germ cell tumors, especially those with serologic or histologic evidence of yolk sac elements, had hematologic neoplasia. The 2 most common hematologic neoplasms were acute megakaryoblastic leukemia and malignant histiocytosis. Although consistent cytogenetic abnormalities were not identified, the marker chromosome isochromosome(12p) was found in the mediastinal germ cell tumor and associated leukemic blasts in 1 patient. This suggests that these tumors may arise from a common progenitor cell.

Conclusions.—Although the pathogenetic mechanisms of the development of this syndrome are not yet clear, there does seem to be an association between mediastinal germ cell tumors and malignant hematopoietic disorders. This rare syndrome may enable observation of the leukemogenetic process. Future research will probably involve additional cell lines from mediastinal germ cell tumors, as well as continued refinement of the clinical and cytogenetic details of the syndrome.

▶ The reported association of primary mediastinal germ cell tumors and hematologic neoplasia is interesting, curious, and probably real!—J.B. Cousar, M.D.

Curschmann's Spirals in Pleural and Peritoneal Effusions

Naylor B (Univ of Michigan)

Acta Cytol 34:474–478, 1990 4–14

Background.—Before 1971, the only reported source of Curschmann's spirals was in secretions of the lower respiratory tract. Since then, these spirals have been found in human cervical smears and endometrial washings in mares. Additional examples of this rare and unexpected phenomenon were encountered.

Patients.—Five patients with Curschmann's spirals in cellular samples of spontaneously developing pleural and peritoneal fluids were seen in the past 11 years. The specimens were 3 pleural fluids obtained by thoracentesis and 2 peritoneal fluids obtained by abdominal paracentesis.

Findings.—The spirals were similar to those occurring in the respiratory tract, although usually much smaller. In 3 cases the fluids also contained mucus-secreting adenocarcinoma cells. The spirals may have formed from mucus secreted by these cells. In the other 2 cases, signs of serosal inflammation were found. These spirals may have developed from submesothelial connective tissue mucosubstances that entered the serosal cavity through a mesothelium of heightened permeability because of the inflammation.

Conclusions.—Several simple explanations have been offered as to how Curschmann's spirals form. None of these explanations, however, seems satisfactory. The mode of spiral formation is presumed to be a complex physical and biochemical phenomenon.

Malignant Cells of Epithelial Phenotype Limited to Thoracic Lymph Nodes

Gould VE, Warren WH, Faber LP, Kuhn C, Franke WW (Rush Med College, Chicago; German Cancer Research Ctr, Heidelberg)

Eur J Cancer 26:1121–1126, 1990 4–15

Background.—Metastases in the lymph nodes characterize the natural history of most epithelial cancers. Three patients had asymptomatic thoracopulmonary lymphadenopathy, but primary carcinomas could not be found, even after extensive examination.

Case 1.—Man, 57, had a 2-week history of coughing up dark clotted blood. He smoked 1 pack of cigarettes a day and had a history of wheezing and bronchodilator and theophylline use. A chest radiograph obtained at admission demonstrated an enlargement in the left hilum, which was verified by tomography.

Case 2.—Man, 44, had a 4-month history of sputum intermittently streaked with blood. He had smoked 1 pack of cigarettes a day for 30 years and had a history of untreated hypertension. A chest radiograph demonstrated a smooth nodule at the left hilum.

Case 3.—Man, 61, with non–insulin-dependent diabetes was to undergo preoperative testing for cataract surgery to correct impaired vision. He smoked 2 packs of cigarettes a day. A chest radiograph showed an asymptomatic right hilar mass.

Findings.—Highly atypical, pleomorphic nonlymphoid cells with large nuclei and prominent nucleoli were found in lymph node samples from all 3 patients. Mitoses occurred frequently. In patients 1 and 2, the cells were large and often closely packed. Immunohistochemical tests in all 3 cases found atypical cells stained uniformly and strongly with antibodies reactive to cytokeratins 8 and 18, to desmoplakin and desmoglein antibodies, and to other cytokeratins. Electron microscopy demonstrated neoplastic cells with numerous and prominent tonofilament bundles in all 3 cases. Neoplastic cells were found only in the thoracic lymph nodes. All 3 patients appeared well at 111, 39, and 13 months after the initial findings, with no additional lymphadenopathy or tumor detected to date.

Conclusion.—These 3 cases show an unusual clinical course and distinct intranodal distribution and marker expression patterns. In the absence of any detectable primary carcinoma, however, a cancer diagnosis followed by extensive surgery and/or aggressive chemotherapy is not warranted.

▶ The report describes the occurrence of lymphoepithelioma-like carcinomas (LLCs) limited to thoracic lymph nodes in 3 patients. During the past decade, LLCs have been described in the thymus, salivary glands, cervix, skin, tonsil, and lung. Most recently, LLCs have also been described in the stomach (1, 2). Many of these cases have been associated with Epstein-Barr virus. After study of these 3 cases by a panel of monoclonal antibodies and electron microscopy, these authors suggest that the malignant cells may have originated in the lymph nodes.—A.J. Garvin, M.D., Ph.D.

References

1. Burke AP, et al: *Mod Pathol* 3:377, 1990.
2. Min K, et al: *Am J Clin Pathol* 96:219, 1991.

Pleural Plaques Do Not Predict Asbestosis: High-Resolution Computed Tomography and Pathology Study

Ren H, Lee DR, Hruban RH, Kuhlman JE, Fishman EK, Wheeler PS, Hutchins GM (Johns Hopkins Med Insts)

Mod Pathol 4:201–209, 1991 4–16

Objective.—Pleural plaques may represent asbestos exposure, but their value for predicting a diagnosis of pulmonary asbestos remains uncertain. The ability of high-resolution CT to accurately detect asbestosis also is unclear. The findings in 29 autopsied patients who had bilateral parietal pleural plaques were compared with those in the same number of age- and sex-matched subjects without pleural plaques.

Observations.—Seven patients with pleural plaques had a definite history of asbestos exposure, whereas none of the controls had such a history. High-resolution CT showed no significant differences between the 2 groups, although it was able to distinguish between lungs with and those without plaques. There were no significant histologic differences between the 2 groups. Asbestos fiber counts were higher in the group with plaques, but not to a significantly significant degree. Both patients with asbestosis had known exposures to asbestos.

Conclusions.—Pleural plaques alone do not predict asbestosis. High-resolution CT accurately demonstrates interstitial and parenchymal lung disease but has not been able to definitively diagnose asbestosis.

▶ The rather weak association between typical parietal pleural plaques and asbestos fiber counts, and the relatively low fiber counts described in this study, suggest the need for a more refined technique. Pleural plaques of the type examined here are traditionally viewed as being associated with greater than background asbestos exposure in most cases. The finding of histologically identifiable asbestosis in only 2 of these patients (7%) also was surprising.

High-resolution CT (HRCT) produces images that pathologists appreciate as being remarkably like the gross appearance of lung. The radiologists in this study were able to see abnormalities, but could not find a pattern that would differentiate their 2 cases of asbestosis from other diseases. Perhaps future studies of more cases of asbestosis combining HRCT findings with more detailed clinical information, pulmonary function, and the results of bronchoalveolar lavage and transbronchial biopsy will improve results. For the time being, HRCT will be considered an adjunct to the clinical diagnosis of asbestosis, and the present study will have to be regarded as a valiant effort.—R.A. Harley, M.D.

Multilocular Thymic Cyst: An Acquired Reactive Process: Study of 18 Cases

Suster S, Rosai J (Yale Univ)

Am J Surg Pathol 15:388–398, 1991 4–17

Background.—Thymic cysts are relatively rare. Some have a multilocular gross appearance and a prominent inflammatory and fibrotic component. These "multilocular thymic cysts" (MTCs) may be difficult to diagnose because of their apparently invasive appearance on gross inspection, variegated microscopic features, and the fact that they may be associated with certain thymic neoplasms.

Methods.—Eighteen MTCs of the anterior mediastinum not associated with Hodgkin's disease or seminoma were studied. Most of the patients

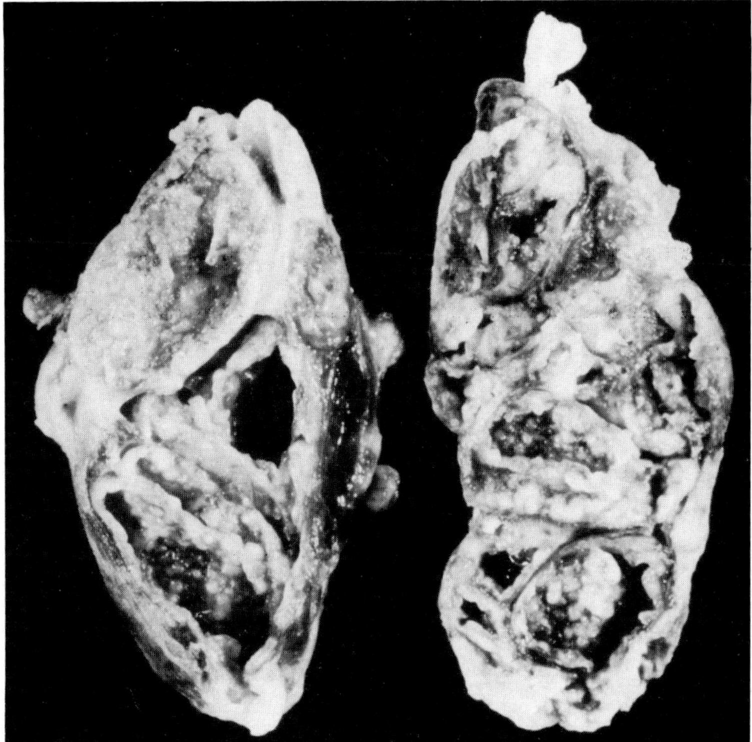

Fig 4–6.—Gross appearance of MTC, with fibrous walls of varying thickness circumscribing multilocular cystic spaces. (Courtesy of Suster S, Rosai J: *Am J Surg Pathol* 15:388–398, 1991.)

were asymptomatic, the MTC being discovered incidentally on routine chest x-ray examination. Presenting symptoms included acute chest pain or discomfort, sometimes associated with dyspnea. Two patients had an incidental thymoma. Another 2 had an incidental thymic carcinoma.

Results.—Histologically, the MTCs had multiple cystic cavities partially lined by squamous, columnar, or cuboidal epithelium. Some had features of Hassall's corpuscles. Another main histologic feature was the presence of scattered nests and islands of non-neoplastic thymic tissue in the cyst walls, often continuous with the cyst lining. There was also severe acute and chronic inflammation, accompanied by fibrovascular proliferation, necrosis, hemorrhage, and cholesterol granuloma formation. Reactive lymphoid hyperplasia with prominent germinal centers also was seen (Figs 4–6 and 4–7).

Conclusions.—These histologic findings suggest that MTC probably results from the cystic transformation of medullary duct epithelium-derived structures induced by an acquired inflammatory process. These changes are similar to those sometimes occurring in thymic Hodgkin's disease and thymic seminoma, which also probably result from the inflammation accompanying these tumors instead of from the tumors

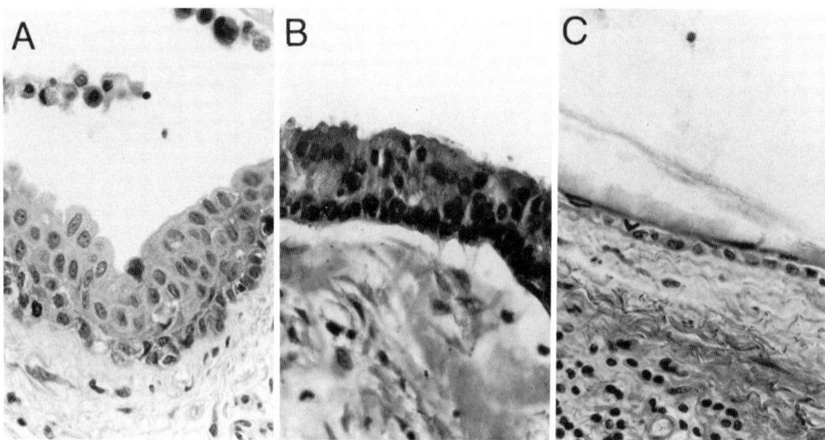

Fig 4–7.—Cyst wall lined by squamous epithelium (**A**), by ciliated columnar epithelium (**B**), and by flattened cuboidal epithelium (**C**). (Courtesy of Suster S, Rosai J: *Am J Surg Pathol* 15:388–398, 1991.)

themselves. Further, the MTC appears to be pathogenetically analogous to a variety of cystic conditions of the head and neck region. The common denominator of these conditions seems to be induction of cystic transformation in ductular epithelial formations of branchial pouch or related derivation by an acquired inflammatory process.

▶ This paper reports a large series of thymic cysts and includes a good discussion of cystic lesions of the mediastinum and their pathogenesis.—A.J. Garvin, M.D. Ph.D.

5 Head and Neck

Laryngeal Paragangliomas and Neuroendocrine Carcinomas

Milroy CM, Rode J, Moss E (Univ College, Middlesex School of Medicine, London)

Histopathology 18:201–209, 1991 5–1

Background.—Reports of paragangliomas and neuroendocrine carcinomas, rare laryngeal tumors, have appeared in the literature mostly as single case studies. There is confusion about the diagnosis and classification of these tumors. Studies were made of a large group of laryngeal tumors initially classified as paragangliomas, many of which gave rise to metastases, and tumors classified as neuroendocrine carcinomas.

Findings.—Of 48 neuroendocrine tumors of the larynx examined, 41 were classified as large cell neuroendocrine carcinomas. Most occurred in the supraglottic larynx. Most of the patients were males, and a third of the patients overall had intense pain. These carcinomas metastasized, often to the skin, giving rise to painful secondary lesions.

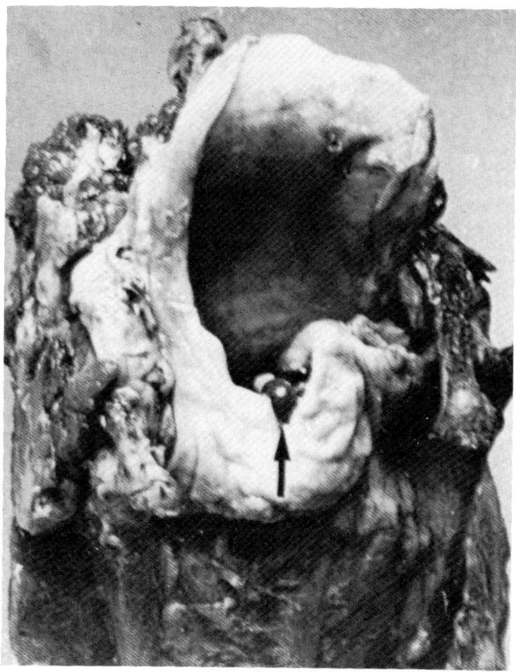

Fig 5–1.—Laryngectomy specimen showing a small nodular large cell neuroendocrine carcinoma on the aryepiglottic fold *(arrow)*. (Courtesy of Milroy CM, Rode J, Moss E: *Histopathology* 18:201–209, 1991.)

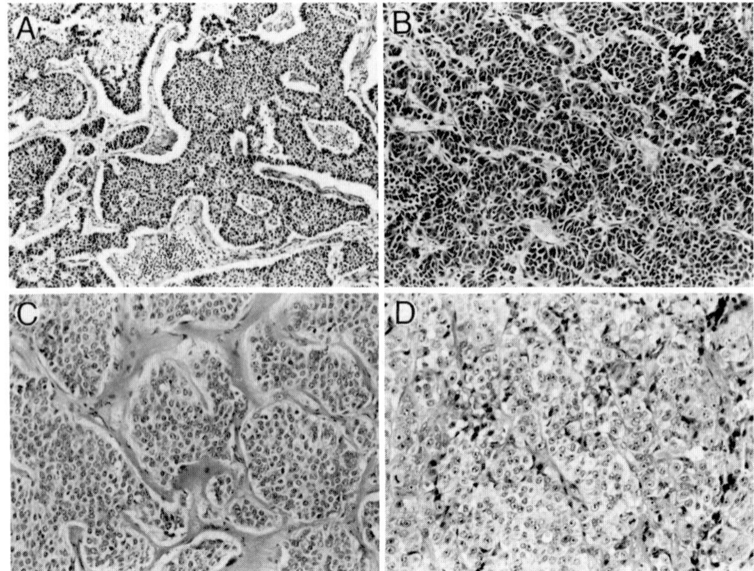

Fig 5–2.—Histologic patterns of large cell neuroendocrine carcinoma. **A,** insular pattern; **B,** trabecular and pseudoacinar pattern; **C,** "Zellballen" pattern mimicking paraganglioma; **D,** large-cell neuroendocrine carcinoma originally diagnosed as malignant paraganglioma. Note large cells with prominent nucleoli (hematoxylin-eosin). (Courtesy of Milroy CM, Rode J, Moss E: *Histopathology* 18:201–209, 1991.)

Histopathology.—Histologically, large cell neuroendocrine carcinomas had several characteristics seen in neuroendocrine tumors at other sites. One such feature was grouping into "Zellballen," which mimics paraganglioma. Four tumors that appeared benign were definitely paragangliomas. Three tumors were small cell neuroendocrine carcinomas; this tumor is identical histologically to its counterpart in the bronchus and is very aggressive. All 3 tumor types expressed general neuroendocrine markers. Only large cell neuroendocrine carcinoma marked for cytokeratin and calcitonin. Sustentacular cells were identified and marked for S-100 protein and glial fibrillary acidic protein in the paragangliomas (Figs 5–1 and 5–2).

Conclusions.—Pathologists should be aware of the histopathologic patterns observed in neuroendocrine carcinomas and paragangliomas. The combination of conventional histologic assessment and immunohistochemistry permits accurate diagnosis and appropriate treatment.

▶ This report provides an excellent reference for separation of the 3 groups of tumors: paraganglioma, small cell neuroendocrine carcinoma, and large cell neuroendocrine carcinoma. This distinction is important because paragangliomas should be treated with adequate local excision, and small cell neuroendocrine carcinoma should be treated with chemotherapy and radiotherapy, whereas large cell neuroendocrine carcinomas require surgical excision as these tumors do not appear to be chemosensitive or radiosensitive.—A.J. Garvin, M.D., Ph.D.

Teflonomas of the Larynx and Neck

Wenig BM, Heffner DK, Oertel YC, Johnson FB (Armed Forces Inst of Pathology, Washington, DC; George Washington Univ)

Hum Pathol 21:617–623, 1990 5–2

Introduction.—Surgical trauma to the recurrent laryngeal nerve and tumors in the vocal cord or in the recurrent laryngeal nerve represent the major causes of vocal cord paralysis. Paralysis of the vocal cord can result in aspiration problems related to open glottic incompetence, ineffective cough, and reduced voice production. Patients with vocal paralysis can be treated by injecting paraffin into the paralyzed cord, but this procedure can produce a "paraffinoma," a lesion caused by extravasation of the paraffin into surrounding tissue. Teflon paste can be used instead of

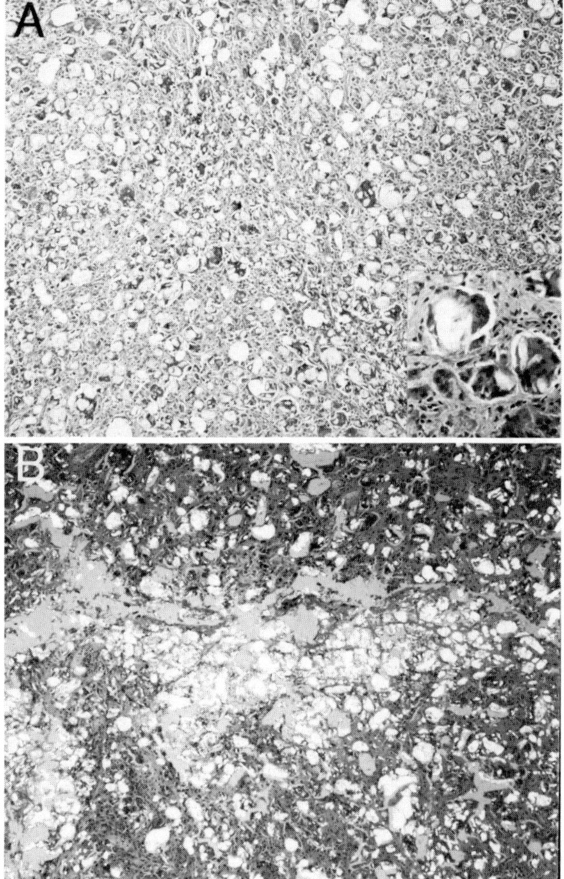

Fig 5–3.—**A,** neck mass composed entirely of foreign body giant cell reaction. Hematoxylin-eosin; original magnification, ×59. Giant cells contain glassy-appearing foreign material. Hematoxylin-eosin; original magnification, ×160. **B,** polarization of foreign material demonstrates its birefringent qualities. Polarized hematoxylin-eosin; original magnification, ×59. (Courtesy of Wenig BM, Heffner DK, Oertel YC, et al: *Hum Pathol* 21:617–623, 1990.)

paraffin; however, "Teflonomas" can also form; these are difficult to distinguish from neoplasms.

Methods.—The records of 7 patients in whom a laryngeal lesion or neck mass developed as a reaction to a Teflon injection were reviewed. An additional case of "Teflonoma" in a patient treated for vocal cord paralysis in another institution was also studied.

Findings.—The 5 women and 3 men were aged 31–72 years. The initial causes of their vocal cord paralysis included surgical trauma, postviral neuritis, and primary or metastatic carcinoma. The cause of paralysis remained unknown in 1 patient. Symptoms such as persistent hoarseness or a neck mass were present from 1 month to 15 years after Teflon injection. Five patients underwent surgical removal of the Teflon-induced lesion, which improved or eliminated all symptoms. One patient had the material aspirated from the mass.

Histopathology.—The tumors were described as polyploid lesions within the submucosal compartment of the vocal cord. In microscopic analysis of the masses a glassy-appearing material was observed that was birefringent under polarized light within the multinucleated giant cells (Fig 5–3). Scanning electron microscopy of the material demonstrated many ovoid-to-spherical particles having a flaky appearance.

Conclusions.—Teflon injection is still the treatment of choice for unilateral vocal cord paralysis. Although it appears to be a safe procedure, physicians should be aware of the possible complications that sometimes mimic the presence of a neoplasm.

▶ Conclusive identification of an unusual foreign substance in histopathologic material usually requires knowledge of its existence as an injectable material or application of a relatively sophisticated technique, e.g., energy dispersive x-ray analysis. The authors have served us well by calling our attention to the problem and analyzing the substance by the methods described above to prove its composition. The brilliantly polarizable material contained in giant cells appears to have a unique microscopic appearance that has not been described previously in the pathology literature.—G.F. Worsham, M.D.

Interpretation of Head and Neck Biopsies in Wegener's Granulomatosis: A Pathologic Study of 126 Biopsies in 70 Patients

Devaney KO, Travis WD, Hoffman G, Leavitt R, Lebovics R, Fauci AS (Bethesda Naval Hosp Md; Natl Cancer Inst; Natl Inst of Allergy and Infectious Disease; Natl Inst of Deafness and Communicative Disorders, Bethesda)

Am J Surg Pathol 14:555–564, 1990 5–3

Background.—Symptoms of head and neck disease are the most common presentation in classic Wegener's granulomatosis (WG). Biopsy specimens from these sites must be interpreted accurately for correct diagnosis. To better define the diagnostic criteria for WG, 126 head and neck biopsy specimens from 70 patients were studied.

Methods.—The patients were 36 men and 34 women (average age, 36). There were 60 nasal, 27 paranasal sinus, 17 laryngeal, 5 periorbital,

Parenchymal Histologic Changes in Head and Neck Biopsy Specimens in Wegener's Granulomatosis

Site	No.	Geographic necrosis	Poorly formed granulomas	Scattered giant cells	Microabscesses	Microabscesses with granulomas
		N (%)				
Nasal	60	12 (20)	28 (47)	28 (47)	20 (33)	12 (20)
Paranasal sinuses	27	15 (56)	16 (59)	16 (59)	10 (37)	9 (33)
Larynx	17	3 (18)	4 (23)	4 (23)	3 (18)	3 (18)
Periorbital	5	0	0	0	3 (60)	0
Oral	5	0	1 (20)	1 (20)	0	0
Mastoid	3	2 (67)	2 (67)	2 (67)	1 (33)	1 (33)
Middle ear	4	1 (25)	1 (25)	1 (25)	1 (25)	0
External ear	2	1 (50)	2 (100)	2 (100)	0	0
Salivary gland	3	2 (67)	2 (67)	2 (67)	2 (67)	0

(Courtesy of Devaney KO, Travis WD, Hoffman G, et al: *Am J Surg Pathol* 14:555–564, 1990.)

5 oral, 4 middle ear, 3 mastoid, 3 salivary gland, and 2 external ear specimens. Both parenchymal and vascular changes were sought. Patients were divided into groups based on whether they had associated lung or kidney involvement.

Results.—Parenchymal changes included geographic necrosis, poorly formed granulomas, scattered giant cells, and microabscesses with and without granulomas (table). Vasculitis was found in 26% of specimens, necrosis in 33%, and granulomatous inflammation in 42%. Only 16% of the specimens showed vasculitis, necrosis, and granulomatous inflammation. Twenty-one percent of specimens showed both vasculitis and granulomatous inflammation, and 23% vasculitis and necrosis. At least 1 of these features was found in the paranasal sinsuses in 55% of patients, in the nose in 20%, and in the larynx in 18%.

Conclusions.—A criterion for diagnosis of WG can be based on analysis of biopsy specimens from the head and neck. Because many midline granulomatous diseases mimic the pathologic features of WG, the clinical and serologic parameters must be correlated.

Nasal Lymphoma: A Clinicopathologic Study With Immunophenotypic and Genotypic Analysis

Ferry JA, Sklar J, Zukerberg LR, Harris NL (Massachusetts Gen Hosp; Brigham and Women's Hosp, Boston)

Am J Surg Pathol 15:268–279, 1991 5–4

Background.—Malignant lymphomas that originate in the nasal cavity are rare in Western medicine, whereas many series of this disorder have been reported from the Orient. American and European studies have combined nasal malignant lymphoma with paranasal disease, precluding an independent analysis of the former condition. Studies were made in non-Oriental patients with nasal lymphoma classified as malignant and the findings compared with reported Oriental and other Western patients with nasal lymphoma.

Methods.—Nasal lymphoma determined histologically to be malignant

Clinical and Histologic Features

Case	Age (yr)	Sex	Extranasal disease	Stage	Histological subtype: WF	Histological subtype: Kiel	Angioinvasion	Immuno-phenotype	Outcome
1	41	F	None	IE	Immunoblastic polymorphous	Pleomorphic large cell	+	T	NED, 2 yr 2 mo
2	78	F	PNS	IE	Immunoblastic polymorphous	Pleomorphic large cell	+	T	NED, 2 yr
3	59	F	Alveolar ridge	IE	Immunoblastic polymorphous	Pleomorphic large cell	+	T	NED, 1 yr 5 mo
4	50	F	PNS, frontal lobe	IV	Large cleaved cell	Pleomorphic large cell	+	s/o T	Relapse, 13 mo chemo. NED, 2 yr 8 mo later
5	29	M	PNS, NP, palate	IE	Immunoblastic polymorphous	Pleomorphic medium cell	+	s/o T	Relapse, 11 mo. cytoxan + prednisone. DOD, 1 wk later
6	60	M	PNS, NP, orbit	IE	Large cleaved (multilobated)	Centroblastic (multilobated)	+/−	B	Local recurrence, 7 yr 11 mo CHOP + RT. NED, 1 yr later

7	51	M	None	IE	Immunoblastic polymorphous	Pleomorphic large cell	+	NA	NED. died of other causes, 11 yr 5 mo
8	70	M	None	IE	Immunoblastic polymorphous	Pleomorphic large cell	+/−	NA	NED, 1 yr 1 mo
9	78	M	PNS, palate, alveolar ridge, axillary nodes	II	Large cleaved (multilobated)	Centroblastic (multilobated)	−	B	Relapse, 2 yr 6 mo CHOP. NED, 3 yr later
10	55	F	Palate, alveolar ridge	IE	Immunoblastic	Immunoblastic	−	NA	Relapses, starting <1 yr. CHEMO + RT. AWD, 5 mo later
11	27	F	NP	IE	DML	Pleomorphic medium cell	+	s/o T	NED, 10 yr
12	92	F	PNS	IE	DSCL	Pleomorphic small cell	−	T	NED. died of unknown causes, 9 mo
13	38	M	PNS	IE	NA	NA	+	NA	NED, 22 yr 9 mo

Abbreviations: AWD, alive with disease; *DML,* diffuse mixed small- and large-cell lymphoma; *DOD,* dead of disease; *DSCL,* diffuse small cleaved-cell lymphoma; *NA,* not available; *NED,* no evidence of disease; *NP,* nasopharynx; *PNS,* paranasal sinus; *RT,* radiation therapy; *s/o,* suggestive of; *WF,* working foumulation.

(Courtesy of Ferry JA, Sklar J, Zukerberg LR, et al: *Am J Surg Pathol* 15:268–279, 1991.)

lymphoma with predominant or exclusive involvement of the nasal cavity was documented in 13 patients between 1965 and 1989. Twelve of the 13 were American and 1 was Venezuelan. The clinical data were gathered from the patients' medical records, and light microscopy and immunohistochemistry were used to further analyze these patients' specimens. Genomic DNA analysis via Southern blot hybridization was performed on fresh-frozen tissue from 2 patients.

Findings.—Six men and 7 women participated in the study. Their mean age was 56 years (range, 27–92 years). Their symptoms had been present from several months to 1 year before the diagnosis of nasal lymphoma was made. Three patients had lymphoma confined to the nasal cavity, whereas 7 had involvement of 1 or more of the paranasal sinuses. Based on the Working Formulation for Clinical Usage classification, 10 patients had malignant lymphoma, diffuse large cell type; 1 had diffuse mixed type; and 1 had diffuse small cleaved cell type (table). The tumor in 1 patient could not be subclassified. When subclassified as T cell lymphomas in the Kiel classification based on light microscopy alone, 6 tumors were pleomorphic large cell type, 1 was immunoblastic, 2 were pleomorphic medium cell type, and 1 was pleomorphic small cell type. Invasion of blood vessels by the tumor cells was observed in 10 patients. Of 7 specimens analyzed immunohistochemically, 6 had or appeared to have a T cell immunophenotype. The specimen from a patient with diffuse large cell lymphoma demonstrated no evidence of clonal rearrangement, whereas that from the patient with a cleaved cell tumor showed apparent clonal rearrangement of the β- and α-chain genes of the T cell receptor. All patients received local radiation therapy and 3 had additional chemotherapy. All 13 experienced complete remission. Five patients had relapse, all with large cell disease.

Conclusions.—The 13 tumors evaluated in this report were characterized by a high proportion of angiocentric nasal lymphomas usually with a T cell lineage. The patients appeared to have a good prognosis after radiation therapy.

▶ Most true nasal lymphomas demonstrate angioinvasion and a T cell phenotype. The pseudoepitheliomatous hyperplasia observed in some cases is interesting and awaits a biological explanation.—J.B. Cousar, M.D.

Acinic Cell Carcinoma: Clinicopathologic Review

Lewis JE, Olsen KD, Weiland LH (Mayo Clinic and Found, Rochester, Minn; Mayo Clinic, Scottsdale, Ariz)

Cancer 67:172–179, 1991 5–5

Background.—Acinic cell carcinoma is an uncommon tumor of salivary glands with a propensity for local recurrence and metastasis. No histologic features that predict tumor progression have been identified. A large series of patients was followed to evaluate the natural history and clinical and pathologic features of this neoplasm.

Patients.—Ninety patients with histologic material available for review were identified. All were followed for at least 10 years or until death. The series included 55 females and 35 males aged 14–79 years. Sixty-three patients were seen for initial consultation and treatment, and 27 had recurrent disease. The peak incidence occurred in the sixth decade in the primary group; the age at first treatment was more evenly distributed in the recurrent group. The tumor arose from the right parotid gland in 50 patients and from the left parotid gland in 38. A painless mass was the most common initial presentation in both groups, pain being more common in the primary group. Gross invasion into adjacent tissue was noted in 25% of the primary group and 63% of the recurrent group.

Findings.—On histologic examination, the tumors were found to be composed of serous acinar cells resembling intercalated duct-type cells. Solid, microcystic, follicular, and papillary-cystic patterns were seen. Local recurrence developed in 44% of the primary group, metastasis in 19%, and death from the tumor in 25%. Initial local recurrences were seen as long as 30 years after presentation and death occurred as long as 38 years after presentation. Pain or fixation was a poor prognostic feature, as were excision as the initial treatment and the microscopic features of desmoplasia, atypia, or increased mitotic activity. The morphological pattern and cell composition had no predictive value.

Conclusions.—Clinical features and certain pathologic features predictive of survival were identified. Superficial parotidectomy is probably sufficient treatment for a small, well-circumscribed tumor, with total parotidectomy for grossly invasive tumors or those with deep lobe involvement.

▶ This study is the largest review of acinic cell carcinoma since 1983 (1). Their findings support and add detail to previous studies of this entity and emphasize the lengthy period between initial presentation and recurrence or metastases, as well as the usefulness of clinical features at the time of presentation to predict outcome. The special pathologic features that these authors identified as useful predictors of progression were stromal desmoplasia, nuclear atypia, and increased mitotic rate. These features support earlier findings (2) and should be useful in the pathologic evaluation of these uncommon tumors.—G.F. Worsham, M.D.

References

1. Ellis GL, Corio RL: *Cancer* 52:542, 1983.
2. Perzin KH, LiVolsi VA: *Cancer* 44:1434, 1979.

Central Mucoepidermoid Carcinoma of the Jaws: Report of Four Cases With Analysis of the Literature and Discussion of the Relationship to Mucoepidermoid, Sialodontogenic, and Glandular Odontogenic Cysts

Waldron CA, Koh ML (Emory Univ)

J Oral Maxillofac Surg 48:871–877, 1990 5–6

Introduction.—Intraosseous salivary gland tumors in the jaw are rare. Mucoepidermoid carcinoma appears to be the most common form.

Patients.—Four patients with central mucoepidermoid carcinoma of the jaw bring the total thus far reported to 66. Three lesions were diagnosed as low-grade mucoepidermoid carcinomas and 1 as a high-grade tumor with substantial cellular pleomorphism and nuclear hyperchromatism.

Discussion.—These tumors are about threefold more frequent in the mandible than in the maxilla. The radiographic findings are varied and not diagnostic. Both mucous metaplasia of the epithelial lining of an odontogenic cyst and embryologic or developmental entrapment of salivary gland tissue have been implicated in the histogenesis of the disease. The rate of local recurrence is appreciable, possibly approaching 25%. There is evidence that some definite central mucoepidermoid carcinomas arise from epithelial proliferation in a preexisting odontogenic cyst, implying a common odontogenic origin for both. Distinction between a mucoepidermoid cyst and a low-grade, predominantly cystic central mucoepidermoid carcinoma depends largely on the degree of epithelial proliferation.

▶ Surgical pathologists should be aware that epithelial tumors may arise from an intraosseous location. Central mucoepidermoid carcinoma must be distinguished from an odontogenic cyst.—A.J. Garvin, M.D., Ph.D.

6 Alimentary System

Oral Hairy Leukoplakia: A Histopathologic Study of 32 Cases
Fernández JF, Benito MAC, Lizaldez EB, Montañés MA (Univ Autónoma, Madrid; Hosp La Paz, Madrid)
Am J Dermatopathol 12:571–578, 1990 6–1

Introduction.—Hairy leukoplakia (HL) may be seen in the oral cavity as whitish patches with a corrugated or "hairy" surface, usually on the lateral borders of the tongue. Oral HL occurs almost exclusively in patients infected by HIV. Among 32 patients with a clinical diagnosis of HL 7 had AIDS and 25 were seropositive for HIV but lacked clinical features of AIDS. Most of the patients were intravenous drug users or homosexuals.

Histopathology.—Acanthosis and parakeratosis of varying extent were noted in all cases. Various forms of herpes-type intranuclear inclusions were observed, including eosinophilic inclusions surrounded by a halo and eosinophilic or basophilic structures that gave a ground-glass appearance to the entire nuclear surface. Most cells with intranuclear inclusions exhibited large and clear cut ballooning of the cytoplasm or slightly eosinophilic, homogenized cytoplasm with a dense border. Occasionally intranuclear viral inclusions were observed in keratinocytes without cytoplasmic alterations. Cytoplasmic ballooning was seen in keratinocytes in the lower two thirds of the epithelium in 15 cases. In 23 cases there were *Candida* spores and hyphae in superficial areas of parakeratosis.

Immunohistochemical studies for human papillomavirus (HPV) were positive in all but 1 of 26 cases. The HPV-positive nuclei correlated closely with intranuclear inclusions. Ultrastructural studies demonstrated herpesvirus particles in the kerastinocytes of the upper spinous layer in 17 of 20 cases. In all, 30 patients had positive immmunohistochemical or ultrastructural findings.

Conclusions.—The most prominent histologic feature in identifying HL is the presence of herpetic-type intranuclear inclusions in keratinocytes of the stratum spinosum. Representative biopsy findings preclude the need for ultrastructural, immunohistochemical, and DNA hybridization studies.

▶ Earlier reports on oral HL have included herpes, Epstein-Barr virus, human papillomavirus (HPV), and candida as agents for this condition. This study as well as another study (1) found intranuclear inclusions characteristic of the herpesvirus family to be the hallmark of HL. Each study used electron microscopy to verify the nature of the intranuclear inclusions, and each group of authors concluded that they were consistent with Epstein-Barr virus inclusions. An interesting observation in the study abstracted above was the presence of positive immunohistochemistry for HPV, which the authors conclude was secondary to a cross reaction between the antiserum used against HPV. Supporting this conclusion was the absence of usual histopathologic hallmarks of HPV and the absence of HPV on ultrastructural examination. Each study found a high (approximately 70%) incidence of superficial infestation by *Candida sp.*, which they interpreted as colonization.

The characteristic features noted above should enable the recognition of this lesion in most cases in routinely stained biopsy material. Its presence is strongly suggestive of HIV infection.—G.F. Worsham, M.D.

Reference

1. Araqües M, et al: *Clin Exper Dermatol* 15:335, 1990.

Hyaline Ring Granuloma: A Distinct Oral Entity

Chou L, Ficarra G, Hansen LS (Univ of California, San Francisco School of Dentistry)

Oral Surg Oral Med Oral Pathol 70:318–324, 1990 6–2

Introduction.—The hyaline ring granuloma is a distinct entity, also described as chronic periostitis, giant cell hyaline angiopathy, and pulse granuloma.

Case Report.—Man, 55, who wore a full denture, reported recurrent swelling and discomfort in the left molar area of the mandible where a draining sinus tract was present. Radiographs showed central bone resorption and a destructive radiolucency in the area of the second molar. Excisional biopsy showed multinucleated giant cells associated with rings of pale-staining hyaline material and granular calcification. Similar features were noted in the biopsy specimen from a mass that recurred a year later.

Literature Review.—The 64 patients reviewed had a mean age of 43 years. Usually the premolar-molar area of the mandible was involved. Lesions were in edentulous areas in more than 80% of patients. Most patients had a history of tooth extraction and many of the remaining patients reported a deep periodontal pocket, trauma, or surgery.

Discussion.—The origin of hyaline ring granuloma remains uncertain. Both intraosseous and extraosseous lesions are encountered. Treatment is by curettage or excision. Recurrences are rare and probably result from incomplete removal of the lesion.

▶ Although lesions with similar histology have been noted in other sites, the distinctive morphology of these hyaline rings would seem to be unique to the oral cavity.—W.A. Gardner, Jr., M.D.

Adenoid Cystic Carcinoma of the Esophagus: A Clinicopathologic Study of Three Cases

Cerar A, Juteršek A, Vidmar S (Univ of Ljubljana & Univ Clinical Center, Ljubljana, Yugoslavia)

Cancer 67:2159–2164, 1991 6–3

Background.—Adenoid cystic carcinoma (ACC) usually occurs in the salivary glands; the esophagus is a rare site for this tumor. Adenoid cystic carcinoma of the esophagus reportedly is more aggressive and spreads more widely than lesions of the salivary glands. Three patients with ACC among 245 patients with primary esophageal carcinomas seen in 1979–1988 were studied.

Clinical.—The patients were 2 men and 1 woman aged 49–74 years. All of the tumors were in the midesophagus. One patient lived for 15 months after surgery and another, with early ACC, was alive at last follow-up 4½ years after operation without specific symptoms. The third patient did not have surgery and died 13 months after the start of dysphagia.

Pathologic Findings.—The tumors exhibited tubular, cribriform, and solid areas and corresponded to grade 2 lesions. Hyaline substance in the tubular and adenoid structures was strongly periodic acid–Schiff-positive. Cells about tubular and cribriform structures tended to react positively with epithelial membrane antigen, carcinoembryonic antigen, and wide-spectral keratin. Reactivity to S-100 protein was variable.

Conclusions.—There are biological and pathologic similarities between ACC of the esophagus and tumors in the salivary glands. Both synchronous tumors of the esophagus and the site of esophageal ACC make the prognosis worse than for ACC of the salivary glands. Most reported patients with esophageal ACC have had aggressive tumors, but some have lived for 2 years or longer after operative treatment.

▶ In this series of 245 cases of carcinoma of the esophagus, 3 (1.2%) exhibited a predominant pattern of ACC. Squamous cell carcinomas with focal areas of ACC were excluded. The histologic, histochemical, and immunohistochemical findings appeared similar to those of salivary gland ACC. Because of the rarity in the esophagus, the prognostic significance of this histologic variant is uncertain. Interestingly, all 3 cases were contiguous with either squamous cell carcinoma, and 1 merged into an area of tubular adenocarcinoma. In 1 case, a separate primary squamous cell carcinoma of the esophagus was also present.—J.A. Tucker, M.D.

An Extensive Morphogical and Comparative Study of Clinically Early and Obvious Squamous Cell Carcinoma of the Esophagus

Anani PA, Gardiol D, Savary M. Monnier P (Univ of Lausanne, Switzerland)

Pathol Res Pract 187:214–219, 1991 6–4

Introduction.—Squamous cell carcinoma of the esophagus does not become clinically obvious until the tumor has become invasive. Developments in vital staining techniques have gradually improved the endoscopic diagnosis of very early esophageal carcinoma in its dysplastic stage. The morphological and histologic features of 28 esophagectomy specimens obtained from patients with esophageal carcinoma were compared.

Methods.—Between 1979 and 1987, 28 patients underwent esophagectomy in the treatment of squamous cell carcinoma. None of the patients received radiation therapy or chemotherapy before operation. Twelve men and 3 women with a mean age of 55 years had multiple early lesions detected by endoscopy; 10 men and 2 women with a mean age of 59 years had clinically obvious solitary carcinomas; and 1 man, aged 55 years, had a clinically obvious bifocal carcinoma. All specimens were stained with toluidine blue.

Results.—All 15 early lesions were histologically multicentric and were composed of areas containing various degrees of epithelial dysplasia. These dysplastic areas were either confluent or separated from one another by strips of healthy mucosa. However, the dysplastic areas were always associated with 1 or more foci of either in situ, microinvasive, superficial, or even invasive carcinoma. Lymph node metastases were found at operation in 4 (26%) of the 15 patients. Of the 12 obvious solitary invasive carcinomas, 2 (16.6%) were in direct contiguity with dysplastic areas, and 4 (33%) were in direct contiguity with in situ carcinoma. Six patients (50%) had lymph node metastases detected at operation. In the patient with a double well differentiated invasive carcinoma, the 2 tumors were separated from one another by 2.5 cm of healthy mucosa, and there was no evidence of either adjacent dysplasia or adjacent in situ carcinoma.

Discussion.—Invasive squamous cell esophageal carcinoma is always preceded by dysplastic lesions, followed by in situ carcinoma. However, the early carcinomas seen in this study all appeared as multicentric areas, whereas the clinically obvious invasive carcinomas all were solitary masses. There may be 2 different paths of evolution for esophageal carcinoma. Thus, a solitary invasive esophageal carcinoma may not necessarily represent the final evolution of early multifocal esophageal carcinoma.

▶ A toluidine blue staining method was applied to esophagectomy specimens to accentuate subtle lesions. Histologic sections of the entirety of the mucosa were taken in a grid pattern that enabled correlation with the gross specimen and mapping of dysplastic epithelial changes. This technique revealed a geographic distribution of seemingly separate areas of dysplasia with multiple foci of carcinoma in situ and microinvasive carcinoma. Such a distribution of lesions in the cases of esophagectomy for clinically early disease is somewhat unexpected, because the group of clinically obvious tumors exhibited dysplasia in continuity with the main mass and did not exhibit a multifocal pattern. The authors therefore hypothesize that multifocal in situ to microinvasive cancers may represent a different pathogenetic process than solitary invasive carcinomas, though this concept remains speculative. At a practical level, the staining method for gross examination of esophagectomy specimens may be very useful for gross detection of subtle early lesions.—J.A. Tucker, M.D.

Prominent Mononuclear Cell Infiltrate is Characteristic of Herpes Esophagitis

Greenson JK, Beschorner WE, Boitnott JK, Yardley JH (Johns Hopkins Univ)
Hum Pathol 22:541–549, 1991 6–5

Introduction.—Herpes is a common but often underdiagnosed cause of esophagitis. One factor that contributes to esophagitis is the inability to demonstrate the characteristic nuclear inclusions and/or multinucleate giant cells of herpesvirus infection in small endoscopic biopsy specimens. Aggregates of large mononuclear cells with convoluted nuclei adjacent to infected epithelium have been observed in the exudates of herpetic esophagitis. Esophageal biopsy specimens obtained from patients with ulcerative herpetic esophagitis and nonherpetic esophageal ulcers were studied to test the hypothesis that this prominent mononuclear cell infiltrate is a characteristic inflammatory response to herpesvirus infection.

Methods.—Biopsy specimens obtained from 22 patients with herpes esophagitis and 44 control patients with nonherpetic esophageal ulcers, including 9 with candidal and 5 with bacterial esophagitis, were reviewed. The estimated percentage of mononuclear cells present in the specimen was ranked independently by 2 reviewers using coded photomicrographs of exudate.

Findings.—All but 1 of the specimens from patients with herpes contained aggregates of large mononuclear cells with convoluted nuclei

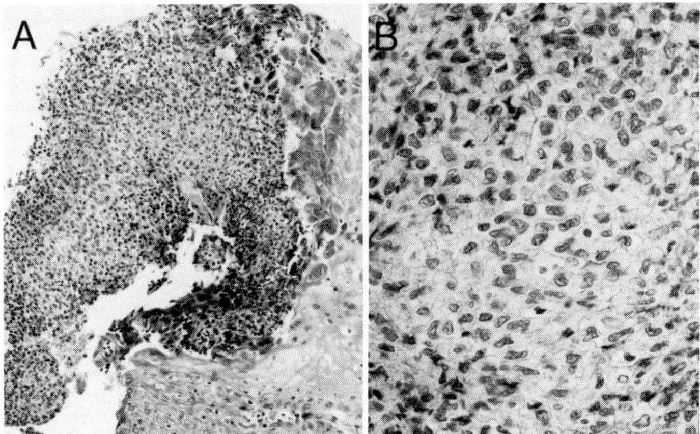

Fig 6–1.—Examples of herpes esophagitis with prominent aggregates of large mononuclear cells. **A,** low-power view of herpetic ulcer with "island" of mononuclear cells. (Hematoxylin-eosin; original magnification, ×180.) **B,** high-power view of mononuclear cells from patient shown in **A.** (Hematoxylin-eosin; original magnification, ×600.) (Courtesy of Greenson JK, Beschorner WE, Boitnott JK, et al: *Hum Pathol* 22:541–549, 1991.)

(Fig 6–1). These aggregates were often quite prominent with well-defined geographic borders and an organized appearance. Wilcoxon rank-sum analysis showed a significant correlation between the presence of herpes and increased mononuclear cells. In 11 patients, immunoperoxidase studies on Hollande-Bouin's fixed paraffin-embedded material showed strong cytoplasmic staining of the mononuclear cells for the macrophage marker KP1 (CD68). Some of the cells also showed focal staining for MT-1 (CD43), UCHL1 (CD45RO), and LN-3, indicating the presence of activated T cells. In contrast, prominent aggregates of macrophages were absent in most control specimens.

Conclusions.—Prominent aggregates of large mononuclear cells with convoluted nuclei are characteristic of the inflammatory response in ulcerative herpetic esophagitis. The presence of these mononuclear cells in esophageal biopsy specimens that do not show diagnostic herpes inclusions or epithelial giant cells warrant further studies to rule out herpesvirus infection.

Prevalence of Columnar-Lined (Barrett's) Esophagus: Comparison of Population-Based Clinical and Autopsy Findings

Cameron AJ, Zinsmeister AR, Ballard DJ, Carney JA (Mayo Clinic and Found, Rochester, Minn)

Gastroenterology 99:918–922, 1990 6–6

Background.—In Barrett's esophagus, columnar epithelium replaces the normal squamous lining of the distal esophagus. This disorder is thought to be acquired and is associated with severe gastroesophageal reflux. It is also believed to be a premalignant condition. The prevalence of Barrett's esophagus was estimated in the general population.

Methods.—A population-based study of clinically diagnosed cases of Barrett's esophagus was done in Olmsted County, Minnesota. Following this, a prospective search of Mayo Clinic autopsy material for the disorder was done using the diagnostic criteria used in the clinical study.

Results.—In the first part of the study, 25 residents of Olmsted County with Barrett's esophagus were identified. The patients had undergone endoscopy and biopsy between 1969 and 1986. The age- and sex-adjusted prevalence rate in this county was 22.6 cases per 100,000. In the second part of the study, 7 cases of Barrett's esophagus were found among 733 unselected autopsies. In 5 of these cases, Barrett's esophagus was first discovered at autopsy. Using the age- and sex-specific prevalence from the first part of the study, the authors expected to find only .19 cases of Barrett's esophagus of the 226 autopsies performed. The approximate 21-fold increase observed corresponded to an autopsy-estimated prevalence of 376 cases per 100,000.

Conclusions.—These findings suggest that most patients with Barrett's esophagus, a premalignant condition, remain unidentified. Until a simple, noninvasive technique for diagnosing Barrett's esophagus is found, this condition is likely to remain undiscovered in most cases.

▶ This demonstration of Barrett's esophagus in the general population may put into perspective some of the clinical interpretations of this microscopic finding. This study, unfortunately, did not note the degree of glandular dysplasia in the esophagi. In a mean of 44 months of follow-up, Berke et al. (1) found no carcinomas in 34 patients with low-grade dysplasia on initial biopsy, whereas in 15 of 43 patients with high-grade dysplasia, invasive carcinoma was diagnosed within 1 year of original endoscopy. The high-grade dysplasias with ulceration were especially likely to be associated with invasion.—W.A. Gardner, Jr., M.D.

Reference

1. Burke AP, et al: *Mod Path* 4:336, 1991.

Lymphoid Infiltrates of the Stomach: Evaluation of Histologic Criteria for the Diagnosis of Low-Grade Gastric Lymphoma on Endoscopic Biopsy Specimens

Zukerberg LR, Ferry JA, Southern JF, Harris NL (Massachusetts Gen Hosp, Boston; Harvard Med School)

Am J Surg Pathol 14:1087–1099, 1990 6–7

Background.—On examination of endoscopic biopsy specimens, it may be difficult to distinguish low-grade gastric lymphomas from benign inflammatory lymphoid infiltrates. It has been suggested that infiltrations of lymphocytes into glandular epithelium, or "lymphoepithelial lesions," are characteristic of primary gastric lymphomas. The presence and prominence of lymphoepithelial lesions, as well as other histologic features, were evaluated in specimens of low-grade gastric lymphoma and benign lymphoid infiltrate.

Methods.—Twenty-five low-grade lymphomas and 50 benign inflammatory infiltrates were studied. Twenty-one of the lymphomas were primary tumors. Tissue was prepared for light microscopic examination, and specimens were investigated for lymphoepithelial lesions, Dutcher bodies, cytologic atypia, the density of lymphoid infiltrate, ulceration, invasion of the muscularis mucosae, germinal centers, crypt abscesses, reactive epithelial atypia, and acute inflammation.

Results.—Seventy-two percent of lymphomas had at least one of the following features: prominent lymphoepithelial lesions, Dutcher bodies, and moderate cytologic atypia. None of these was seen in inflammatory infiltrates. Dense lymphoid infiltrates, rare or questionable lymphoepithelial lesions, muscularis mucosae invasion, ulceration, and mild cytologic atypia were seen more often in lymphomas but were also seen in inflammatory infiltrates. Features seen with equal frequency in the 2 groups were germinal centers, crypt abscesses, and reactive epithelial atypia. Acute inflammation was seen more often in inflammatory infiltrates.

Conclusions.—Histologic findings suggestive of gastric lymphoma include dense lymphoid infiltrates with either prominent lymphoepithelial lesions, moderate cytologic atypia, or Dutcher bodies. About 70% of endoscopic biopsy specimens of low-grade gastric lymphoma have these features. Most of these lymphomas can be included in the category of low-grade lymphomas of mucosa-associated lymphoid tissue, but some are lymphomatous polyposes of the gastrointestinal tract.

▶ The diagnosis of lymphoma is usually a challenging experience on a small biopsy specimen of the gastrointestingal tract. The authors delineate useful criteria for the distinction between low grade malignant lymphomas and benign inflammatory infiltrates in the stomach. This study is particularly important because of the inclusion of the control group of benign cases in the same study, a feature not present in the previous studies of primary gastric lymphoma.

Using the most specific of the above criteria, the authors were able to identify confidently 70% of lesions that subsequently proved to be gastric lymphoma, although in the discussion they imply that only about 50% of gastric lymphomas can be diagnosed by paraffin section analysis. Finally, they recommend an approach that should be of practical use: dense lymphoid infiltrates that meet their criteria can be confidently diagnosed as lymphoma; dense infiltrates without the minimal criteria noted above require paraffin section immunostaining for monotypic immunoglobulin. This technique should be diagnostic in 55% of cases of lymphoma. If immunostaining is nondiagnostic, frozen section immunostaining may be undertaken. The authors caution that the presence of germinal centers, acute inflammation, and *Helicobacter pylori* infection does not exclude a diagnosis of malignant lymphoma.—G.F. Worsham, M.D.

Gastric Carcinoids and Their Precursor Lesions: A Histologic and Immunohistochemical Study of 23 Cases

Bordi C, Yu J-Y, Baggi MT, Davoli C, Pilato FP, Baruzzi G, Gardini G, Zamboni G, Franzin G, Papotti M, Bussolati G (Univ of Parma, Italy; Arcispedale S Maria Nuova, Reggio Emilia, Italy; Univ of Verona, Italy; Veneto Region Hosp, Verona, Italy; Univ of Turin, Italy)

Cancer 67:663–672, 1991 6–8

Introduction.—Far from being a pathologic curiosity, gastric carcinoids now make up as many as one third of all carcinoid tumors of the gut. These lesions may arise in patients with pernicious anemia and during long-term treatment with inhibitors of gastric acid secretion. In hypergastric patients, tumors develop through a sequence of hyperplasia, dysplasia, and neoplasia.

Objective.—Histologic and immunohistochemical analysis was undertaken in 23 unselected patients with nonantral gastric carcinoid tumors. None of the patients had Zollinger-Ellison syndrome and none had symptoms suggesting carcinoid syndrome, ulcer disease, or gastric acid hypersecretion.

Findings.—Ten of the 23 patients had multiple gastric carcinoids. Four tumors were entirely intramucosal. One patient had nodal metastases. All but 4 patients had evidence of chronic atrophic gastritis in the extratumoral fundic mucosa. The 4 exceptional patients had single, diffusely infiltrating tumors. Proliferating endocrine cells were limited to the areas of tumor in these cases. In contrast, endocrine cell changes were prevalent in patients with gastritis. The tumor cells were immunoreactive for chromogranin A and synaptophysin, but were usually negative for chromogranin B. Ten tumors contained scattered serotonin cells.

Summary.—This study distinguished 2 variants of nonantral gastric carcinoid tumor: a more aggressive variety not associated with extratumoral endocrine cell proliferation or gastrin hypersecretion, and a type of tumor, often multiple, that is associated with chronic atrophic gastritis and tends to be limited to the mucosa and submucosa.

▶ Of the 23 nonantral gastric carcinoids in this study, 4 occurred in nonatrophic gastric mucosa and 19 occurred in a setting of chronic atrophic gastritis (CAG). There appear to be distinct differences between the 2 groups. The 4 non-CAG associated tumors were single, not associated with hypergastrinemia, and were diffusely infiltrative. The 19 CAG-associated tumors were relatively small, either single or multiple, nonaggressive histologically, and were associated with precursor lesions of endocrine cells in adjacent, nontumoral gastric mucosa. These lesions were thought to be induced by hyperplastic gastric cells in the gastric antrum.

These findings are evidence that carcinoids associated with CAG may be treated by simple endoscopic extirpation, or in the instance of multiple occurrence, by antrectomy to eradicate the hyperplastic gastric cells causing the hypergastrinemia.

The findings of this study may ultimately affect the choice of surgical procedure for these patients. In such instances, the pathologist is afforded the opportunity to act as a consultant. Reporting "carcinoid tumor" on a gastric biopsy is not enough. The report should include whether or not the tumor is associated with CAG in addition to its depth of invasion.—J.M. Harmon, M.D.

Gastric Antral Vascular Ectasia ("Watermelon Stomach"): Radiologic Findings

Urban BA, Jones B, Fishman EK, Kern SE, Ravich WJ (Johns Hopkins Univ)
Radiology 178:517–518, 1991 6–9

Introduction.—Gastric antral vascular ectasia is a rare source of potential gastrointestinal bleeding. It is characterized endoscopically by a distinct appearance of prominent red vascular folds traversing the gastric antrum and radiation to the pyloric sphincter.

Case Report.—Man, 74, was seen with a history of fatigue and melena of several years' duration. Physical examination was negative. His stools were guaiac positive and he was anemic. Gastric analysis with pentagastrin stimulation was consistent with gastric achlorhydria. A double-contrast upper gastrointestinal series showed prominent, scalloped folds in the antrum radiating to the pyloric sphincter and suggesting antral gastritis. Focal thickening of the gastric wall in the antrum was shown on CT. Upper endoscopy revealed thick, friable, actively bleeding antral folds radiating to the pyloric sphincter. Biopsy of the antral folds showed thrombosed, dilated capillaries at the apices of the folds. The diagnosis was established as gastric antral vascular ectasia. He underwent antrectomy and vagotomy with Billroth I anastomosis. The patient developed postoperative complications of outlet obstruction secondary to anastomotic ulceration and bezoar formation, which was treated with further partial gastrectomy several months later. The patient had no evidence of recurrent vascular ectasia.

Conclusion.—Prominent antral folds and antral thickening in an elderly patient with chronic anemia should alert the radiologist to the possibility of gastric antral vascular ectasia. Patients with severe recurrent bleeding can be treated with curative surgery.

▶ Watermelon stomach or gastric antral vascular ectasia (GAVE) may not be well known to general pathologists because there are few references to this entity in the pathologic literature (1,2). The case report outlines the clinical and radiologic findings and notes the characteristic but subtle findings in small biopsy specimens. Previously, Suit et al (1) have noted that mean vascular crossectional area, fibromuscular hyperplasia, and architectural distortion are useful in the differential diagnosis between GAVE and gastritis or normal findings. The origin of this peculiar condition is not clear, but mucosal trauma, specifically prolapse of the mucosa through the pyloric valve has been suggested (3).—G.F. Worsham, M.D.

References

1. Suit PF, et al: *Am J Surg Pathol* 11:750, 1987
2. Gardner GW, et al: *J Clin Pathol* 38:317, 1985.
3. Rawlinson WD, et al: *Med J Aust* 144:709, 1986.

Deceptive Bizarre Stromal Cells in Polyps and Ulcers of the Gastrointestinal Tract

Shekitka KM, Helwig EB (Armed Forces Inst of Pathology, Washington, DC)
Cancer 67:2111–2117, 1991 6–10

Background.—Pseudomalignant lesions, or atypical cellular proliferation in the stroma, may occur in ulcers and in inflammatory polyps. With the increasing use of gastrointestinal endoscopy, these lesions are being encountered more frequently. Histologic features, immunohistochemical profiles, and clinical follow-up data were compared for a series of patients with gastrointestinal pseudomalignant lesions.

Methods.—Histologically pseudomalignant stromal lesions of the gastrointestinal tract from 33 patients were reviewed. Markers for various histologic characteristics were selected, and immunostains for detection of cytomegalovirus were performed. Clinical and follow-up information was collected when available.

Results.—Lesions were identified in ulcers in 7 patients and in polyps in 26 patients. In 3 patients in each group, malignant neoplasm was wrongly diagnosed. The patients commonly had a history of gastrointestinal bleeding and/or inflammatory bowel disease. Bizarre stromal cells appeared as atypical spindled, epithelioid, or large round cells in the lamina propria or in granulation tissue. In 20 of 23 lesions the cells stained strongly for vimentin, and in 7 of 23 lesions they stained for muscle-specific actin. The cells appeared to be fibroblasts or myoblasts. Follow-up information was available for 24 patients, including the 6 in whom a malignancy was initially diagnosed. At an average follow-up of 13 months, 12 patients were alive with no evidence of a gastrointestinal lesion, and 2 had died of other causes.

Conclusions.—Bizarre stromal cells in gastrointestinal ulcers and in inflammatory cells must be correctly recognized to avoid serious diagnostic pitfalls. Immunohistochemical stains may be helpful, particularly with small biopsy specimens and an indefinite clinical picture. The reactive nature of the lesions should be established by conservative local incision of the entire lesion, histologic examination, and careful follow-up.

Gastrointestinal Stromal Tumours: Correlation of Immunophenotype With Clinicopathological Features

Newman PL, Wadden C, Fletcher CDM (St Thomas's Hosp, London; Univ Hosp of Wales, Cardiff)

J Pathol 164:107–117, 1991 6–11

Introduction.—The histogenesis and biological behavior of stromal tumors of the gastrointestinal tract remain controversial. A retrospective study was conducted to define the correlation of immunophenotype to prognosis in stromal tumors of the gastrointestinal tract.

Methods.—Formalin-fixed, paraffin-embedded blocks from 60 patients with gastrointestinal stromal tumors were studied. Immunohistochemistry was done using the avidin-biotin-peroxidase technique, with a panel of 7 antibodies directed at identifying smooth muscular or neural differentiation. Immunophenotype was correlated with the site of the lesions and clinical behavior.

Findings.—Whereas 36% of the tumors showed neural differentiation, only 6.6% expressed S-100 protein. Another 31% showed smooth muscle differentiation, of which 73.6% expressed both desmin and smooth muscle actin. The other 20% reacted with both neural and smooth muscle markers other than S-100, and 13% were negative with all antibodies. All tumors that stained with S-100 were located outside the stomach. In contrast, 17 of 18 tumors that stained for neuron-specific enolase and/or PGP 9.5, in the absence of S-100, were located within the stomach, including 9 tumors with the distinctive syncytial, palisading pattern. There was no correlation between histologic appearance and immunophenotype. Forty-two patients were followed for a mean 5 years. Only 1 of 22 with purely neural markers died. The expression of desmin and smooth muscle actin with up to 4 mitoses per 30 high-power field was associated with a benign course.

Implication.—Larger studies are warranted to further assess the value of immunophenotyping in stromal tumors of the gastrointestinal tract.

▶ Although failing to provide a correlation of immunophenotype with either clinical behavior or histologic appearance, the abstracted paper disclosed an example of a lesion similar to the highly malignant "plexosarcoma" described by Herrera et al. (1). All of the cases reported here, however, proved to be benign.—W.A. Gardner, Jr., M.D.

References

1. Herrera GA, et al: *Arch Pathol Lab Med* 113:846, 1989.

Depressed Adenoma of the Stomach, Revisited: Histologic, Histochemical, and Immunohistochemical Profiles

Xuan ZX, Ambe K, Enjoji M (Kyushu Univ, Fukuoka, Japan)

Cancer 67:2382–2389, 1991 6–12

Background.—Histologic features alone cannot easily differentiate the malignant potentials of depressed and nondepressed adenomas. A further qualification was made of depressed adenomas by histochemical and immunohistochemical methods.

Methods.—Fifty-six depressed adenomas from 52 patients were studied (Fig 6–2). Forty-four well-differentiated, grossly depressed early gastric carcinomas and 57 nondepressed adenomas were also studied. Histopathologic studies were done on all of these tumors, and immunohistochemical studies were conducted on 43 depressed gastric adenomas, 41 early gastric carcinomas, and 53 nondepressed adenomas.

Results.—Seventy-three percent of the depressed adenomas involved the entire thickness of the stomach mucous membrane with tubules of atypical epithelium. Epithelial atypia was severe in 41% of depressed adenomas, and Paneth's cells were found in 61%, significantly more often than in nondepressed adenomas. Argyrophil cells were found in 63% of depressed adenomas, 36% of nondepressed adenomas, and 32% of early gastric carcinomas. Carcinoembryonic antigen and carbohydrate antigen 19-9 were found immunohistochemically in 28% of depressed adenomas and in 6% of benign nondepressed adenomas. The frequencies were 71% for carcinoembryonic antigen and 66% for carbohydrate antigen 19-9 in early gastric carcinomas. Lectin reactivity and mucin content were the same in both depressed and nondepressed adenomas. In the early depressed carcinomas, tumor cells had higher lectin reactivities and lower mucin contents than did adenomas.

Conclusions.—Depressed adenomas appear to be benign neoplastic lesions. However, based on their immunoreactivity to tumor markers and

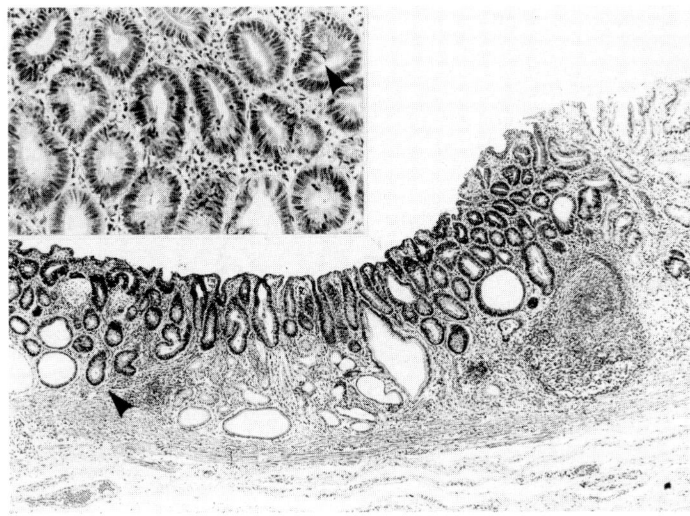

Fig 6–2.—Depressed adenoma. Adenomatous tubules partly extending to a deeper portion of the mucosa (*arrowhead*) with few dilated pyloric glands underneath. Hematoxylin and eosin; original magnification, ×50. **Inset,** some mucin goblets are present in atypical tubules (*arrowhead*). Hematoxylin and eosin; original magnification, ×190. (Courtesy of Xuan ZX, Ambe K, Enjoji M: *Cancer* 67:2382–2389, 1991.)

in previously reported follow-up results, their malignant potential may be greater than that of nondepressed adenomas.

▶ Japanese colleagues have greater familiarity than we do with early gastric cancers and their precursor lesions. This paper follows the original recognition of this morphological pattern by one of the authors (1).—W.A. Gardner, Jr., M.D.

Reference

1. Nakamura K, et al: *Cancer* 62:2197, 1988.

Carcinoid Tumors of the Duodenum: A Clinicopathologic Study of 99 Cases

Burke AP, Sobin LH, Federspiel BH, Shekitka KM, Helwig EB (Armed Forces Inst of Pathology, Washington, DC)
Arch Pathol Lab Med 114:700–704, 1990 6–13

Background.—Duodenal carcinoids are rare and are usually discovered on endoscopy. There is little available information about affected patients, particularly those who have had endoscopic biopsy only. A study was done to determine which pathologic parameters predict metastasis.

Patients.—Ninety-nine patients with carcinoid tumors of the duodenum were studied. There were 59 men and 40 women, with a mean age of 59. The initial diagnosis was made by endoscopic biopsy in 41 patients. Seventy-seven patients were followed for an average of 65 months. Twenty tumors were found at autopsy, and 2 patients were unavailable for follow-up. Metastases were present in 21% of patients and all were discovered initially. Four percent of patients died of metastatic disease at a mean 37 months after surgery. Twelve patients were managed by biopsy only, and none died of tumor-related disease.

Findings.—Involvement of the muscularis propria, tumor size greater than 2 cm, and the presence of mitotic figures were associated with risk of metastasis. In 51 tumors, no correlation was seen between immunohistochemical somatostatin positivity and a history of diarrhea, cholelithiasis, or diabetes mellitus (the components of the somatostatin syndrome). Five patients had Zollinger-Ellison syndrome with immunohistochemical gastrin positivity, but none of the others showed any correlation between ulcer disease and gastrin positivity.

Conclusions.—Duodenal carcinoids are indolent, particularly when they are small and confined to the submucosa. The lesions commonly contain gastrin and somatostatin, but this appears to have little clinical relevance.

▶ Investigators previously have recommended surgical removal of all gastrointestinal carcinoids, because of the unpredictable behavior of such tumors. The recommendation has often been based on data collected before the impact of advanced endoscopic technology. Newer technology has resulted in the discovery of much smaller tumors to which this recommendation may not apply. This change appplies particularly to those tumors involving the duodenum where a surgical procedure near or involving the ampulla may not be feasible.

This study reports the findings of 99 duodenal carcinoids and shows the association of increased metastatic potential with tumor size greater than 2 cm, the presence of mitosis, and involvement of the muscularis propria. The report offers data that can be used by pathologists when advising clinicians about therapy for this entity. This study also confirms the previously documented association of von Recklinghausen's disease and ampullary carcinoids and offers this advice: In the jaundiced patient with von Recklinghausen's disease, think ampullary carcinoid.—J.M. Harmon, M.D.

Granulomatous Vasculitis in Crohn's Disease

Wakefield AJ, Sankey EA, Dhillon AP, Sawyerr AM, More L, Sim R, Pittilo RM, Rowles PM, Hudson M, Lewis AAM, Pounder RE (Royal Free Hosp; Univ College and Middlesex Hosp, London)

Gastroenterology 100:1279–1287, 1991 6–14

Background.—Recently, an inflammatory microvascular occlusion, which appears to be mediated by a mesenteric vasculitis, has been implicated in the pathogenesis of Crohn's disease. It was hypothesized that the granulomas in Crohn's disease could be of vascular origin, and that a granulomatous vasculitis may play an important role in the spectrum of vascular inflammation in Crohn's disease.

Methods.—Twenty-four consecutive resected specimens of small and large intestinal Crohn's disease were studied to evaluate the possible vascular origin of granulomas in this condition. To preserve a normal vascular shape, the tissues were preserved by arterial perfusion-fixation with 100% formol saline solution at mean arterial pressure of 100 mm Hg. On histopathologic examination of sections stained with hematoxylin and eosin, 15 specimens contained granulomas. Sections were stained immunohistochemically using polyclonal antibodies against fibrinogen and macrophages and monoclonal antibodies against collagen type IV (a constituent of vascular basal lamina) and QB-end-10 (which binds to the CD34 antigen expressed specifically by vascular endothelial cells).

Results.—Of the 15 specimens containing granulomas, 485 granulomas were identified. The majority of these (77%) were found deep to the mucosa, particularly in the submucosa (42%). A majority of the granulomas (85%) involved damaged blood vessels directly. The damage was characterized by disintegration or reduplication of the vascular basal lamina, adherence of chronic inflammatory cells to the damaged endothelium, and fibrin deposition. Immunostaining with collagen type IV clearly established the focus of vascular mural injury in relation to the normal adjacent vascular-basal lamina, and immunostaining for QB-end-10 confirmed the vascular origin of the mucosal and submucosal granulomas. In advanced granulomatous vasculitis, in which the vascular origin of the granulomas was not apparent on sections stained with hematoxylin and eosin, the combination of perfusion-fixation and immunostaining for vascular structures showed the intimate association of granulomas and blood vessels along the course of the affected vessel, as demonstrated by a computer-generated 3-dimensional reconstruction of serial sections.

Conclusion.—This study shows the frequent vascular origin of granulomas in Crohn's disease. However, although granulomatous vasculitis is an integral part of the pattern of vascular inflammation in Crohn's disease, the findings do not provide conclusive evidence that vasculitis is essential to the pathogenesis of this condition.

▶ The presence of granulomas in Crohn's disease has long been recognized but poorly understood. Routine histologic examination of cases of Crohn's disease reveals lymphocytic and granulomatous vasculitis in a minority of cases, but most granulomas are not observed to be associated with vessels. In this study, by combining a careful perfusion fixation method with immunostaining for vascular basement membrane and endothelial cells, the authors showed that most of the granulomas (85%) were directly involved with damaged blood vessels, an association not usually demonstrable without these special techniques. Computer reconstruction demonstrated that granulomas followed the course of blood vessels. Further, the granulomas of Crohn's disease were compared with those from 2 cases of Wegener's granulomatosis, and no difference in the pattern of granulomatous vascular injury was identified. Granulomatous vasculitis was identified in 15 of 24 cases of Crohn's disease examined by these methods, and a lymphocyte-predominant vasculitis was identified in the other 9 cases. This study appears to represent an exciting advance in the understanding of Crohn's disease. Although the basic causative agent remains unknown and the vasculitis may not represent a primary process, the histologic findings in Crohn's disease, including transmural inflammation, mucosal ulceration, and granulomatous inflammation, could all be explained on the basis of a granulomatous vasculitis. This study, then, raises the interesting possibility that granulomatous vasculitis represents the basic lesion of Crohn's disease.—J.A. Tucker, M.D.

Intestinal Ganglioneuromatosis: Mucosal and Transmural Types. A Clinicopathologic and Immunohistochemical Study of Six Cases

D'Amore ESG, Manivel JC, Pettinato G, Niehans GA, Snover DC (Univ of Minnesota; Istituto Nazionale per la Ricerca sul Cancro, Genova, Italy; Universita di Napoli, Naples; Minneapolis VA Hosp)

Hum Pathol 22:276–286, 1991 6–15

Background.—Intestinal ganglioneuromatosis (GN) consists of a massive proliferation of nerve fibers, ganglion cells, and supporting cells belonging to the enteric nervous system. In 6 cases of GN, a variety of clinical signs and morphological characteristics were observed.

Methods.—Formalin-fixed, paraffin-embedded transmural sections (5 cases) and bioptic material (1 case) were available for immunohistochemical analysis, which was performed using a panel of antibodies against specific intestinal neurotransmitters and markers.

Findings.—The microscopic findings from cases 1 through 3 demonstrated similar morphological characteristics, including involvement of all layers of the bowel wall. The marked and diffuse hyperplasia in the myenteric plexus consisted of aggregates of nerve fibers, ganglion cells, and

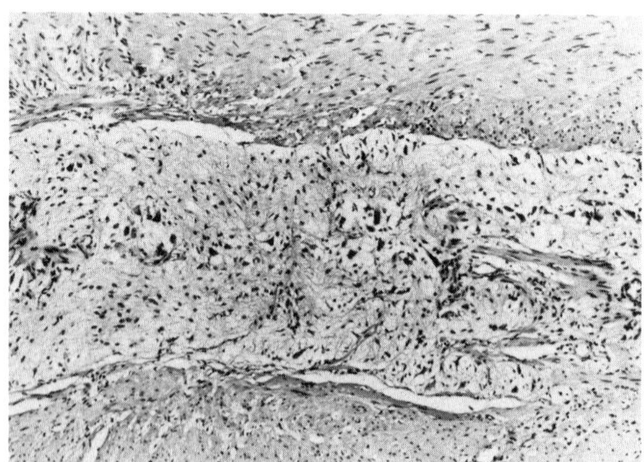

Fig 6–3.—Marked hyperplasia of the myenteric plexus in transmural GN associated with MEN IIb syndrome. (Hematoxylin-eosin; original magnification ×30). (Courtesy of D'Amore ESG, Manivel JC, Pettinato G, et al: *Hum Pathol* 22:276–286, 1991.)

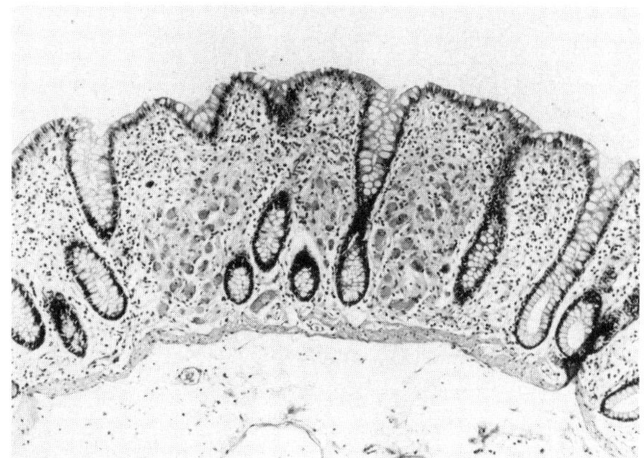

Fig 6–4.—Clusters of ganglion cells and supportive cells in the lamina propria. (Hematoxylin-eosin; original magnification ×300). (Courtesy of D'Amore ESG, Manivel JC, Pettinato G, et al: *Hum Pathol* 22:276–286, 1991.)

supportive cells, forming a nearly continuous band between the circular and longitudinal muscle layers (Fig 6–3). The proliferation in the submucosal plexus appeared diffuse but less intense. In case 6, microscopic findings demonstrated a markedly dilatated colon with multiple tubular adenomas and a focal GN in the mucosa. Clusters of large ganglion cells and a small number of supporting cells were distributed among normal areas of mucosa and sometimes extended into the muscularis mucosae (Fig 6–4). The submucosal and myenteric plexuses appeared not to be affected.

Immunohistochemical/Histochemical Data.—A high degree of heterogeneity and increased reactivity for vasoactive intestinal polypeptide, opioid peptides leu-enkephalin and met-enkephalin, and substance P in those patients who had transmural involvement. A mild increased immunoreactivity for tyrosine hydroxylase in the myenteric plexus was observed in 4 of 4 patients with this involvement. Histochemical analyses showed hyperplasia of the parasympthetic fibers and neurons in 1 patient with transmural GN. Electron microscopic results suggested that several neurotransmitters were present in at least 1 sample.

Conclusions.—Hyperplasia of various peptidergic fibers and neurons occurs in GN. In addition, GN consists of some heterogeneous immunohistochemical reactivity of the proliferating neural aspects. The exact understanding of the physiopathology of GN requires further research.

▶ This detailed study illustrates the clinical and histologic findings in the unusual entity of intestinal GN. The authors place a useful emphasis on the distinction between transmural GN, as associated with multiple endocrine neoplasia IIb, and mucosal GN. Ganglioneuromatosis remains a poorly understood entity. This work, however, illustrates a heterogeneous immunohistochemical distribution of neurotransmitters, providing evidence that the lesion does not develop as a selected growth of any single type of ganglion cell or nerve fiber, but appears to have a more complex cause. Ultrastructural study was also performed on 1 case and revealed heterogeneous neurosecretory granules. The authors were able to expand the range of neurotransmitter localization using histochemical determination of acetylcholinesterase activity in 1 case in which frozen tissue was available, and they speculate that further research using frozen tissue and an expanded battery of histochemical and immunohistochemical stains might be useful.—J.A. Tucker, M.D.

Obstructive Colitis: Ulceroinflammatory Lesions Occurring Proximal to Colonic Obstruction

Toner M, Condell D, O'Briain DS (St James's Hosp, Dublin; Trinity College, Dublin)

Am J Surg Pathol 14:719–728, 1990 6–16

Background.—Obstructive colitis, the presence of ulceroinflammatory lesions in the colon proximal to an obstructing or potentially obstructing lesion, has been studied mainly from surgical and radiologic viewpoints. Resected colon tissue from patients with disease of varying severity was investigated to define the pathologic spectrum of this condition.

Methods.—Nine patients were studied over a 9-month period. There were 8 women and 1 man (mean age, 73). All but 1 patient had hypertension, diabetes, or some other chronic illness. Resected colon tissue was examined by gross and microscopic methods, and follow-up information was gathered from medical records. Follow-up ranged from 24 to 32 months.

Results.—Seven obstructions resulted from adenocarcinoma and 2 from diverticular disease. Circumscribed ulcers .5 to 2 cm in diameter

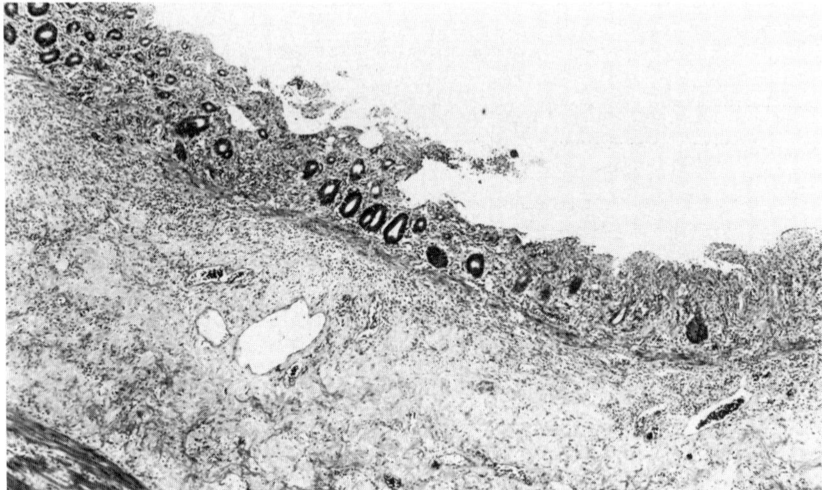

Fig 6–5.—Obstructive colitis. There is loss of the upper half of the mucosa and a moderate mucosal inflammatory infiltrate. The muscularis mucosae and muscularis propria are intact, and the submucosa is expanded by a hyaline edematous exudate. (Courtesy of Toner M, Condell D, O'Briain DS: *Am J Surg Pathol* 14:719–728, 1990.)

were seen in 3 bowels, and confluent circumferential lesions 8 to 25 cm long were found in 6. A 2.5- to 35-cm segment of normal colon was always found between these lesions and the more distal obstructing lesions. Dilation was generally mild, with moderate thickening of the wall and a granular luminal surface with occasional deep longitudinal or transverse ulcers. Scattered pseudopolyps were sometimes seen, and the margins of diseased tissue were well demarcated and irregular. The lesions comprised granulation tissue with a mixed acute and chronic inflammatory infiltrate in place of the mucosa and often the submucosa (Fig 6–5). When this infiltrate extended to the muscularis propria, peritonitis and perforation were seen.

Conclusions.—Obstructive colitis can usually be distinguished pathologically from Crohn's disease and other forms of colitis. Ischemia may be responsible for many of the features of obstructive colitis, probably resulting mainly from pressure-induced hypoperfusion. Alterations in fecal flora may have a synergistic effect. Peritonitis may occur, as may perforation and breakdown of anastomoses through involved colonic segments, which may appear normal at operation.

▶ As clinicians expand the patient base of coloscopic biopsy, newly recognized patterns of inflammation enable the pathologist to move the diagnoses from descriptive or nonspecific to diagnoses that are specific, or at least characteristic. Nine cases identified by the authors in resected specimens delineate a range of features that the authors term "obstructive colitis." They raise the possibility of an ischemic injury on the basis of both the morphologic findings and the probable pathophysiology involved in the development of the lesions. Knowledge of this pattern of mucosal injury may also be useful in small biopsy specimens when inflammatory bowel disease is in the clinical or pathologic differential diagnosis.—G.F. Worsham, M.D.

Pitfalls in the Diagnosis of Collagenous Colitis: Experience With 75 Cases From a Registry of Collagenous Colitis at The Johns Hopkins Hospital

Lazenby AJ, Yardley JH, Giardiello FM, Bayless TM (Johns Hopkins Med Insts)

Hum Pathol 21:905–910, 1990 6–17

Background.—The clinical entity of collagenous colitis has been defined since 1976, but misconceptions and interpretive difficulties accompany the diagnosis of this rare disorder. The histologic and clinical characteristics of collagenous colitis were reviewed.

Clinical Aspects.—The major signs and symptoms of collagenous colitis include chronic watery diarrhea. The condition occurs most often in middle-aged, white women. Endoscopy and radiography do not help in the diagnosis. A biopsy of normal-appearing mucosa is usually the only method of obtaining a definitive diagnosis.

Histology.—The condition is characterized by collagenous thickening and colitis of the mucosa. A moderate to marked increase in mononuclear cells is seen in the lamina propria (Fig 6–6), which shows clusters

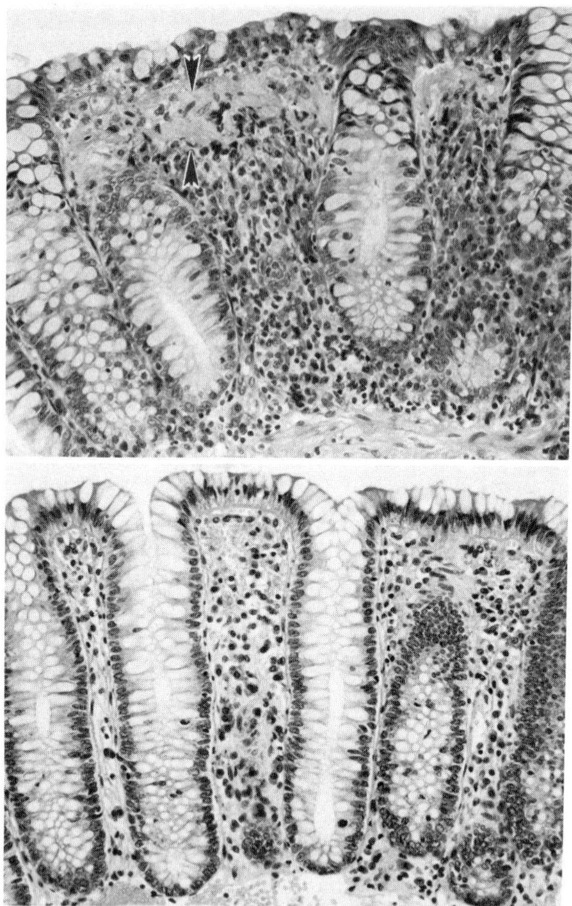

Fig 6–6.—Increased mucosal inflammation is prerequisite for a diagnosis of active or untreated collagenous colitis. **Top,** in addition to the thickened subepithelial collagen band (**between arrows**), this case of collagenous colitis has prominent intraepithelial lymphocytes as well as increased mononuclear cells in the lamina propria. Hematoxylin-eosin; original magnification, ×260. **Bottom,** in this histologically normal colon, the modest numbers of inflammatory cells in both the lamina propria and epithelium contrast sharply with the increased inflammation of collagenous colitis. Hematoxylin-eosin; original magnification, ×220. (Courtesy of Lazenby AJ, Yardley JH, Giardiello FM, et al: *Hum Pathol* 21:905–910, 1990.)

of plasma cells at the base of the crypts. Increased mucosal inflammation is a key characteristic of this disorder, but it may be decreased by anti-inflammatory treatment or during spontaneous remission. The subepithelial collagenous thickening can produce a mean thickness of 15–20 μm in most patients. The basement membrane located under the surface epithelium is defined by sharp, distinct edges (Fig 6–7). However, in early cases the basement membrane can have a lacy appearance.

Diagnostic Difficulties.—The appearance of increased mucosal inflammation is a prerequisite in untreated patients. Normal structures can be

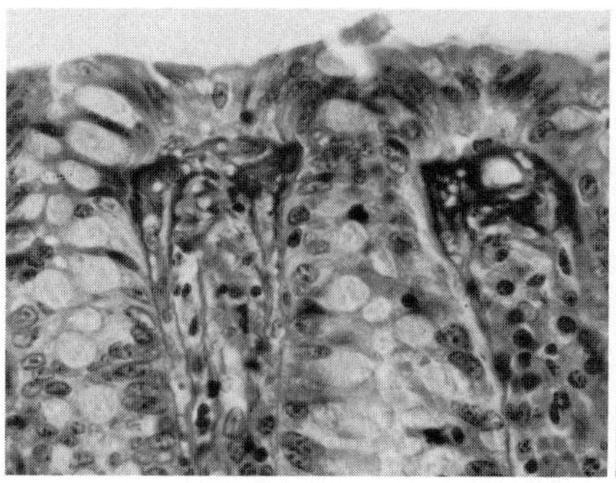
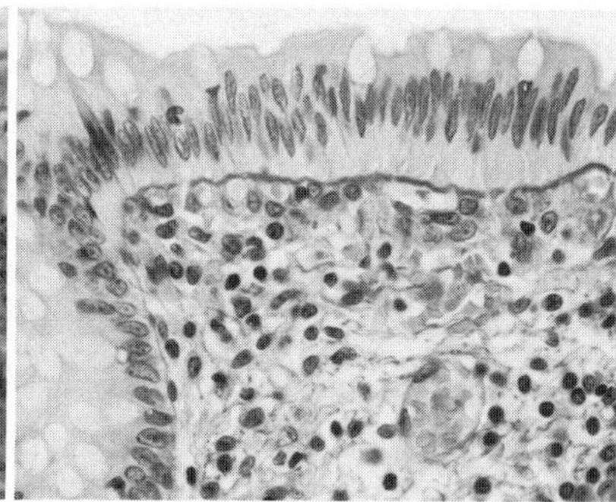

Fig 6–7.—Trichrome stains are useful for highlighting increased subepithelial collagen. **Left,** in this case of collagenous colitis, the increased subepithelial collagen is relatively subtle and characterized as much by qualitative as quantitative changes. Strands of collagen extend down into the upper lamina propria, giving the lower border of the subepithelial collagen layer an irregular, spiculated appearance. **Right,** in this histologically normal colon, the sharp, distinct, lower border of the basement membrane is qualitatively different from that of collagenous colitis. Masson's Trichrome, red filter; original magnification, ×450. (Courtesy of Lazenby AJ, Yardley JH, Giardiello FM, et al: *Hum Pathol* 21:905–910, 1990.)

interpreted as a thickened subepithelial collagen band when they do not warrant such a description. If the basement membrane has a smooth lower edge or if inflammation is not present, the patient does not have collagenous colitis. Finally, the biopsy site should be in the area of the proximal descending colon, which can be accomplished using a flexible sigmoidoscope.

▶ Collagenous colitis and the related condition, microscopic or lymphocytic colitis, are important pathologic considerations in the patient who has a normal colonoscopy with a clinical history of chronic watery diarrhea. Although I suspect that this clinical differential diagnosis has meant an increase in the number of biopsies we have performed, the present study emphasizes the rarity of this condition, which was diagnosed only 6 times in 1,469 cases. The authors also call attention to an unusually high rate of collagenous colitis in their consultation material from southern Florida and raise the possibility of substantial regional variations in the prevalence of this condition.

The authors emphasize a major pitfall in diagnosis (i.e., interpreting tangential sectioning of the subepithelial membrane as being abnormally thickened). They recommend making the diagnosis of collagenous colitis only in the presence of the inflammatory changes they describe.—G.F. Worsham, M.D.

Aberrant Crypts: Putative Preneoplastic Foci in Human Colonic Mucosa
Pretlow TP, Barrow BJ, Ashton WS, O'Riordan MA, Pretlow TG, Jurcisek JA, Stellato TA (Case Western Reserve Univ)
Cancer Res 51:1564–1567, 1991 6–18

Introduction.—Colorectal cancer is the second most common cause of death from cancer in the United States. A study was conducted to deter-

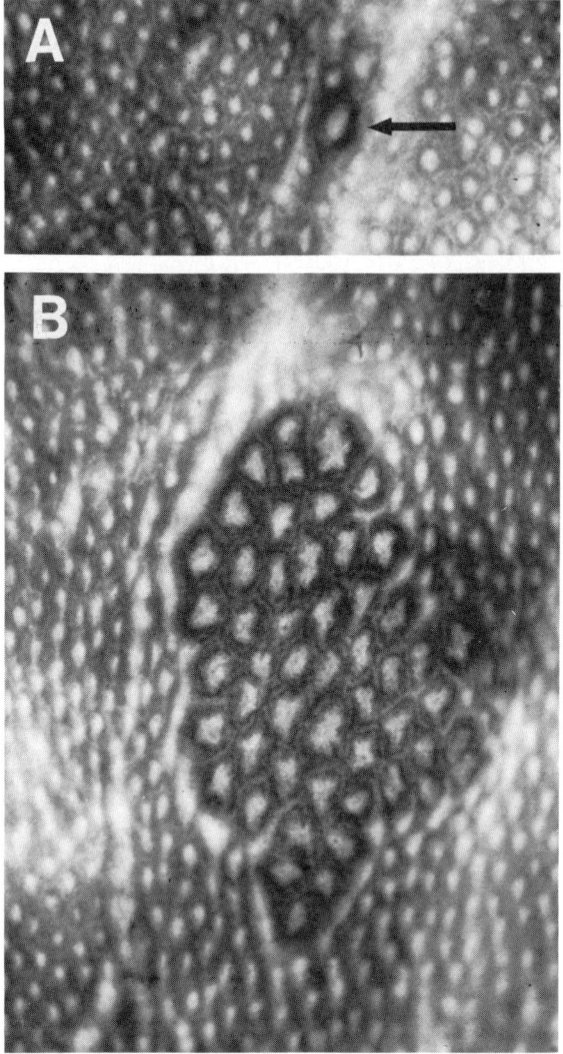

Fig 6–8.—Whole-mount segments of grossly normal human colonic mucosa from patients with colon cancer. **A,** single aberrant crypt (*arrow*); **B,** larger focus or plaque of aberrant crypts. Elevation of the plaque above the mucosal surface is apparent from the fact that it is in a different focal plane. Methylene blue; original magnification, ×29. (Courtesy of Pretlow TP, Barrow BJ, Ashton WS, et al: *Cancer Res* 51:1564–1567, 1991.)

mine whether preneoplastic lesions can be identified in the colons of humans with colon cancer. Aberrant crypts were identified in grossly normal human colonic mucosa.

Methods.—Mucosa samples were obtained from the walls of grossly normal colons from 22 consecutive patients with sporadic colonic carcinoma. Control samples were obtained from 1 colonic carcinoma patient with Gardner's syndrome, from 1 patient with a recurrent tubulovillous polyp, from 1 patient with Crohn's disease, from 1 with diverticulitis, and from 1 with clinically redundant colon free of pathologic abnormalities. The 22 patients with colon cancer had a mean age of 69. There were 10 women and 12 men. Aberrant crypts found on whole mounts were marked with permanent ink.

Outcome.—Figure 6–8 shows aberrant crypts in grossly normal human colonic mucosa stained with methylene blue. These aberrant crypts were identified in tissue from 9 of 9 left colons, from 0 of 1 transverse colon, and from 4 of 12 right colons of samples taken from patients with colon cancer. No aberrant crypts were found in the mucosa from the surgically resected descending colon of the patient with recurrent tubulovillous polyp, from the surgically resected left colon of the patient with clinically redundant colon, or in autopsy samples from the right colons of 13 individuals without colon cancer. All aberrant crypts appeared 3 times larger in diameter than normal crypts, and most had oval or slit-shaped lumina. The frequency of aberrant crypts in the patient with Crohn's disease was very similar to that found in colon cancer patients. In the patient with Gardner's syndrome, the aberrant crypts occurred more frequently and occupied more space than those found in the patients with colon cancer. Methacrylate-embedded sections studied histologically (Fig 6–9) and histochemically showed that some of the aberrant crypts had nuclei varying from normal to dysplastic.

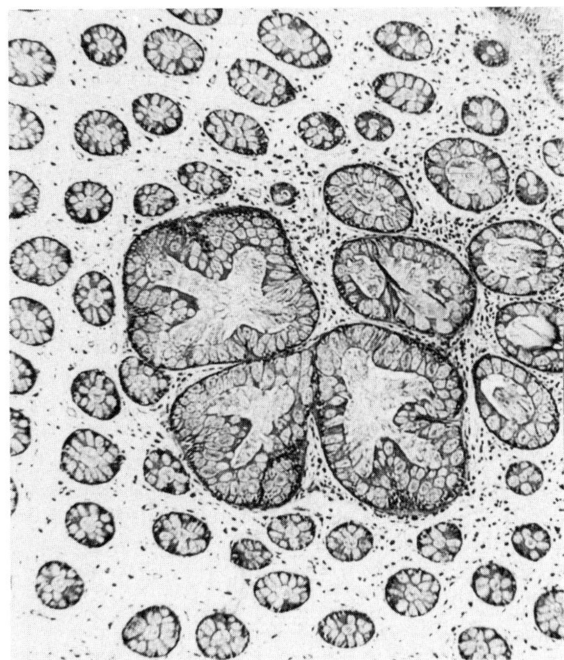

Fig 6–9.—Cross-section of a focus of aberrant crypts surrounded by normal crypts from a colon of a patient with sporadic colon cancer. Section is embedded in methacrylate and cut at 3 μm. Hematoxylin-eosin and azure II; original magnification, ×64. (Courtesy of Pretlow TP, Barrow BJ, Ashton WS, et al: *Cancer Res* 51:1564–1567, 1991.)

Implications.—Preneoplastic lesions may exist in the grossly normal colonic mucosa of patients with colon cancer. These lesions resemble those previously reported in rodents, supporting the use of animal models in the study of this disease. Further study of many more samples of grossly normal mucosa from patients with and without colon cancer is required to establish the conditions that predispose to cancer.

▶ At the same time that a picture is emerging of the sequence of molecular biological changes involved in colonic neoplasia, morphological counterparts of these premalignant transformations are being recognized. The lesions illustrated in this paper constitute the first demonstration of colonic lesions comparable to those observed by these authors (1) and others in the colons of both rats and mice receiving colon carcinogens.—W.A. Gardner, Jr., M.D.

Reference

1. Pretlow TP, et al: *Am J Pathol* 136:13, 1990.

Deciduosis of the Appendix

Suster S, Moran CA (Yale Univ)

Am J Gastroenterol 85:841–845, 1990 6–19

Background.—The presence of extrauterine or ectopic decidua is usually an asymptomatic and incidental finding. Rarely, however, it may cause abdominal symptoms, particularly pain and intraperitoneal hemorrhage. Six patients with ectopic decidua of the appendix were identified from a review of surgical pathology files for an 11-year period.

Methods.—Hematoxylin- and eosin-stained slides were reviewed and periodic acid-Schiff stains were done. Immunohistochemical studies were done on the ectopic decidua and on 10 endometrial currettings containing decidua. The patients' records were reviewed for clinical information and follow-up.

Results.—The 6 patients were pregnant women, ranging in age from 18 to 40. Signs and symptoms of acute appendicitis were seen in 4 of the patients between their 26th and 31st weeks of pregnancy. Lesions were discovered in the other 2 women incidentally in appendectomy specimens obtained during cesarean section and tubal ligation at term. Histologic examination showed multiple irregularly distributed submesothelial deposits of decidualized cells in the serosa of the appendix. No associated evidence of endometriosis was seen. On immunohistochemical study, strong labeling of the decidualized cells with vimentin antibodies was seen, consistent with their stromal origin. Two patients had coexpression of vimentin and desmin intermediate filaments, suggesting myoid differentiation.

Conclusions.—The term "deciduosis of the appendix" is proposed because of the diffuse multifocal nature of the lesions. Deposits may be found in association with acute appendicitis during pregnancy or unassociated with clinical symptoms. It is unknown whether the decidual deposits are responsible for the development of peritoneal irritation.

▶ In the absence of a history of pregnancy, the principal differential diagnosis would probably be benign or malignant mesothelial proliferation. Ectopic decidua have been described in many other loci of the peritoneal surface. These are usually incidental. The pathogenesis of a clinical picture of appendicitis could be explained by either mechanical or chemical mechanisms, e.g., smooth muscle stimulation by decidual prostaglandin.—W.A. Gardner, Jr., M.D.

Intraepithelial Bodies in Colorectal Adenomas: Leuchtenberger Bodies Revisited

Rubio CA, Alm T, Aly A, Poppen B (Karolinska Hosp, Stockholm)
Dis Colon Rectum 34:47–50, 1991 6–20

Background.—Epithelial inclusion bodies may occur in great numbers in adenomas from patients with familial adenomatous polyposis (FAP). In adenomas from patients without FAP, only occasional inclusion granules were noted. The frequency of intraepithelial inclusion bodies, or Leuchtenberger bodies, was investigated in rectal or colonic specimens from 130 patients with and without FAP.

Methods.—The study material comprised 50 consecutive renal biopsy specimens from FAP patients, 5 consecutive prophylactic colectomy specimens from FAP patients, 5 colonic specimens with adenoma from non-FAP patients, 50 specimens containing rectal adenomas from non-FAP patients, 10 rectal specimens from active chronic ulcerative colitis patients, and 10 rectal specimens showing epithelial dysplasia from colitic patients. Additionally, 5 adenomas from FAP patients and 5 from non-FAP patients were stained with Feulgen stain to specifically label DNA.

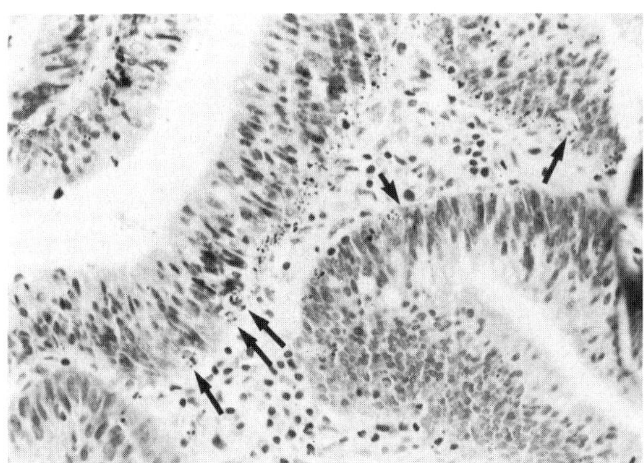

Fig 6–10.—Tubular adenoma of the rectum from a patient with FAP. Note multiple intraepithelial granules at the base of the dysplastic epithelium and intraepithelial macrophages containing debris (*arrows*). Hematoxylin-eosin; original magnification, ×250. (Courtesy of Rubio CA, Alm T, Aly A, et al: *Dis Colon Rectum* 34:47–50, 1991.)

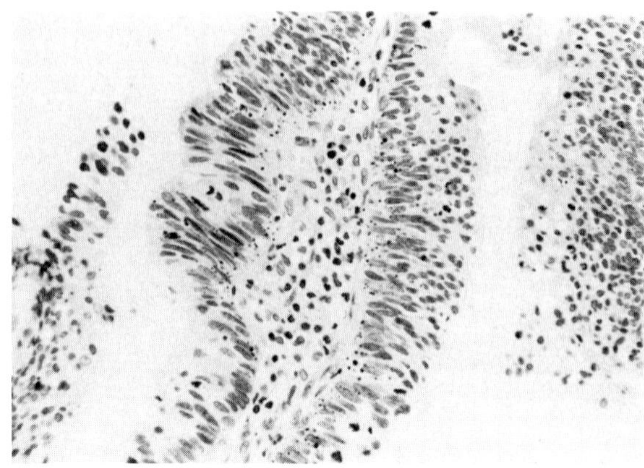

Fig 6–11.—Adenoma showing DNA-positive intraepithelial granules. Feulgen; original magnification, ×250. (Courtesy of Rubio CA, Alm T, Aly A, et al: *Dis Colon Rectum* 34:47–50, 1991.)

Results.—Of 55 colorectal adenomas from patients with FAP, a large to moderate number of intraepithelial bodies were found in 81.8% (Fig 6–10). The intraepithelial granules were positive on Feulgen staining (Fig 6–11) and were probably nuclear fragments of destroyed lymphocytes. Granular material was not found in 1 FAP patient, but intraepithelial lymphocytosis was (Fig 6–12). Of the 55 non-FAP adenomas and the 20 specimens from patients with ulcerative colitis, none had large or moderate amounts of intraepithelial granules.

Conclusions.—Large to moderate numbers of intraepithelial bodies in colorectal adenomas strongly suggest FAP. The pathogenesis of this phenomenon is unclear, but other cells may be involved.

▶ Given the inevitable malignant transformation in familial adenomatous polyposis, any morphologic clue to this diagnosis is welcomed, especially one that

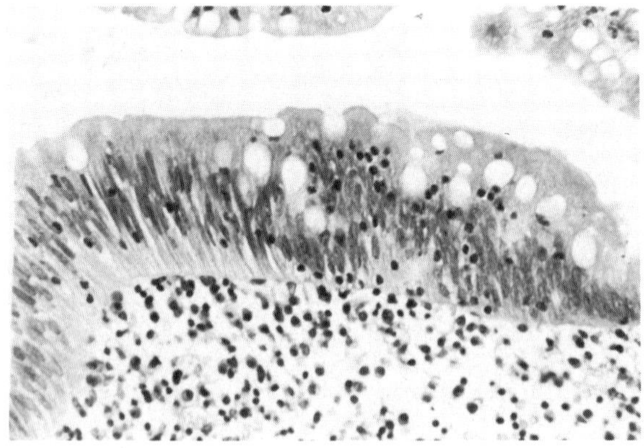

Fig 6–12.—Rectal adenoma from a patient with FAP. Note the intraepithelial lymphocytic infiltration with absence of intraepithelial granules. Hematoxylin-eosin; original magnification, ×250. (Courtesy of Rubio CA, Alm T, Aly A, et al: *Dis Colon Rectum* 34:47–50, 1991.)

can be found on routinely processed light microscopic slides. The precise nature of these distinctive bodies remains a mystery.—W.A. Gardner, Jr., M.D.

Intraepithelial Neoplasia of the Anal Canal in Hemorrhoidal Tissue: A Study of 19 Cases

Foust RL, Dean PJ, Stoler MH, Moinuddin SM (Univ of Tennessee–Baptist Mem Hosp, Memphis; Midsouth Pathology Group, Inc, Memphis; Univ of Rochester)

Hum Pathol 22:528–534, 1991 6–21

Introduction.—Unanticipated abnormalities may be discovered incidentally in routinely excised hemorrhoidal tissues. The clinical and path-

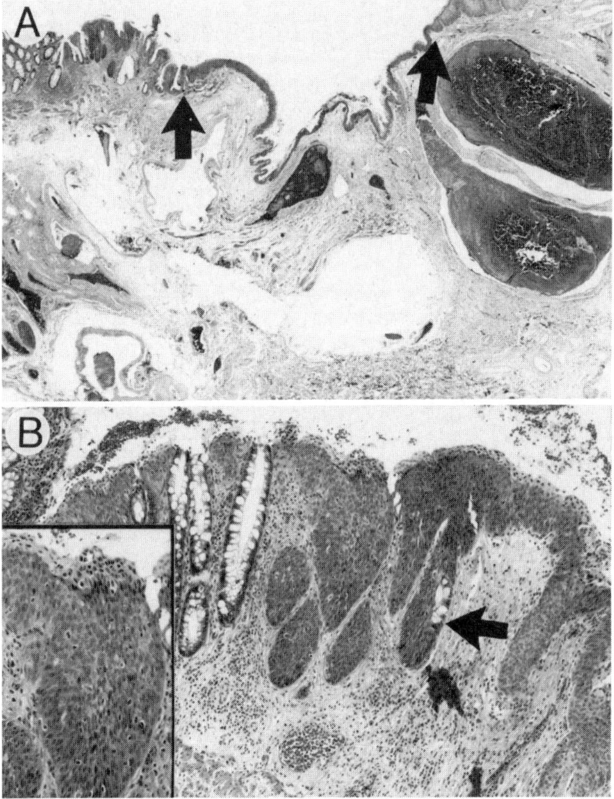

Fig 6–13.—**A,** transition zone of the anal canal, shown by *arrows*, flanked by colorectal zone mucosa in the left and squamous zone mucosa on the right. To the right of the field are dilated blood vessels of the hemorrhoidal venous plexus. Intraepithelial neoplasia involves the entire transition zone mucosa. This is shown at higher magnification in **B.** (Hematoxylin-eosin; original magnification, ×10.) **B,** high-grade intraepithelial neoplasia of the anal canal transition zone epithelium abuts and replaces glands of the colorectal zone mucosa (*arrow*). (Hematoxylin-eosin; original magnification, ×60.) *Inset*, the intraepithelial neoplasia resembles cloacogenic carcinoma but retains surface keratinization. (Hematoxylin-eosin; original magnification, ×110.) (Courtesy of Foust RL, Dean PJ, Stoler MH, et al: *Hum Pathol* 22:528–534, 1991.)

ologic features of 19 patients with intraepithelial neoplasia occurring in the anal canal mucosa of routinely excised hemorrhoidal tissue seen from 1965 to 1987 were reviewed.

Clinical Features.—The series included 12 women and 7 men aged 21–74 years (mean, 48 years). Two patients had coexistent anogenital condylomato acuminata, and another 2 patients had leukoplakia of the hemorrhoidal surface (Bowen's disease). During a mean follow-up of 6.6 years after hemorrhoidectomy, 18 patients had no clinical evidence or recurrent or progressive disease. One patient had repeated recurrences up to 49 months post hemorrhoidectomy and was treated with local excisions, with no recurrence for 7 years.

Pathologic Features.—Intraepithelial neoplasia arose in the transition zone of the anal canal in 11 patients, in the squamous zone in 5, and in both zones in 3. All tumors demonstrated high-grade epithelial atypism, including moderate to severe dysplasia in 1 patient, severe dysplasia-carcinoma in situ in 17 patients, and microinvasive carcinoma in 1 patient. The neoplastic epithelium often abutted and spread over the proximal colorectal zone mucosa (Fig 6–13) involving the distal anal skin in 3 patients. In 6 patients, preinvasive cloacogenic carcinoma was observed; 5 had keratinizing squamous epithelial proliferation, and 3 had both features. Koilocytotic atypia was present in 16 patients. In situ hybridization for human papillomavirus (HPV) messenger RNA showed HPV RNA sequences in 7 of 9 neoplasms, including 5 HPV type 16, 1 HPV type 18, and 1 coinfection with HPV types 6 and 18.

Discussion.—Incidentally discovered high-grade intraepithelial neoplasia in routinely excised hemorrhoidal tissue is clinically nonaggressive, with hemorrhoidectomy providing curative resection in most patients. Intraepithelial neoplasia is frequently associated with HPV infection, but more recently its incidence appears to be increasing among homosexual men.

▶ This is another disease for which the profile is likely to be changing (i.e., becoming more common) and to be increasingly found in association with AIDS.—W.A. Gardner, Jr., M.D.

Histological Diagnosis of Intestinal Microsporidiosis in Patients With AIDS

Peacock CS, Blanshard C, Tovey DG, Ellis DS, Gazzard BG (Westminster Hosp, London; London School of Hygiene and Tropical Medicine)

J Clin Pathol 44:558–563, 1991 6–22

Introduction.—Intestinal microsporidiosis is increasingly diagnosed in patients with HIV infection and diarrhea in whom no other pathogens are detected. Because diagnostic serologic tests are not yet available, the currently recommended method for detecting microsporidiosis is by electron microscopy of duodenal and jejunal biopsy specimens, a technique that is both time-consuming and expensive. Whether microsporidiosis in HIV-positive patients with diarrhea could be diagnosed reliably by light microscopy was determined.

Patients.—Two groups of patients were studied. The first group consisted of 59 HIV-positive patients with diarrhea, 14 of whom had no other pathogens identified on microbiologic studies of stool samples, duodenal aspiration, rigid sigmoidoscopy, and rectal biopsy. The second group consisted of 20 HIV-positive patients without diarrhea who were being investigated for malabsorption because of weight loss. Duodenal, jejunal, and rectal biopsy specimens were examined for microsporidiosis using both light and electron microscopy.

Results.—Microsporidiosis was identified by both electron and light microscopy in 8 patients; in 5 of these, it was the sole pathogen found. No microsporidia were found in any patient without diarrhea. None of the rectal biopsy specimens had evidence of microsporidiosis by either microscopy technique. All stages of the life cycle other than the sporoplast were identified with either technique. The stages were best seen in 1 μm resin sections stained with Giemsa, but spores could be easily detected in 5 μm sections stained with hematoxylin-eosin. Both light and electron microscopy showed extrusion of necrotic cells containing large numbers of spores, a method of shedding and transmission of the parasite not previously recorded. Microsporidia were identified both in duodenal pinch and jejunal "Crosby" capsule biopsy specimens.

Conclusion.—In the absence of serologic testing methods, light microscopic examination of a duodenal pinch biopsy specimen is the optimal method for detecting intestinal microsporidiosis in HIV-positive patients with diarrhea. Identification of individual microsporidia species requires electron microscopy.

▶ The illustrations in this paper would seem to indicate a clear advantage to methacrylate embedding for evaluation of these specimens.—W.A. Gardner, Jr., M.D.

Neuroendocrine Carcinoma of the Colon and Rectum: A Clinicopathologic, Ultrastructural, and Immunohistochemical Study of 24 Cases

Gaffey MJ, Mills SE, Lack EE (Univ of Virginia; City of Hope Nat Med Ctr, Duarte, Calif; Georgetown Univ)

Am J Surg Pathol 14:1010–1023, 1990 6–23

Introduction.—Small cell undifferentiated carcinomas (SCUCs) of the colon and rectum are rare, aggressive neoplasms. The first documented series of colonic SCUCs with ultrastructural evidence of neuroendocrine differentiation was reported in 1978. A clinicopathologic, ultrastructural, and immunohistochemical study was made of a group of patients with neuroendocrine carcinoma of the colon and rectum.

Methods.—Twenty-four patients had carcinomas subtyped as small cell neuroendocrine, oat cell variant; small cell neuroendocrine, intermediate cell variant; or moderately differentiated neuroendocrine. Five of 6 oat cell variants, 14 of 16 intermediate variants, and both moderately differentiated tumors were assessed with antibodies to cytokeratin, vimentin, epithelial membrane antigen, neuron-specific enolase, chromogranin, synaptophysin, neurofilament, S-100 protein, carcinoembryonic antigen, and Leu-7.

Findings.—All tumors were immunoreactive for cytokeratin. Most were also positive for epithelial membrane antigen and neuron-specific enolase. Positivity for specific neuroendocrine markers was not common. Synaptophysin reactivity was noted in 1 oat cell variant and 4 intermediate cell variants, and chromogranin positivity was found in 4 intermediate cell variants and 1 moderately differentiated tumor. Ultrastructural examination of 4 oat cell variants, 8 intermediate cell variants, and 1 moderately differentiated tumor showed neurosecretory-type, dense-core granules in all lesions except 2 oat cell variants studied from paraffin-retrieved material. Five of 6 oat cell, 8 of 16 intermediate, and both moderately differentiated tumors had hepatic and regional lymph node metastases. Only 2 of 17 patients followed up were alive after 1 year. No differences could be found in survival or response to treatment between morphologic subtypes.

Conclusions.—The prognosis for patients with colorectal neuroendocrine carcinoma seems worse than for those with adenocarcinoma of similar stage. Thus, the distinction is important. The intermediate cell variants and moderately differentiated tumors may be misinterpreted as forms of adenocarcinoma.

▶ Twenty-four cases of colorectal carcinoma with neuroendocrine differentiation are discussed. The tumors are divided into 3 groups: small neuroendocrine oat cell variant, small cell neuroendocrine intermediate cell variant, and moderately differentiated neuroendocrine carcinoma. The study shows that the diagnosis of neuroendocrine carcinoma of the lower gut, regardless of subtype, is a disastrous one. Of the 24 cases, 3 were stage 3 and 17 were stage 4 at the time of diagnosis, a combined rate of 83%. This is in contrast to a 35% rate of stage 3 or 4 disease at time of diagnosis for the usual adenocarcinoma of the colon and rectum. Also, the prognosis of neuroendocrine carcinoma appears to be much worse than that of stage-matched colorectal adenocarcinoma. The study shows only 2 of 20 (10%) patients with stage 3 or 4 disese were alive after 1 year, which contrasts with a 45% 2-year survival and a 22% 5-year survival for stage 3 or 4 adenocarcinoma reported in other studies. The aggressiveness of the tumor is demonstrated by liver and lymph node metastases in 2 cases that showed only superficial submucosal invasion at the primary site.

The differential diagnosis of small cell neuroendocrine carcinoma includes lymphoma, and for those in the rectum, melanoma and cloacogenic carcinoma. Because of its very poor prognosis, neuroendocrine carcinoma should be clearly distinguished from adenocarcinoma. The oat cell variant represents a fairly easy diagnosis, but the intermediate cell variant and the moderately differentiated neuroendocrine carcinoma may be overlooked. Last, the consultant pathologist need not be reminded to be sure that the patient has no previous history of lung carcinoma. A case of oat cell carcinoma of the lung with a rectal metastasis has been seen in our hospital.—J.M. Harmon, M.D.

7 Hepatobiliary System

Detection of Hepatitis B Virus DNA in Formalin-Fixed, Paraffin-Embedded Liver Tissue by the Polymerase Chain Reaction

Lampertico P, Malter JS, Colombo M, Gerber MA (Univ of Milan, Italy; Tulane Univ)

Am J Pathol 137:253–258, 1990 7–1

Objective.—Coupling Southern blot (SB) hybridization to the polymerase chain reaction (PCR-SB) allows detection of very low levels of target DNA in paraffin-embedded tissue samples. With a modified PCR-SB technique, the prevalence of hepatitis B virus (HBV) DNA in hepatocellular carcinoma was studied in formalin-fixed, paraffin-embedded liver tissues.

Methods.—With 4 sets of primers, 2 specific for the surface gene and 2 for the core gene, 22 paraffin blocks from 9 patients with hepatocellular carcinoma and from 6 controls were screened for HBV DNA by a modified PCR-SB technique. The results wer correlated with histologic, immunohistochemical, and serologic findings.

Results.—All tissues from patients with an established HBV etiology were positive by PCR-SB, as were 3 patients with negative HBV markers in serum and tissues. Despite this great sensitivity, amplification was not observed with all primer sets. There was selective amplification with 1 primer set; in 2 patients, smaller than expected amplification products were produced, suggesting HBV DNA deletions. In some unpurified paraffin-extracted DNA samples known to be positive for HBV DNA, the presence of a potent PCR inhibitor that could be removed by Sephadex G-50 chromatography was confirmed.

Conclusion.—The PCR-SB technique is a highly sensitive method for the diagnosis and follow-up of patients with HBV infection. Its use may provide insights into viral hepatocarcinogenesis.

▸ The use of immunohistochemical procedures such as immunoperoxidase extended our diagnostic abilities on tissue sections further than most pathologists would have dreamed possible when these studies were initially described. In a similar vein, the PCR, especially when combined with Southern blot hybridization of amplification products, can go far beyond the small quantities of antigens detectible by immunoperoxidase. In this study, Lampertico et al. used a combination of PCR and Southern blot to detect as little as 100 attograms of viral DNA (approximately 5 copies). The degree to which this technology can expand our knowledge of the role of various infectious agents (e.g., HBV) in development of disease is almost beyond the scope of imagination. These techniques can also be used to demonstrate copies of oncogenes, identify previously undetectable cell products allowing better classification of neoplasms, etc. Applied to serum, the PCR is a sensitive and potentially rapid technique for detecting HBV DNA in patients with very early and very late infection (1). Although these techniques are currently used as research tools only, we can expect within a short time to see them available as routine procedures in histology and chemistry laboratories and to be succeeded in research laboratories by even more sensitive and specific procedures.—B.D. Bennett, M.D., Ph.D.

Reference

1. Kaneko S, et al: *Gastroenterology* 99:799, 1990.

The Effect of Ethanol on the Uptake, Binding, and Desialylation of Transferrin by Rat Liver Endothelium: Implications in the Pathogenesis of Alcohol-Associated Hepatic Siderosis

Mihas AA, Tavassoli M (VAMC, Jackson Miss; Univ of Mississippi)
Am J Med Sci 301:299–304, 1991 7–2

Background.—Chronic alcoholism is associated with a decreased carbohydrate content of transferrin, especially its reduced sialylation state. Low transferrin sialylation state is currently used as an objective marker of chronic alcohol abuse. The pathophysiologic significance of this finding was examined in relation to hepatic siderosis, which is also commonly associated with chronic alcoholism.

Methods.—The effect of ethanol on the uptake, binding, and desialylation of transferrin by isolated rat liver endothelium in vitro was documented. Transferrin labeled with ^{125}I or ^{3}H was incubated with isolated, fractionated liver endothelium with and without ethanol and supernates were subjected to column chromatography in pulse-chase experiments.

Results.—Endothelium incubation with increasing levels of ethanol resulted in a progressive rise in the desialylation rate of transferrin. This rate was highest when 160-mM concentration of ethanol was used.

Conclusions.—Ethanol clearly promotes desialylation of transferrin by rat liver endothelium. This may be the first step in the cascade of events that result in iron overload in alcoholics. Desialylated transferrin can subsequently enter hepatocytes through asialoglycoprotein receptors.

▶ Despite the frequency of alcohol-induced liver disease, the mechanisms by which ethanol produces liver cell injury remain a mystery. This paper supports previous hypotheses that ethanol produces a change in the iron transport protein transferrin, which increases the uptake of iron by hepatocytes via a route that promotes intracellular deposition. Studies indicate a similar mechanism is probably operative in humans. The demonstration that ethanol can alter intracellular handling of a glycoprotein by extracellular modification of its carbohydrate content has implications far beyond transferrin and iron deposition. This study shows that rat liver endothelium provides a suitable model for evaluation of this process and should be applied to other substances.—B.D. Bennett, M.D., Ph.D.

The Predictive Value of Donor Liver Biopsies for the Development of Primary Nonfunction After Orthotopic Liver Transplantation

D'Alessandro AM, Kalayoglu M, Sollinger HW, Hoffmann RM, Reed A, Knechtle SJ, Pirsch JD, Hafez GR, Lorentzen D, Belzer FO (Univ of Wisconsin)

Transplantation 51:157–163, 1991 7–3

Background.—Primary nonfunction (PNF) after liver transplantation causes significant morbidity and mortality in patients undergoing this procedure. Improved preservation methods, the use of UW solution in particular, have allowed histologic analysis of liver tissue before transplantation. Data on 124 liver transplantations using UW solution were reviewed.

Methods.—Between June 1987 and May 1990, 147 patients underwent 170 liver transplants in which donor livers were divided into 3 groups: Group 1 consisted of 77 biopsy specimens obtained within 2–4 hours after revascularization; group 2, 19 biopsy specimens obtained before dissection but not examined until after transplantation; and group 3, 28 biopsy specimens obtained before dissection but examined before transplantation. All livers were preserved in UW solution for a mean preservation time of 12.5 hours (13.1 hours for livers with a biopsy specimen available).

Findings.—Histology was normal in 89 livers. Primary nonfunction developed in 3 of these, with macrovesicular steatosis observed (Fig 7–1). In 1 of the 26 specimens that had a minimal or moderate amount of fatty infiltration, PNF developed. Primary nonfunction also occurred in 3 livers

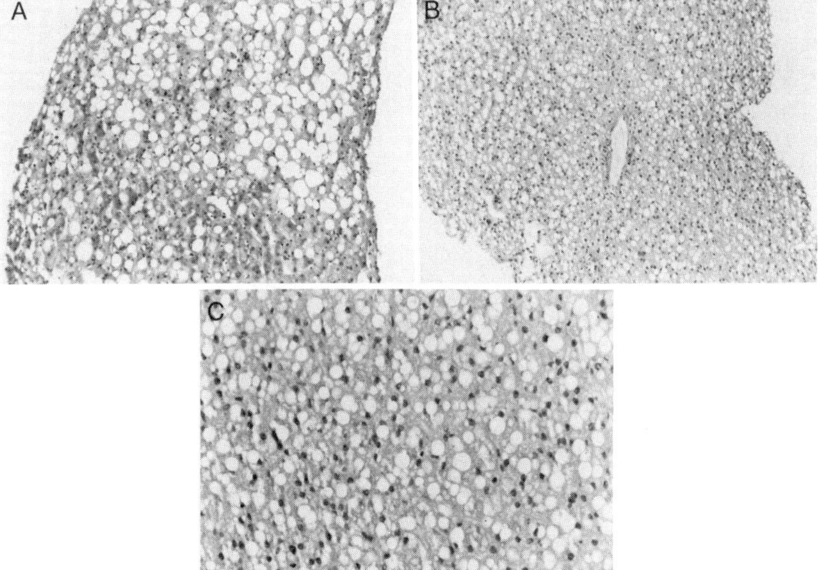

Fig 7–1.—Severe fatty infiltration in 3 livers in which PNF developed after transplantation. Note the widespread macrovesicular steatosis with very few normal-appearing hepatocytes (hematoxylin-eosin; original magification: **A and B**, ×100; **C**, ×250). (Courtesy of D'Alessandro AM, Kalayoglu M, Sollinger HW, et al: *Transplantation* 51:157–163, 1991.)

with severe fatty infiltration, in 3 with hydropic degeneration, and in 1 with centrilobular necrosis. A fourth liver of the 89 that had hydropic degeneration and poor function eventually required retransplantation after 8 weeks. Donor age and weight were significantly higher in those livers found to have fatty infiltration when compared with normal organs.

Conclusions.—Prospective liver biopsy specimens are important in assessing abnormal hepatic pathology in livers available for transplantation. Severe fatty infiltration and hydropic degeneration in these organs indicate a high degree of PNF. Thus livers with these histologic features should not be used. Although the cost of discarding the organ is high, it is ultimately much less than retransplantation after PNF develops in the initial liver transplant.

▶ Despite improvements in organ retrieval, preservation, and recipient implantation, PNF occurs in 2% to 12% of transplanted livers (1). Along with the usual criteria, frozen-section biopsy specimens obtained from livers before transplant have been used. This paper reports the association of severe fatty infiltration and hydropic degeneration with an increased failure to function. These morphological criteria do not always hold true, and it is apparent that additional methods of assessing donor livers along with biopsy specimens are necessary to decrease PNF.—A.J. Garvin, M.D., Ph.D.

Reference

1. Cooper J, et al: *Transplant Proc* 22:477, 1990.

Hepatic Fibrin-Ring Granulomas: A Clinicopathologic Study of 23 Patients

Marazuela M, Moreno A, Yebra M, Cerezo E, Gómez-Gesto C, Vargas JA (Hosp Puerta de Hierro, Madrid; Hosp Ramón y Cajal, Madrid)

Hum Pathol 22:607–613, 1991 7–4

Introduction.—The fibrin-ring or "doughnut" hepatic granuloma is characterized by eosinophilic fibrinoid material surrounding a central fat vacuole. It is considered to be the hallmark of acute Q fever, but it is described in other disorders as well.

Patients.—Nine of 23 patients with typical hepatic fibrin-ring granulomas had acute Q fever. Five others had visceral leishmaniasis, and 2 had boutonneuse fever. Other diagnoses included Hodgkin's disease, toxoplasmosis, and a reaction to allopurinol. No causative agent was identified in 3 instances.

Pathologic Findings.—In most patients few granulomas were present. They tended to be small and intralobular, with fibrinoid material usually arranged in a ring about a central space but sometimes intermixed with the cellular components of the lesion. Multinucleated giant cells were present in 5 patients. There was a broad range of nongranulomatous changes.

Discussion.—Acute Q fever was the most common cause of hepatic fibrin-ring granuloma in this series, followed by visceral leishmaniasis. The pathogenesis of these granulomas is uncertain. Immunologically mediated vasculitis has been proposed. Many different mechanisms may produce a similar histologic pattern of vascular inflammation.

▶ This unusual form of granuloma appears to result from vasculitis-related conditions by many different pathogenic mechanisms.—A.J. Garvin, M.D., Ph.D.

Immunohistochemistry in the Differential Diagnosis of Liver Carcinomas
Hurlimann J, Gardiol D (Univ of Lausanne, Switzerland)
Am J Surg Pathol 15:280–288, 1991 7–5

Objective.—The contribution of immunohistology to the differential diagnosis of hepatic carcinomas was analyzed in 177 hepatic tumors.

Methods.—A selective panel of markers was used to define the phenotype of 60 typical hepatocellular carcinomas (HCCs), 26 probable HCCs, 31 possible HCCs, 12 cholangiocarcinomas, 20 combined hepatocholangiocarcinomas, 13 adenocarcinomas of unknown origin, and 15 metastatic carcinomas as defined on routine sections.

Immunohistology.—The association of positivity for C-reactive protein, α-fetoprotein, factor XIII_a, and keratins 8 and 18, and negativity for Lewis a, vimentin, keratin 19, carcinoembryogenic antigen (CEA) (monoclonal), and CA 19-9, was considered the immunohistologic phenotype typical for HCC. Keratins 1, 5, 10, 11, 19, and true CEA were absent from HCC. Because C-reactive protein was found in 84% of HCCs, it thus appears to be more sensitive than α-fetoprotein. In addition to histiocytes, factor XIII_a was also expressed by hepatocytes and hepatocytic tumor cells. As a result of this immunohistochemical analysis, the diagnosis was reclassified in 21 HCCs, particularly among histologically possible HCC. Several cases were found to be intermediate between HCC and cholangiocarcinoma, and some tumor cells expressed keratins of bile duct type in 12 cases. Except in 2 cases, immunohistochemical methods were useless in differentiating between cholangiocarcinoma and metastatic carcinoma.

Conclusion.—Immunohistochemistry appears to be an important tool in the diagnosis of hepatic tumors. Immunohistology is useful in correcting possible histologic errors, revealing intermediate cases, and strongly reducing the number of histologically uncertain diagnoses.

▶ At this point in time, there is no one specific immunohistochemical marker for hepatocytes or HCC. This article demonstrates a profile of immunohistochemical stains for the identification of HCC. The most sensitive and specific marker was C-reactive protein. In contrast, cholangiocarcinomas demonstrate CEA and a keratin profile of epithelial cells.—A.J. Garvin, M.D., Ph.D.

"Neuroendocrine" Differentiation in Primary Neoplasms of the Liver
Wang J, Dhillon AP, Sankey EA, Wightman AK, Lewin JF, Scheuer PJ (Royal Free Hosp and School of Medicine, London)
J Pathol 163:61–67, 1991 7–6

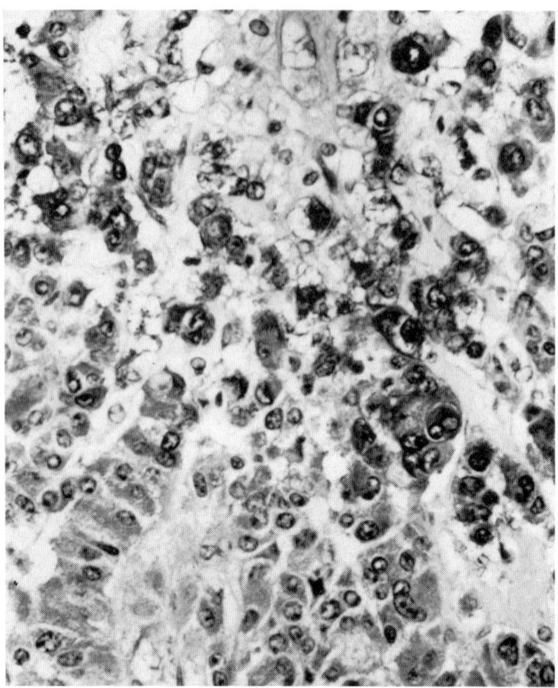

Fig 7–2.—Tumor cells immunostaining for NSE in fibrolamellar carcinoma. (Courtesy of Wang J, Dhillon AP, Sankey EA, et al: *J Pathol* 163:61–67, 1991.)

Introduction.—A systematic study of neuroendocrine differentiation may help to distinguish primary from metastatic liver tumors. Thirty primary hepatic neoplasms were examined for expression of the general neuroendocrine markers neuron-specific enolase (NSE) and protein gene product 9.5 (PGP 9.5). The tumors (16 hepatocellular carcinomas, 9 biliary tumors, and 5 epithelioid hemangioendotheliomas) also were studied for neurosecretory granules, S100 protein, HMB-45, vasoactive intestinal polypeptide (VIP), and calcitonin.

Results.—All 6 fibrolamellar carcinomas stained for PGP9.5, 3 stained for NSE (Fig 7–2), and 3 stained for HMB-45. Five of 10 classic hepatocellular carcinomas, regardless of morphological differentiation, stained for PGP9.5 and 5 stained for VIP. Three of these tumors stained for HMB-45 and 3 stained for neurosecretory granules. Several epithelioid hemangioendotheliomas stained for PGP9.5 or NSE. Two of 3 biliary adenocarcinomas stained for PGP9.5 and NSE, and 2 of 6 cholangiocarcinomas stained for neurosecretory granules.

Conclusion.—Neuroendocrine differentiation is observed in a significant proportion of primary liver tumors.

▶ The significance of this article lies in the fact that a significant percentage of primary tumors of the liver demonstrate neuroendocrine differentiation. Therefore this property cannot be used to distinguish primary from metastatic tumors.—A.J. Garvin, M.D., Ph.D.

Neuroendocrine Differentiation in Hepatoblastoma: An Immunohistochemical Investigation

Ruck P, Harms D, Kaiserling E (Eberhard-Karls Univ, Tübingen, Germany; Christian-Albrechts Univ, Kiel, Germany)

Am J Surg Pathol 14:847–855, 1990 7–7

Background.—Hepatoblastoma, the most common malignant liver tumor of childhood, follows a wide range of epithelial and mesenchymal lines of differentiation, but neuroendocrine differentiation has not been documented.

Methods.—A large panel of antibodies against epithelial, mesenchymal, neural, and neuroendocrine markers was used to characterize 7 he-

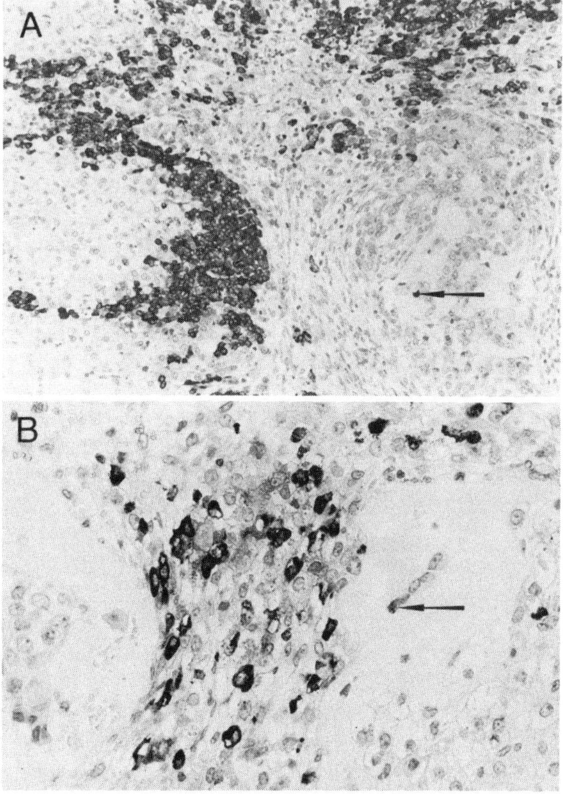

Fig 7–3.—Mixed hepatoblastoma. **A,** embryonal area shows tumor cells immunoreactive for chromogranin A. These are found in large groups and scattered irregularly. Area of osteoid-like material on right also contains chromogranin A-reactive cell (*arrow*). **B,** chromogranin A-reactive cell in area of osteoid-like material at higher magnification (*arrow*). (Antichromogranin A, ABC method.) (Courtesy of Ruck P, Harms D, Kaiserling E: *Am J Surg Pathol* 14:847–855, 1990.)

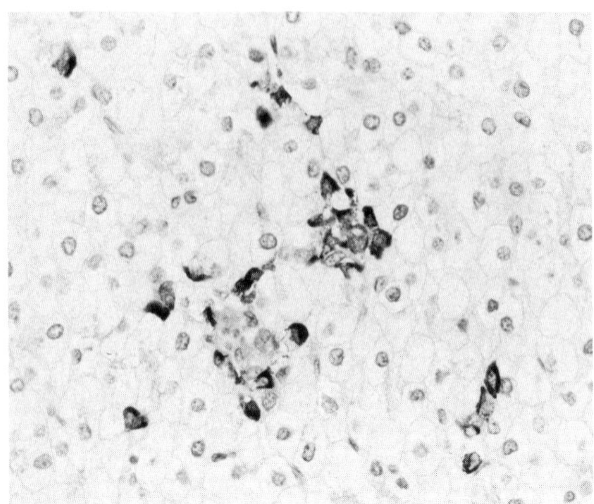

Fig 7–4.—Mixed hepatoblastoma. Clustered and solitary cells in fetal area are intensively stained by antibody against chromogranin A. (Antichromogranin A, ABC method.) (Courtesy of Ruck P, Harms D, Kaiserling E: *Am J Surg Pathol* 14:847–855, 1990.)

patoblastomas. These included 5 pure epithelial lesions and 2 mixed tumors with a primitive mesenchymal component.

Findings.—Antikeratin antibody produced cytoplasmic staining in most neoplastic epithelial cells. Most tumor cells in the primitive mesenchymal and osteoid areas of mixed hepatoblastomas stained with antibody against vimentin. Most cells in osteoid-like material stained for S-100 protein. A large proportion of epithelial cells in 5 tumors stained from carcinoembryonic antigen. Most embryonal cells and many fetal cells reacted with antibodies against α-1-antitrypsin and α-1-antichymotrypsin. Cells in both of the mixed tumors stained for chromogranin A (Figs 7–3 and 7–4). Fetal- and embryonal-type cells in these tumors also stained for serotonin and somatostatin.

Conclusions.—Hepatoblastomas can exhibit neuroendocrine differentiation. Cells in the osteoid-like material of mixed hepatoblastomas may well be of epithelial origin.

▶ Neuroendocrine cells occur in the intrahepatic biliary tree of the normal liver (1). Primary carcinoid tumors of the liver with neuroendocrine features have been described in adults (2) and children (3). This series reports the immunohistochemical identification of neuroendocrine cells in 2 mixed hepatoblastomas. Neuroendocrine cells have been found in other embryonal tumors, e.g., pulmonary blastomas and Wilms' tumors. The presence of neuroendocrine differentiation is of unknown significance.—A.J. Garvin, M.D., Ph.D.

References

1. Kurumaya H, et al: *Arch Pathol Lab Med* 113:143, 1989.
2. Barsky SH, et al: *Hum Pathol* 15:892, 1984.
3. Smith AL, et al: *J Pediatr Gastroenterol Nutr* 3:801, 1984.

Hepatic Vascular Disease and Portal Hypertension in Polycythemia Vera and Agnogenic Myeloid Metaplasia: A Clinicopathological Study of 145 Patients Examined at Autopsy

Wanless IR, Peterson P, Das A, Boitnott JK, Moore GW, Bernier V (Univ of Toronto; Cornell Univ; Johns Hopkins Univ)

Hepatology 12:1166–1174, 1990 7–8

Introduction.—Liver biopsy findings frequently show minimal changes in patients with myeloproliferative disorders in whom portal hyperten-

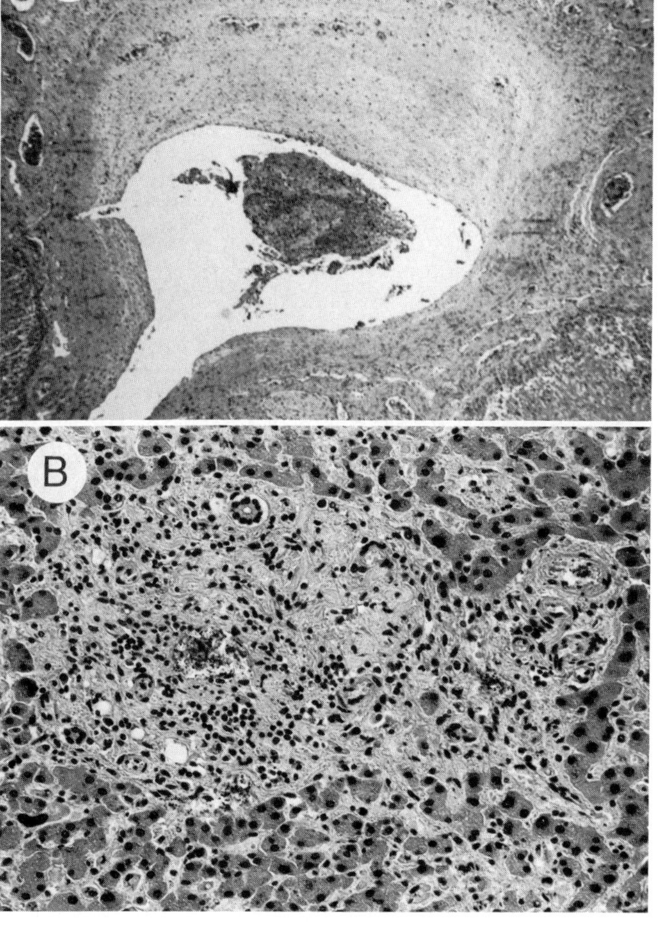

Fig 7–5.—Photomicrographs of portal tracts from man aged 67 years with esophageal varices and AMM. Extrahepatic portal vein was severely narrowed by organized thrombus at hilum. **A,** large portal vein 2 mm in diameter showing organized and partially recanalized thrombus. Hematoxylin-phloxine-saffron; original magnification, ×35. **B,** example of microvascular disease in small portal tract showing marked attenuation of portal vein with lumen measuring 35 μm. Original vein would have measured approximately 80μm. Hematoxylin-phloxine-saffron; original magnification, ×212. (Courtesy of Wanless IR, Peterson P, Das A, et al: *Hepatology* 12:1166–1174, 1990.)

sion develops, making the cause of the hypertension difficult to understand. Increased splenic blood flow, hepatic infiltration with hematopoietic cells, and sinusoidal fibrosis may be important factors. To correlate portal hypertension with hepatic histologic findings, autopsy findings in 97 patients were reviewed.

Methods.—The autopsy and clinical records of 97 patients with polycythemia vera (PV) and 48 patients with agnogenic myeloid metaplasia (AMM) were examined. Liver slides ere studied without knowledge of the clinical findings.

Findings.—Autopsy showed that 7 patients had cirrhosis; 1 of the 7 had bleeding varices and 2 had more than 500 mL of ascites. Seven patients with PV and 3 with AMM without cirrhosis had clinical evidence of esophageal varices. Lesions of the small- or medium-sized portal veins were present in all 10 patients, and stenosis of the extrahepatic portal vein and histologic findings compatible with organized thrombi were present in 4. Photomicrographs of portal tracts from a patient with esophageal varices and AMM are shown in Figure 7–5. Overall, 14.6% of patients had nodular regenerative hyperplasia. This finding correlated closely with the presence of portal vein lesions. More than 500 mL of ascites was found in 30 patients; 7 of this group had varices and 6 had hepatic vein thrombosis. A correlation was noted between ascites and hepatic vein disease confined to small intrahepatic branches. No correlation was seen between infiltration of the liver by hematopoietic or leukemic cells and signs of portal hypertension.

Discussion.—Esophageal varices appear to be common in patients with myeloproliferative disorders in whom portal hypertension develops, and they are almost always associated with microscopic portal vein lesions. These lesions, as well as the secondary effects of nodular regenerative hyperplasia and portal hypertension, probably result from portal vein thrombosis. Moderate to severe obliteration of small and large veins is a sensitive, but not specific, predictor of portal hypertension.

▶ This detailed study of the liver in patients with myeloproliferative disorders gives the best evidence to date that thrombi within the small or medium-sized portal veins account for the portal hypertension observed in these patients.—A.J. Garvin, M.D., Ph.D.

8 Kidney

So-Called Embryonal Hyperplasia of Bowman's Capsular Epithelium: An Immunohistochemical and Ultrastructural Study

Ogata K, Hajikano H, Sakaguchi H (Keio Univ, Tokyo; Tokyo Metropolitan Higashikurume Health Ctr)

Virchows Arch [A] 418:143–147, 1991 8–1

Introduction.—Embryonal hyperplasia of Bowman's capsular epithelium (EHBCE) is a fairly specific lesions seen in the kidneys of patients maintained on chronic dialysis. In EHBCE, poorly differentiated cells proliferate around sclerosed or obsolescent glomeruli.

Case Report.—Boy, 4 years, had hematuria and proteinuria. Renal function deteriorated, and a biopsy specimen obtained 8 months after onset showed end-stage kidney disease. Peritoneal dialysis was instituted 4 months later and was continued for a year. Bilateral nephrectomy was carried out in preparation for renal transplantation. Marked renal atrophy was noted; there were very few functioning nephrons. Small undifferentiated cells with round, hyperchromatic nuclei proliferated to form clusters around solidified or obsolescent glomeruli. The cluster cells were arranged in a papillary or tubular pattern. Undifferentiated cells were found mostly within Bowman's parietal wall. The cells of EHBCE stained with antivimentin antibody. With electron microscopy, specialized junctions were visible between cells and microvillus-like structures were seen on the cell surfaces.

Discussion.—The cause of this unusual proliferative process remains uncertain, but EHBCE may develop against the same background in which neoplasms develop in end-stage kidneys of adults on long-term dialysis.

▶ Since the original article by Hughson et al. (1), there have been few descriptions of this intriguing proliferative lesion of "embryonal cells." Is this an attempt by the kidney to regenerate? Are these blastemal cells or stem cells that have arisen from proliferative stimuli and/or growth factors in the end-stage kidney? This is the first immunohistochemical staining of these cells and their intermediate filament profile resembles blastemal cells. Further studies on this lesion are needed to identify these cells.—A.J. Garvin, M.D., Ph.D.

Reference

1. Hughson M.D., et al: *Am J Pathol* 91:71, 1978.

Two Cases of a Renal Epithelial Tumour Resembling Immature Nephron

Nagashima Y, Arai N, Tanaka Y, Yoshida S, Sumino K, Ohaki Y, Matsushita K, Morita T, Misugi K (Yokohama City Univ; Fujisawa Municipal Hosp; Chigasaki Municipal Hosp, Japan)

Virchows Arch [A] Pathol Anat 418:77–81, 1991 8–2

Background.—The definition of renal epithelial tumors is still being debated. Two renal epithelial tumors were observed that were morphologically and immunohistochemically similar to immature nephrons with glomeruloid bodies.

Patients.—The patients were 2 Japanese women aged 46 years and 66 years. The first complained of abdominal fullness and gross hematuria,

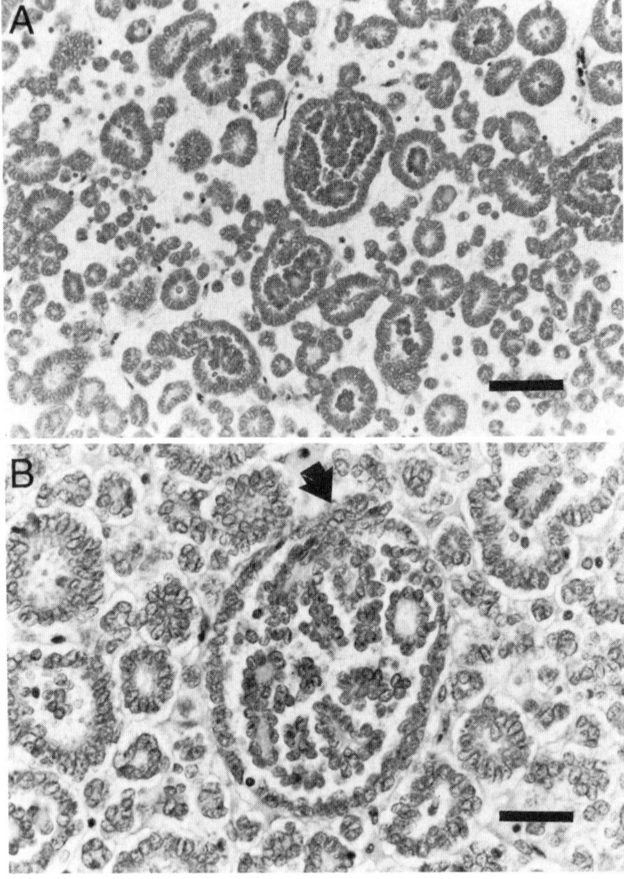

Fig 8–1.—**A,** histopathologic findings. Both tumors were composed of various-sized tubular structures. Glomeruloid bodies are seen in tumors. *Bar* represents 100 μm. **B,** higher magnification of glomeruloid body. *Arrow* indicates connection between glomeruloid body and tubular structure, similar to normal glomeruli and tubules. *Bar* represents 25 μm. (Courtesy of Nagashima Y, Arai N, Tanaka Y, et al: *Virchows Arch [A] Pathol Anat* 418:77–81, 1991.)

and the other complained of persistant diarrhea. Both were found to have large tumors without invasive growth or metastasis.

Histopathology.—The tumors were similar histologically (Fig 8–1). They were composed of immature epithelial cells that formed tubules with abortive glomeruloid structures. Poorly developed polarity and intracytoplasmic organelles were noted on electron microscopy. The immunohistochemical reactions in both tumors were similar to those of developing nephrons, especially those of the S-shaped body. The tumor cell nuclear DNA content was almost euploid.

Conclusions.—These 2 renal epithelial tumors were believed to be epithelial tumors of the kidney that histologically mimicked developing renal parenchyma.

▶ These authors describe 2 renal tumors composed of epithelial cells. The tumors were in the size range of what should be considered renal cell carcinomas. However, the tumors failed to demonstrate the immunohistochemical markers of renal cell carcinoma and contained glomeruloid bodies. The staining pattern of the epithelial cells resembled the S-shaped body, a tubular and glomerular precursor, of the fetal kidney. No blastemal tissue was identified in either tumor. These cases raise the possibility of a monophasic nephrogenic epithelial tumor that may be a differentiated form of Wilms' tumor.—A.J. Garvin, M.D., Ph.D.

Renin Gene Expression in Nephroblastoma

Lindop GBM, Duncan K, Millan DWM, Gibson AAM, Patrick WJA, Leckie BJ, Birnie GD (Univ of Glasgow; Royal Hosp for Sick Children; Western Infirmary; Beatson Inst for Cancer Research, Glasgow)

J Pathol 161:93–97, 1990 8–3

Background.—Both renal cell carcinoma and nephroblastoma may be associated with high plasma renin levels. The renin, which usually is biologically inactive, may serve as a tumor marker. Most nephroblastomas also have a small population of cells containing immunoreactive renin.

Methods.—Renin-specific mRNA was sought in nephroblastoma tissue from 11 patients as direct evidence that these tumors synthesize renin. A cDNA probe and Northern blot analyses were used to analyze RNA purified from snap-frozen tumor tissue taken at nephrectomy.

Findings.—Renin-specific mRNA was identified in 5 of 11 nephroblastomas. Its length was similar to that of the mRNA present in normal kidney tissue and in tissue from kidneys with renal artery stenosis. In 1 tumor the cDNA probe hybridized with an mRNA that was 3 Kb, rather than 1.6 Kb, long.

Conclusion.—Some nephroblastomas evidently synthesize renin. The unusual mRNA identified in 1 case might be a partially processed gene transcript or an aberrant transcript containing part or all of the normal renin mRNA sequence.

▶ Most patients with nephroblastoma have high levels of inactive renin in their blood and, after nephrectomy, their plasma levels fall to normal (1). Because the renin could have been secreted by the tumor or the adjacent normal kidney, its source has been unclear. This study gives the first evidence that some nephroblastomas produce renin.—A.J. Garvin, M.D., Ph.D.

Reference

1. Carachi R, et al: *J Pediatr Surg* 22:278, 1987.

Percutaneous Needle Biopsy Preceding Preoperative Chemotherapy in the Management of Massive Renal Tumors in Children

Saarinen UM, Wikström S, Koskimies O, Sariola H (Univ of Helsinki)
J Clin Oncol 9:406–415, 1991 8–4

Background.—One approach to Wilms' tumor entails accurate staging and in-depth histologic assessment; when possible, operative removal is advocated as the first step. An alternative approach emphasizes the need to operate safely and only when feasible. Biopsy alone has been discouraged because of the risk of abdominal spillage.

Objective.—An operative approach was developed that combines the benefits of both recommended policies. A percutaneous posterior needle biopsy specimen is obtained initially. Chemotherapy and, when necessary, radiotherapy are given preoperatively to reduce tumor bulk and facilitate operative treatment. Small and medium-sized tumors are managed by primary surgery.

Experience.—Seven patients were managed in this way, receiving vincristine and dactinomycin as preoperative chemotherapy. Tumor removal was uneventful. Two tumors were totally or nearly wholly necrotic at the time of surgery. Two patients would have been incorrectly managed without primary needle biopsy. Two patients had subcapsular intratumoral bleeding, and another had multiple small intratumoral bleeds. Four patients may have been septic but not in relation to the time of needle biopsy. All 7 patients were well, without disease, within 7–47 months after diagnosis.

Conclusions.—Percutaneous posterior needle biopsy is a safe procedure in children with massive renal tumors. Chemotherapy is helpful in reducing the size of initially massive Wilms' tumor, facilitating its removal.

▶ More European patients with Wilms' tumors present with high-stage disease than is the case in the United States (1). Patients with massive renal tumors (more than half their body diameter) were biopsied posteriorly with a Tru-Cut needle and given chemotherapy and radiation before attempts at surgical removal. This biopsy technique was safe and accurate, while preventing peritoneal tumor spillage.—A.J. Garvin, M.D., Ph.D.

Reference

1. Tournade M-F: in Voute PA, et al (eds): *Cancer in Children*. New York, Springer Verlag, 1986, p 252.

Tissue, Developmental, and Tumor-Specific Expression of Divergent Transcripts in Wilms Tumor

Huang A, Campbell CE, Bonetta L, McAndrews-Hill MS, Chilton-MacNeill S, Coppes MJ, Law DJ, Feinberg AP, Yeger H, Williams BRG (Hosp for Sick Children, Toronto; Univ of Toronto; Univ of Michigan)

Science 250:991–994, 1990 8–5

Background.—Previous analyses implicated a single recessive oncogene locus in the etiology of Wilms' tumor. It is now thought that mutations in at least 3 loci can cause this tumor. Heterogeneity of tissue types also characterizes the histopathologic findings of Wilms' tumor.

Methods.—The Wilms' tumor locus of chromosome 11p13, which is associated with intralobar Wilms' tumors, was mapped to a region defined by overlapping, tumor-specific deletions. Two complementary DNA clones isolated from a kidney complementary DNA library were found to represent transcripts of 2.5 kb (WIT-1) and 3.5 kb (WIT-2) mapping to this region.

Results.—Fetal kidney and spleen RNA showed both the WIT-1 and WIT-2 transcripts, but they were absent from all other fetal tissue RNAs. Divergent transcription of both WIT-1 and WIT-2, originating from a DNA region of less than 600 bp, were revealed by RNase protection. High concentrations of both transcripts were found in the fetal kidney; greatly reduced amounts were found in 5-year-old and adult kidneys. A series of histopathologically heterologous and homologous Wilms' tumors were investigated for expression of these transcripts. Of 12 heterologous Wilms' tumors, 11 showed absent or reduced WIT-2 expression. Of 14 homologous Wilms' tumors, only 4 showed reduced WIT-2 expression.

Conclusions.—There is a molecular basis for pathogenetic heterogeneity in the pathogenesis of Wilms' tumor. The WIT-1 and WIT-2 genes appear to be regulated coordinately during normal kidney development and tumorigenesis. Methylation may have a central role in regulating the expression of both genes.

▶ The homozygous inactivation of a gene or genes on chromosome 11p13 is thought to predispose to Wilms' tumor. These authors have isolated 2 DNA clones from this region. One of these, WIT-2, is identical to a cDNA clone (WIT-1) previously isolated from this region by 2 other groups (1,2). Northern blots were performed on fetal tissue as well as on Wilms' tumors using these

2 clones. In the Wilms' tumors, the relative abundance of the WIT-2 (WIT-1) transcripts correlated inversely within the degree of heterologous differentiation; i.e., those tumors with heterologous differentiation have, in general, lower levels of transcripts than those without heterologous differentiation. These results suggest a relationship between WIT-2 (WIT-1) expression and cellular differentiation. Alteration of this gene may contribute to the cascade of events responsible for Wilms' tumor development.—A.J. Garvin, M.D., Ph.D.

References

1. Call KM, et al: *Cell* 60:509, 1990.
2. Gessler M, et al: *Nature* 343:774, 1990.

9 Urinary Bladder and Male Genital System

Primary Adenocarcinoma of the Urinary Bladder: A Clinicopathologic Analysis of 72 Cases

Grignon DJ, Ro JY, Ayala AG, Johnson DE, Ordóñez NG (Univ of Texas, Houston)

Cancer 67:2165–2172, 1991 9–1

Background.—Primary adenocarcinomas are uncommon tumors of the urinary bladder, accounting for less than 2% of cases. The importance of differentiating these tumors into urachal and nonurachal types remains controversial. To investigate further, the clinicopathologic features of 72 patients with primary adenocarcinomas of the urinary bladder seen during a 40-year period were reviewed.

Methods.—The stage at presentation, histologic type, and mucin staining were evaluated. Immunohistochemical analysis was performed in 22 patients to determine their reaction to carcinoembryonic antigen (CEA), Leu-M1, prostate-specific antigen (PSA), and prostatic acid phosphatase (PAP).

Results.—There were 24 urachal and 48 nonurachal tumors. The mean age of the patients was 58.3 years. Patients with urachal tumors were younger and had a male-to-female ratio close to 1:1. Hematuria was the most frequent symptom in those with urachal tumors, whereas irritative symptoms were strongly associated with nonurachal tumors. The 5-year survival rate was 61% for patients with urachal tumors and 31% for those with nonurachal tumors, but the difference in survival overall was not significant. Tumor stage was a highly significant predictor of outcome, whereas histologic type was not, although signet-ring carcinoma appeared to be highly aggressive. Mucin staining did not differentiate between tumor types nor were there differences in the immunohistochemical profiles between them. Both tumors reacted similarly to CEA and Leu-M1, but not to PAP, whereas a few tumors showed reactivity to the polyclonal PSA but not to the monoclonal PSA antibody.

Discussion.—Stage at diagnosis is a significant predictor of outcome in patients with primary bladder adenocarcinoma. Mucin histochemistry and immunohistochemistry are not useful markers in differentiating between nonurachal and urachal tumors. Distinction between urachal and nonurachal adenocarcinomas continues to require clinicopathologic correlation.

▶ Because pure adenocarcinoma of the bladder is such an uncommon lesion, this collection of 72 cases provides useful information about the spectrum of this disease. The authors divide these carcinomas into 5 histologic subtypes:

enteric, mucinous, signet-ring cell, mixed, and not otherwise specified. Although the histologic sublcassification did not demonstrate a statistically significant relationship to survival, this system is easily reproducible and provides useful insight into the histologic spectrum of the disease. As one might expect, the signet-ring cell type seemed more aggressive than the others. The mucin produced by these tumors in the 24 cases tested was positive for PAS, mucicarmine, and alcian blue. The cases tested by immunohistochemistry proved CEA positive. Three neoplasms exhibited a positive reaction for polyclonal PSA, although not for monoclonal PSA. Prostate specific antigen has proven to be relatively specific, but this finding emphasizes that no immunoperoxidase reaction should be considered 100% specific. The authors advocate the use of both PSA and PAP when trying to distinguish between a prostatic and bladder adenocarcinoma. This study was limited to cases of pure adenocarcinoma; the significance of adenocarcinoma of the bladder occurring as a component of a transitional cell carcinoma remains controversial.—J.A. Tucker, M.D.

The Prevalence and Character of the Muscularis Mucosae of the Human Urinary Bladder

Weaver MG, Abdul Karim FW (Case Western Reserve Univ; Univ Hosps of Cleveland)

Histopathology 17:563–566, 1990 9–2

Background.—Traditionally, a muscularis mucosae (MM) was not thought to be present in the normal urinary bladder, but recently this

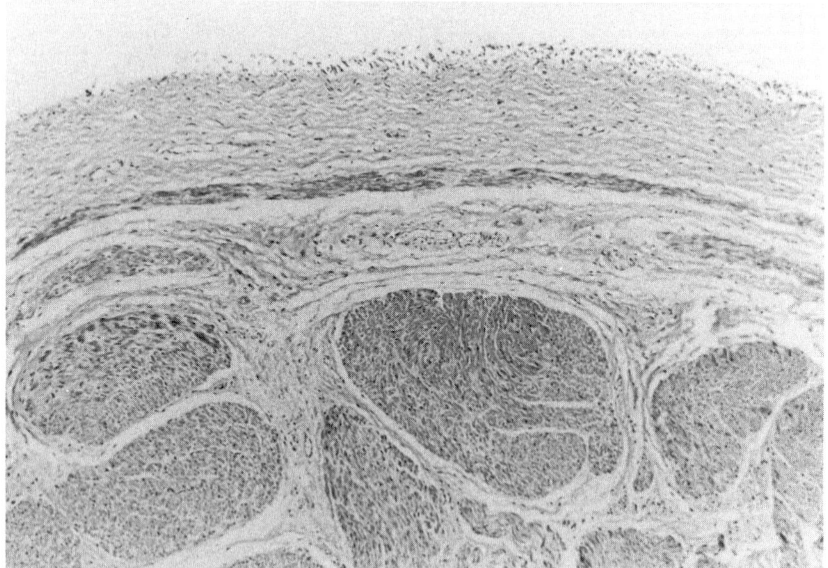

Fig 9–1.—A complete muscularis mucosae is present as a continuous band of smooth muscle, lying below the urothelium, separated from the muscularis propria by loose suburothelial connective tissue. (Courtesy of Weaver MG, Abdul Karim FW: *Histopathology* 17:563–566, 1990.)

structure has been well documented in patients with bladder cancer. Whether a complete or partial MM is present in the normal human bladder was investigated in consecutive autopsy specimens obtained from 335 normal bladders.

Findings.—An MM (Fig 9–1) was identified in 35% of all bladder specimens. Overall, 45% of female bladders and 25% of male bladders contained this structure. No relationship was noted between the presence of an MM and age or any disease process.

Conclusion.—About 35% of normal bladders contain an MM. The structure is found more often in women, for reasons that are not understood. Awareness of the muscularis may help in evaluating bladder biopsy specimens for muscle-invading neoplasms.

▶ This study is of sufficient size and thoroughness as to address the discrepancies previously reported in the literature regarding the presence of a urinary bladder MM. Familiarity with this anatomical landmark is now an important part of evaluating bladder biopsy specimens, as the study reviewed in Abstract 9–3 demonstrates.—W.A. Gardner, Jr., M.D.

The Usefulness of the Level of the Muscularis Mucosae in the Staging of Invasive Transitional Cell Carcinoma of the Urinary Bladder

Younes M, Sussman J, True LD (Yale Univ; VA Hosp, West Haven, Conn)

Cancer 66:543–548, 1990 9–3

Introduction.—The presence of a muscularis mucosae (MM) in most normal bladders raises the possibility that this structure can serve as a landmark for more precise staging of bladder cancers. Biopsy specimens obtained from 50 patients with high-grade invasive transitional cell carcinoma of the bladder were examined. After staging, patients were followed for a median of 4.6 years.

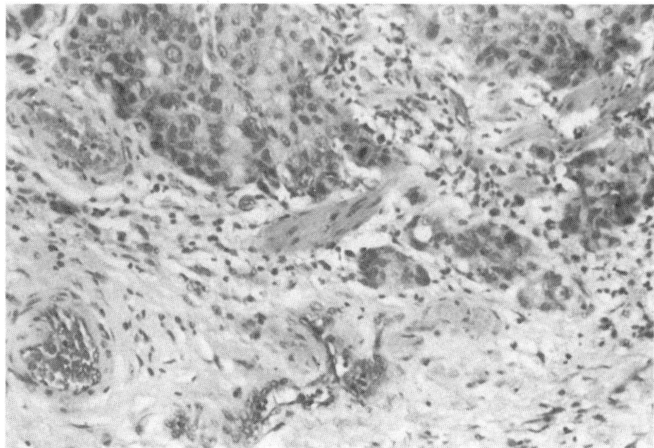

Fig 9–2.—Invasive transitional cell carcinoma interspersed with fibers of MM (stage T1B). (Courtesy of Younes M, Sussman J, True LD: *Cancer* 66:543–548, 1990.)

Staging System.—An MM was identified in 72% of specimens. Stage T1A disease involves connective tissue superficial to the MM; T1B lesions invade to the MM; T1C disease extends through the MM but remains superficial to the muscularis propria; and stage B disease invades the muscularis propria.

Findings:—Fifteen patients had level T1A invasive disease and 3 had tumors invading to the level of the MM (Fig 9–2). Fourteen lesions invaded to level T1C and 19 to level B. Most patients were operated on; 13 received radiotherapy as well, and 2 were given chemotherapy. The 5-year survival was 45% for patients with Jewett-Strong invasive stage A disease and 20% for those with stage B tumors. Using the present staging system, minimally invasive (T1A and T1B) lesions were associated with a 5-year survival of 75%, whereas only 11% of patients with tumors invading deep to the MM lived for 5 years. The distinction was even more marked when only patients having transurethral resection were analyzed.

Conclusion.—It appears prognostically useful to determine the depth of invasion of transitional cell bladder carcinoma in the initial biopsy, even when a muscularis propria is not present.

Inflammatory Pseudotumour of the Urinary Bladder

Coyne JD, Wilson G, Sandhu D, Young RH (Withington Hosp, Manchester, England; Massachusetts Gen Hosp, Boston)

Histopathology 18:261–264, 1991 9–4

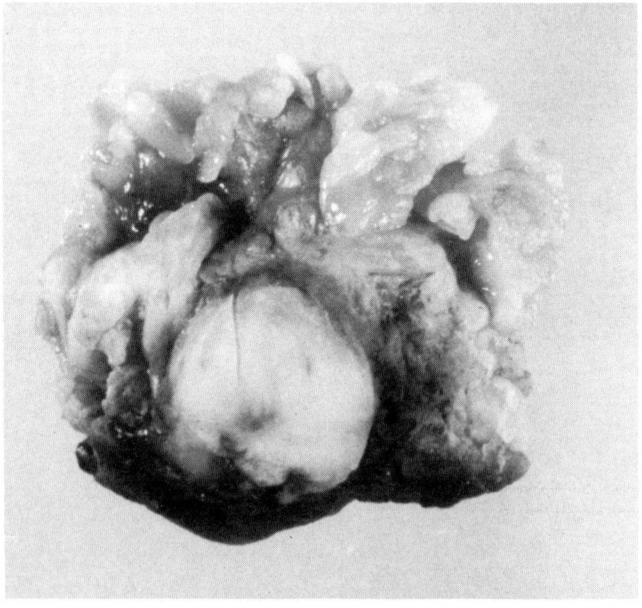

Fig 9–3.—Macroscopic appearance showing the well-circumscribed nature of the lesion. (Courtesy of Coyne JD, Wilson G, Sandhu D, et al: *Histopathology* 18:261–264, 1991.)

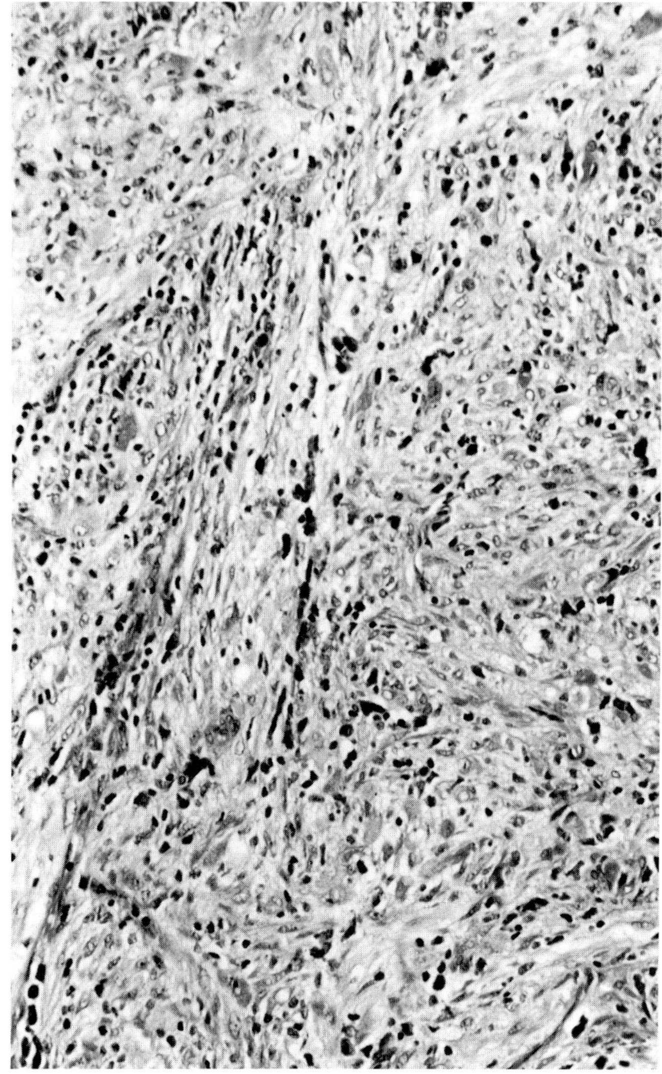

Fig 9–4.—Proliferation of spindle cells with an associated inflammatory cell infiltrate and granulation tissue-like vascularity. (Hematoxylin-eosin; original magnification, ×200.) (Courtesy of Coyne JD, Wilson G, Sandhu D, et al: *Histopathology* 18:261–264, 1991.)

Introduction.—Inflammatory pseudotumor of the urinary bladder is an uncommon, benign lesion that may be mistaken for sarcoma.

Case Report.—Woman, 33, complained of recurrent urinary tract infections and right groin pain. Intravenous urography revealed a space-occupying bladder lesion. Biopsy specimens taken from the lesion identified it as an inflammatory pseudotumor. The patient underwent partial cystectomy for removal of the remainder of the lesion (Fig 9–3). She has remained well after 9 months of follow-up.

Pathologic Findings.—The lesion was characterized by a proliferation of spindle cells that were haphazardly arranged but in some places formed fascicles. The cells had vesicular nuclei with prominent nucleoli but no significant atypia. There was a marked inflammatory cell infiltrate that included lymphocytes, neutrophils, eosinophils, and numerous plasma cells (Fig 9–4). Immunohistochemical staining was negative. Ultrastructural examination revealed spindle-shaped cells with irregular nuclear outlines, abundant rough endoplasmic reticulum, and actin-like myofilaments with dense bodies.

Conclusion.—The inflammatory pseudotumor arising in the urinary bladder has features consistent with myofibroblasts. Recognition of this unusual lesion will prevent misinterpretation.

Pseudosarcomatous Myofibroblastic Proliferations in the Urinary Bladder of Children

Albores-Saavedra J, Manivel JC, Essenfeld H, Dehner LP, Drut R, Gould E, Rosai J (Univ of Miami; Univ of Minnesota; Washington Univ; Hosp de Ninos La Plata, Argentina; Yale Univ)

Cancer 66:1234–1241, 1990 9–5

Introduction.—Recent studies have described spindle-cell nodules resembling sarcomas in the genitourinary tract of adults. However, ultrastructural studies have shown that the predominant proliferating cells are myofibroblasts and fibroblasts, and these structures have therefore been given the name pseudosarcomatous myofibroblastic proliferations (PMP). Although PMP are most often associated with recent surgical procedures, some have appeared spontaneously. The pathologic, immunohistochemical, and ultrastructural features of PMP involving the urinary bladder in children aged 2–16 years were studied to further investigate their resemblance to sarcoma.

Patients.—Seven patients were seen for painless hematuria and 3 others for dysuria. Sarcoma was diagnosed initially in 7 children, whereas the correct pathologic diagnosis was made initially in the other 3. None of the patients had a history of trauma or previous operations. Five children underwent local excision only. Follow-up information was available for 8 patients, none of whom had evidence of local recurrence or metastasis 18 months to 6 years after operation.

Pathologic Findings.—The lesions appeared as polypoid nodular masses of variable size, with myxoid and hemorrhagic areas. All lesions were composed of densely cellular interlacing fascicles of elongated, spindle-shaped cells and minimal atypia. Edematous and myxoid areas of variable extension were interspersed throughout, but they were prominent in the superficial portions of the lesions. Diffuse collagen deposition was uncommon, and only 1 lesion revealed extensive areas of collagen deposition resembling fibromatosis. Despite the striking cellularity of some of the lesions, most showed only minimal mitotic activity. The spindle-shaped cells and the inflammatory cells had infiltrated the muscularis propria of the urinary bladder in 6 patients and the perivesical soft tissues in 2. Subendothelial intravascular growth was detected in 1 patient. The 6 bladder lesions tested were diffusely positive for vimentin and muscle-specific actin. Two lesions expressed desmin and 2 others expressed cytokeratin.

Conclusion.—The findings strongly support a nonsarcomatous nature for PMP.

Post-Surgical Necrobiotic Granulomas of Urinary Bladder

Eble JN, Banks ER (Indiana Univ, Indianapolis; Richard L Roudebush VA Med Ctr, Indianapolis)

Urology 35:454–457, 1990 9–6

Background.—Transurethral surgery of the prostate has for the past 2 decades been considered to be the cause of necrotizing palisading granulomas. The histologic characteristics of these postoperative granulomas have been associated with surgeries at other anatomical locations, including the kidney, uterine cervix, ovary, and fallopian tube. To date, only 1 report has described postsurgical granuloma of the urinary bladder. Palisading necrobiotic granulomas were observed in 3 men who had repeated biopsies for noninvasive urothelial cancer.

Case Report.—Man, 89, underwent initial transurethral resection for noninvasive papillary urothelial carcinoma (grade II/IV) in 1981. Similar procedures were performed in 1982 and 1984 for superficially invasive urothelial carcinoma and a large papillary carcinoma (grade II/IV) of the bladder, respectively. The patient had no history of medical problems or diseases. In 1986, surveillance cytoscopy demonstrated noninvasive urothelial carcinoma (grade II/IV). Autopsy in the same year showed vesical carcinoma and urothelial carcinoma, which had metastasized to the lymph nodes and lung.

Findings.—The specimens obtained at surgery demonstrated microscopic carcinoma composed of papillary structures lined by thickened urothelium with enlarged nuclei. Linear granulomas occurred away from the neoplasm and contained histiocytes and foreign body giant cells around the central eosinophilic, fibrinoid-like tissue in a linear arrangement (Fig 9–5). The centers of the linear granulomas contained focal strands of yellow-brown material. Collagen fibers surrounded the granulomas.

Implications.—Granulomas have only recently been associated with the genital and urinary systems in patients who have undergone surgery. The case histories of the 3 patients described in this report provide no other possible antecedent condition for the granulomas than the endoscopic surgical procedures that each patient underwent over time. The granulomas' characteristic morphology (long, narrow outlines of palisading histiocytes with eosinophilic centers) is specific to this type of lesion, no matter in which organ or tissue it occurs. Postsurgical granulomas

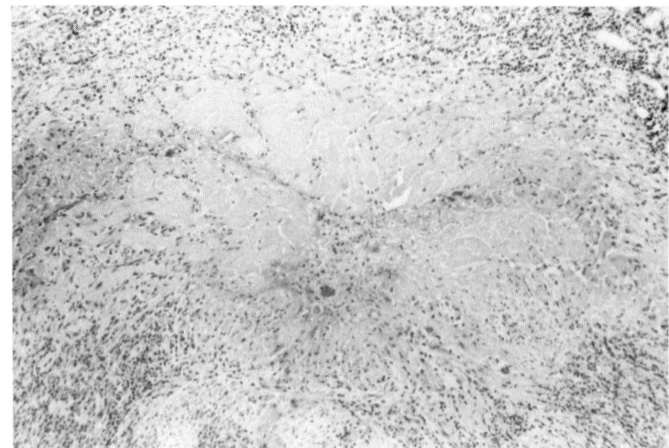

Fig 9–5.—Elongate granuloma with central acellular eosinophilic material and necrotic debris. Note histiocytes in palisade at lower border of lesion (hematoxylin-eosin; original magnification, ×25). (Courtesy of Eble JN, Banks ER: *Urology* 35:454–457, 1990.)

also appear to be linked with electrocautery procedures. Both the surgical pathologist and the urologist should consider the possibility of postsurgical palisading necrobiotic granulomas in patients who have undergone these types of operations.

▶ These 3 papers (Abstracts 9–4, 9–5, and 9–6) illustrate a spectrum of a benign but pseudo-neoplastic reaction to injury in the urinary bladder. These lesions and variations on these morphological themes are being recognized with increasing frequency. The postoperative lesions may lack the characteristic central necrosis and palisading and demonstrate a cellularity more suggestive of sarcoma (1). The inflammatory pseudotumors may [as in the cases reported by Gugliada et al. (2)] reach large size (7 cm), invade local tissues, and recur after incomplete resection. The striking histologic similarities of these lesions to sarcomas as seen on permanent sections suggest that frozen-section diagnoses of such lesions be made with all the more caution.—W.A Gardner, Jr., M.D.

References

1. Vekemans K, et al: *Urology* 35:342, 1990.
2. Gugliada K, et al: *Radiology* 179:66, 1991.

The Histology of Interstitial Cystitis

Lynes WL, Flynn SD, Shortliffe L, Stamey TA (Stanford Univ; Yale Univ)

Am J Surg Pathol 14:969–976, 1990 9–7

Introduction.—There have been several reports of histologic findings in interstitial cystitis (IC) bladder specimens; however, these reports noted considerable histologic variations, probably because of different criteria used to define the condition. The histologic biopsy findings of IC patients were compared with those of controls.

Patients.—The subjects were 22 IC patients and 10 controls; 1 patient in each group was male. This series included 5 IC patients and 3 controls from a previously reported series. For each patient, the right lateral, left lateral, and posterior bladder walls were biopsied twice with cup biopsy forceps. Only 2 IC patients were previously diagnosed as having the condition.

Findings.—Patients with IC had a higher incidence and degree of denuded epithelium, ulceration, and submucosal inflammation; however, none of these findings was pathognomonic, and they occurred only in IC patients who had pyuria or a small bladder capacity. A predominantly lymphocytic inflammatory infiltrate was seen; numbers of plasma cells increased along with the degree of inflammation. The infiltrate showed no specific predilection to be perineural. Associations were seen between submucosal inflammation and denuded epithelium, ulceration, pyuria, and the clinical response to therapy. There were no significant differences between IC patients and controls in epithelial and basement membrane thickness, submucosal edema, vascular ectasia, fibrosis, and detrusor muscle inflammation and fibrosis.

Discussion.—Interstitial cystitis appears to be a chronic submucosal inflammatory disease, especially in patients with pyuria or small bladder capacity. The diagnosis of IC is best made on clinical grounds, as the histologic changes seen in the bladder biopsy specimen play only a supportive role. There is only a limited diagnostic role for mast cells.

▶ These authors have previously noted comparable numbers of mast cells in controls and biopsy specimens of IC, and their view of the importance of histopathologic interpretation represents one pole. The opposite pole is represented by Johansson and Fall (1), who point out that the above authors' method of fixation diminishes visualization of mucosal mast cells. For a diametrically opposed view, i.e., that there are characteristic, specific, morphological features to diagnose and even subtype IC see their article.—W.A. Gardner, Jr., M.D.

Reference

1. Johansson SL, Fall M: *J Urol* 143:1118, 1990.

Ploidy Level Determinations in High-Grade and Low-Grade Malignant Variants of Prostatic Carcinoma

Forsslund G, Zetterberg A (Karolinska Hosp, Stockholm)

Cancer Res 50:4281–4285, 1990 9–8

Background.—An important prognostic aspect of prostate malignancies is the nuclear DNA content. In prostatic and breast tumors with cell DNA in excess of the normal diploid value, tumors with tetraploid cells have a less favorable course than those with aneuploidies. Cytophotometric DNA criteria were defined to distinguish high-grade malignancies from low-grde malignant variants of prostatic cancer by using standard cytologic slides.

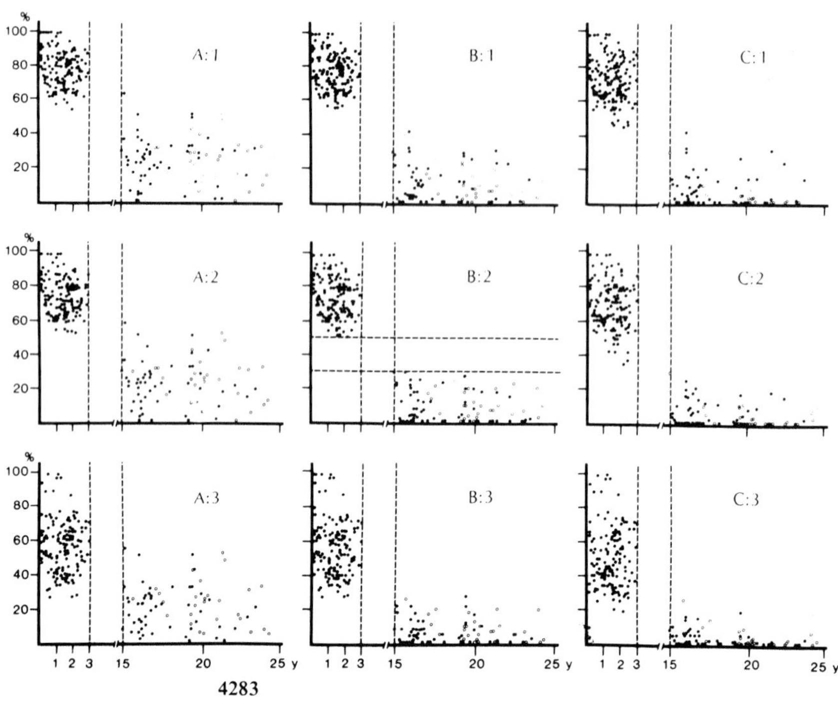

Fig 9–6.—Relationship between survival time (in years) and percentage of tumor cells that are non-2c and non 4-c in 213 cases of prostatic cancer. Extreme group 1 (dead within 3 years), 131 cases; extreme group 2 (alive after 15 years), 82 cases. 2c region: A = 2.25c; B = 2.5c; C = 2.75c. 4c region: 1 = 3.6c–4.4c; 2 = 3.5c–4.5c; 3 = 3.2c–4.8c. (Courtesy of Forrslund G, Zetterberg A: *Cancer Res* 50:4281–4285, 1990.)

Methods.—From a large pool of patients, 213 with primary prostatic carcinoma were selected to represent 2 extremes of survival. The short-survival group consisted of 131 patients who died within 3 years of diagnosis; the long-survival group comprised 82 patients who survived for at least 15 years. To evaluate DNA in benign diseases, DNA histograms were made from 19 cases representing 3 nonmalignant prostatic lesions. A third group of 79 cancer patients with an intermediate range of survival times was used to assess the predictive validity of the criteria derived from analysis of the extreme groups. The May-Grunwald-Giemsa slides used for the original diagnoses were reprocessed for the acid Feulgen procedure and examined cytophotometrically. On each slide, granulocytes were used as internal controls that represented normal diploid DNA content, designated 2c, and compared with tumor cells or benign epithelial cells. The categories used were diploid, in the 2c to 2.5c range of the internal controls: tetraploid, from 3.5c to 4.5c; abnormal, all non-2c and non-4c cells. The most frequent c value within bins of 0.5c width was taken as the modal value.

Results.—The relationship between survival time and percentage of abnormal tumor cells is illustrated in Figure 9–6. Although several ranges were tried, the best separation of the long- and short-survival groups was achieved by using the stated diploid and tetraploid boundaries. In fact, there was a gap of 20% between the lowest percentage of abnormal cells in the short-survival group and the highest percentage in the long-survival group. In addition, in the short-survival group the modal DNA values fell between 2.5c and 7.5c (designated abnormal (A) tumors), contrasting with values clustered around 2c (diploid tumors) or 4c (tetraploid tumors) in the long-survival group. When these criteria were applied to patients with intermediate survival times, classification of a tumor as A type correctly predicted a survival of less than 5 years. Similar to benign prostatic lesions, diploid tumors and tetraploid tumors had DNA patterns mainly in the 2c and 4c regions.

Discussion.—Ploidy level determined from quantitative cytophotometry of tumor cell nuclei can be used effectively to distinguish highly malignant A type tumors from less malignant diploid and tetraploid tumors. The success of this prognostic tool depends heavily on the selection of appropriate ranges for the different ploidy levels. In this study the ranges were based on quantification of ploidy levels in benign prostatic lesions and internal control cells treated with the same histologic procedures.

▶ The presence in urology journals of commercial advertisements for ploidy analysis reflects the widespread acceptance of this prognostic indicator for prostate cancer. Studies by the above authors have emphasized the use of slide ploidy for cytophotometric analysis, i.e., microscopic slides up to 20 years old rather than cell suspensions for flow cytometry. Studies by these authors have been expanded and continue to support the prognostic significance of DNA analysis (1).—W.A. Gardner, Jr., M.D.

Reference

1. Zetterberg A, Forsslund G: *Acta Oncol* 30:193, 1991.

Granulomatous Prostatitis and Poorly Differentiated Prostate Carcinoma: Their Distinction With the Use of Immunohistochemical Methods

Presti B, Weidner N (St Mary Corwin Hosp, Pueblo, Colo; Brigham and Women's Hosp, Boston)

Am J Clin Pathol 95:330–334, 1991 9–9

Background.—Men who have granulomatous prostatitis and those with prostate carcinoma may both have a hard, fixed nodule on rectal examination; when the carcinoma is the poorly differentiated type, light microscopic level histology may not distinguish changes caused by inflammatory versus malignant processes. On 1 hand, histiocytes with reactive nuclear changes but without clear granuloma in granulomatous prostatitis may resemble invasion by poorly differentiated prostate carcinoma; on the other hand, poorly differentiated, infiltrating cancer cells may be mistaken for epithelioid histiocytes. Although the problem is not frequent, misdiagnosis is likely to result in inappropriate treatment.

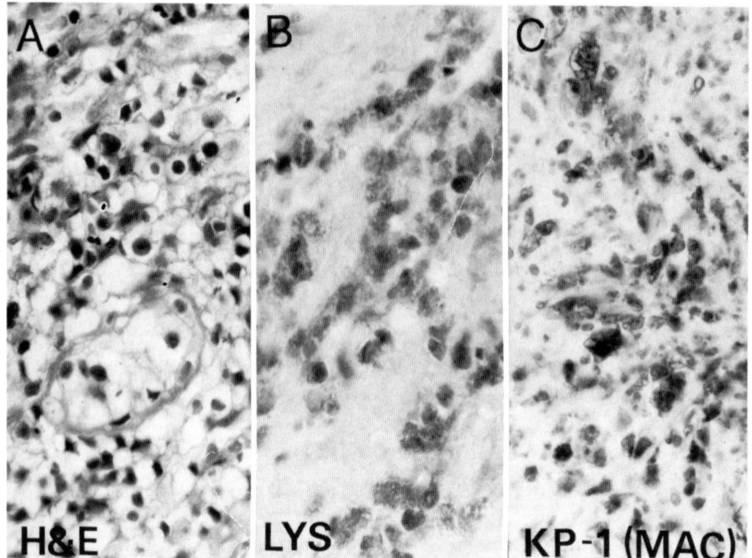

Fig 9–7.—A, epithelioid histiocytes admixed with lymphocytes. Hematoxylin-eosin; ×160. B, epithelioid histiocytes from granulomatous prostatitis are shown with immunoreactivity to antilysozyme (LYS). Peroxidase-antiperoxidase; original magnification, ×160. C, epithelioid histiocytes with immunoreactivity to antimacrophage M (MAC-M). Peroxidase-antiperoxidase; original magnification, ×100. (Courtesy of Presti B, Weidner N: *Am J Clin Pathol* 95:330–334, 1991.)

Whether immunohistochemical techniques can help to resolve cases of ambiguous prostate pathology was investigated.

Methods.—After a retrospective review of all diagnoses of granulomatous prostatitis made during a 10-year period, formalin-fixed tissue samples were taken from 9 cases that resembled poorly differentiated prostate carcinoma. The prostate glands were distorted or destroyed by sheets, clusters, or scattered epithelioid histiocytes in the stroma. These samples were compared with maximally similar tissue from 6 invasive, poorly differentiated carcinomas by using immunoperoxidase labeling for prostatic acid phosphatase (PAP), prostate-specific antigen (PSA), cytokeratins, leukocyte common antigen, lysozyme, and macrophage M antigen.

Results.—All malignant and some benign prostatic glands expressed PAP, PSA, and cytokeratin (Fig 9–7) but none of the epithelioid histiocytes in the 9 cases of granulomatous prostatitis did so. Lysozyme caused a reaction in 100% of the epithelioid histiocytes in the 9 cases of granulomatous prostatitis (Fig 9–8) and in none of the invasive carcinoma cells. Macrophage M was also a good marker, with 7 cases of granulomatous prostatitis, but none of prostate cancer, reacting.

Discussion.—The results indicate that there are sufficient differences in the immunoreactivity of hematopoietic and epithelial determinants to discriminate between these 2 diseases. Although a positive reaction for any epithelial marker eliminates granulomatous prostatitis as the diagnosis, poorly differentiated prostate tumors may not be reactive for PAP and

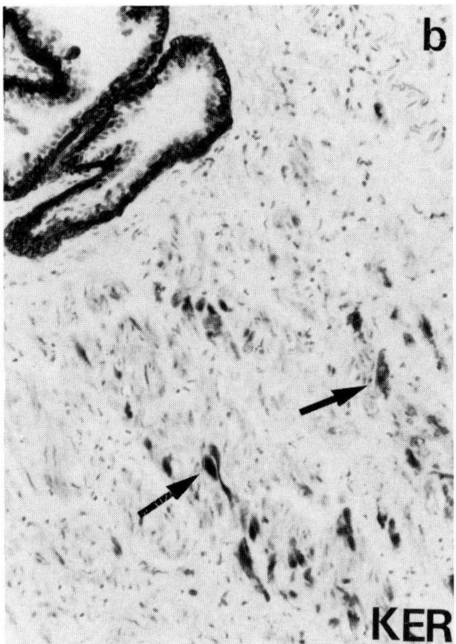

Fig 9–8.—Stromal smooth cells (*arrows*) and benign prostate gland are seen, both demonstrating immunoreactivity to anticytokeratin antibody (KER) (AE1/3). Peroxidase-antiperoxidase; original magnification, ×100. (Courtesy of Presti B, Weidner N: *Am J Clin Pathol* 95:330–334, 1991.)

PSA. When results are ambiguous, antilysozyme is a useful marker for the large lymphoid cells, which can be confused with undifferentiated small cell tumor cells; it is a reliable indicator for the epithelioid histiocytes of granulomatous prostatitis.

▶ One of the more common causes of misdiagnosis of prostate carcinoma is the presence of granulomatous prostatitis with diffusely infiltrating histiocytes. The resemblance to infiltrating epithelial cells is especially noted when there is prominent cytoplasmic clearing of the histiocytes. Histochemical staining with antilysozyme would seem to provide a straightforward differentiation. In most cases of diffuse granulomatous prostatitis the etiology is unknown, although extravasated or altered prostatic secretions have been suggested as providing the antigenic basis for this disease. Dhundee and Maciver (1) investigated the serum proteins PSA and PAP in such cases and found a reduction in PSA and acid phosphatase in granulomatous prostatitis. These authors noted T lymphocytes along with the macrophages, but few B lymphocytes. They postulate that the epithelial destruction caused by cytokines from these inflammatory cells accounts for the loss of PSA and PAP.

Macrophages in granulomatous prostatitis may also take on a spindled appearance (2) and suggest a diagnosis of spindle cell tumor, especially when seen in the fine-needle aspirate.—W.A. Gardner, Jr., M.D.

References

1. Dhundee J, Maciver AG: *Histopathology* 18:435, 1991.
2. Stanley MW, et al: *Diagn Cytopathol* 7:508, 1991.

10 Female Genital System

Assessment of Criteria Used in the Histologic Diagnosis of Human Papillomavirus-Related Disease of the Female Lower Genital Tract

Spitzer M, Chernys AE, Hirschfield L, Spiegel G, Sedlis A, Zuna RE, Steinberg B, Brandsma JL, Krumholz BA (Queens Hosp Ctr, Jamaica, NY; Long Island Jewish Med Ctr, New Hyde Park, NY; State Univ of New York, Stony Brook)

Gynecol Oncol 38:105–109, 1990 10–1

Background.—The diagnosis of human papillomavirus (HPV)-associated disease has commonly been confirmed histologically by the finding of koilocytosis, but lesions without definitive evidence of disease have sometimes been called "early condyloma". Techniques of molecular biology have been used to detect HPV, but hybridization techniques and histologic findings may yield contradictory results.

Study Design.—The histologic criteria for the diagnosis of HPV-associated lesions were evluated in a double-blind study to determine which criteria are reliable. The series included 21 consecutive patients who submitted cervical and vulval biopsy specimens. Each specimen was evaluated with in situ hybridization to both DNA and RNA probes for HPV. In addition, each was evaluated by several pathologists for an overall impression of the histologic diagnosis and afterward was scored for each of 12 histologic criteria commonly associated with HPV infections.

Findings.—Among cervical samples, binucleation and dysplasia correlated well with in situ hybridization results, and koilocytosis correlated strongly with the histologic diagnosis. Among vulval samples, koilocytosis, papillomatosis, elongated rete pegs, binucleation, and hypergranulosis correlated most strongly with hybridization data. Among 5 pathologists, a high level of agreement as to the histologic diagnosis of cervical samples and a low level of agreement as to the diagnosis of vulval samples were found. All pathologists agreed well on the diagnosis of dysplasia, and they agreed moderately well on the finding of binucleation among cervical samples. For samples from the vulva, pathologists agreed well only on the presence of papillomatosis.

Conclusions.—It is impossible to reliably predict the presence of HPV in "borderline" or "early" lesions. Without strong evidence of disease, this diagnosis should be avoided because of its possibly serious psychosocial effects. Instead, patients should be followed clinically without treatment.

Cytologic Correlates of Cervical Papillomavirus Infection

Ward BE, Burkett B, Petersen C, Nuckols ML, Brennan C, Birch LM, Crum CP
(Univ of Virginia)
Int J Gynecol Pathol 9:297–305, 1990 10–2

Background.—Human papillomavirus (HPV) infection is associated with several types of cervical lesions. However, conventional cytologic criteria for recognizing HPV infection on Papanicolaou smear often appear to be inadequate. Screening samples were examined to assess the efficiency of cytologic identification of HPV DNA, especially the criteria for identification of atypical smears.

Methods.—Papanicolaou smears were obtained from 518 women attending a university outpatient clinic. The mean age was 20 years and the mean age at first intercourse, 18 years. The study was conducted in 2 phases. In the first phase, 290 smears were independently classified as being normal, atypical, or diagnostic for condyloma or cervical HPV infection (CIN). These diagnoses were then compared to RNA-DNA hybridization results. Information gained from this analysis was used in the second phase to revise the cytologic criteria, which were applied to the remaining 178 smears and to HPV-positive smears that were cytologically negative.

Results.—In phase 1, 8.6% of smears were cytologically atypical, but only 12% of these showed HPV DNA. Five smears were diagnostic of HPV/CIN, and 4 of these were associated with HPV nucleic acids. Using more stringent criteria in phase 2, only 1.8% of smears were atypical, and 2 of these 3 specimens contained HPV nucleic acids. Prominent nuclear enlargement, with either multiple nuclei or nuclear hyperchromatism, most efficiently correlated with positive HPV-DNA findings. There were 19 HPV-positive and 20 control HPV-negative smears originally diagnosed as cytologically negative; the phase 2 criteria found 3 more positive smears in the HPV-positive group and none in the control group.

Conclusions.—The cytologic abnormalities that indicate "subtle" HPV infection may be difficult to separate from non–HPV-related changes. Continual revision of criteria used to imply suggestive but nondiagnostic HPV infection is needed. A large number of cases must be studied to determine the cost effectiveness of HPV DNA testing.

▶ These studies (Abstracts 10–1 and 10–2) confirm each other, finding a low incidence of HPV genomic material in borderline or equivocal morphological specimens. When multiple biopsy specimens are taken, borderline findings may also be seen adjacent to more well-developed morphological patterns. Therefore, careful reevaluation of the original cytologic material for classic and nonclassic findings of an HPV effect need also be considered in these cases (1).—R.M. Austin, M.D., Ph.D.

Reference

1. Meisels A, Fortin R: *Acta Cytol* 20:505, 1976.

Discrepancy of Cervical Cytology and Colposcopic Biopsy: Is Cervical Conization Necessary?

McCord ML, Stovall TG, Summitt RL Jr, Ling FW (Univ of Tennessee, Memphis)

Obstet Gyncol 77:715–719, 1991 10–3

Background.—Traditionally, cervical conization is done when there is a discrepancy between the cytologic and histologic observations in women with cervical cytologic findings suggestive of cervical intraepithelial neoplasia (CIN). However, some studies have suggested that ablative therapy can be done in place of conization. Records of patients with a discrepancy between the Papanicolaou smear and the colposcopically directed biopsy were studied to determine whether diagnostic cervical conization was necessary.

Methods.—Reocrds of 786 patients from a cervical dysplasia clinic were evaluated to find cases with a discrepancy of at least 2 degrees, (e.g., CIN III cytologic findings and CIN I or less in a colposcopic biopsy specimen, or CIN II cytologic findings with no dysplasia in the biopsy specimen). Eighty-seven such patients were found, for an incidence of 11%. After elimination of 12 pregnant patients and 10 who did not return after their first colposcopic examination, 65 patients remained for analysis. Medical treatment was given to 31% and cryotherapy to 14%; diagnostic cervical conization was done in 55%.

Results.—Microinvasive cervical carcinoma was found in 3 patients who underwent cervical conization. Of 20 patients who had medical therapy, follow-up cytologic studies were negative in only 2; 2 had CIN I, 5 received additional therapy, and 11 were lost to follow-up. Of the latter patients, 7 failed to return for a follow-up Papanicolaou smear and 4 failed to return after the follow-up smear showed persistent dysplasia. Six of 9 patients treated with cryotherapy had a negative Papanicolaou smear at their first follow-up.

Conclusions.—Cervical conization maximizes the chance of making the correct diagnosis in patients with a 2-stage or greater discrepancy between the findings on colposcopically directed biopsy and cervical cytologic study. The risk of missing a microinvasive or invasive carcinoma of the cervix far outweighs the risk of conization. Medical therapy may delay definitive treatment in a high-risk population whose compliance with follow-up is poor.

▶ When significant discrepancies occur between previous cytologic findings and colposcopic biopsy findings, several additional steps need to be taken before considering conization. The original cytologic material needs to be reviewed along with the biopsy material to judge whether, in retrospect, cytologic findings may reasonably account for the histologic biopsy findings. Furthermore, additional step sections of colposcopic cervical biopsy material may, on occasion, reveal previously undetected areas of abnormality. It is our observation that these additional steps, which may resolve many discrepancies, nonetheless are frequently not taken. This type of correlation is enhanced when the cytology and biopsy material are reviewed in a single location. Adequacy of colposcopic transformation zone visualization (1), sometimes enhanced by cervical dilators (2), and endocervical curettage are other factors that may facilitate conservative follow-up. Should discrepancies persist despite additional steps and careful examination of the vagina reveals no source of dysplastic cells, conization may become necessary.—R.M. Austin, M.D.

References

1. Kwikkel HJ, et al: *Gynecol Oncol* 24:162, 1986.
2. Stern JL, et al: *Am J Obstet Gynecol* 163:176, 1990.

Mesonephric Remnants, Hyperplasia, and Neoplasia in the Uterine Cervix: A Study of 49 Cases

Ferry JA, Scully RE (Massachusetts Gen Hosp, Boston; Harvard Med School, Boston)

Am J Surg Pathol 14:1100–1111, 1990 10–4

Introduction.—The embryo's mesonephric, or wolffian, ducts form temporary kidneys that later undergo replacement by the permanent organs. The number of neoplasms originating from the mesonephric duct has been overestimated in the past. Forty-nine cases were examined in which mesonephric-derived cells were found in cervical spec-

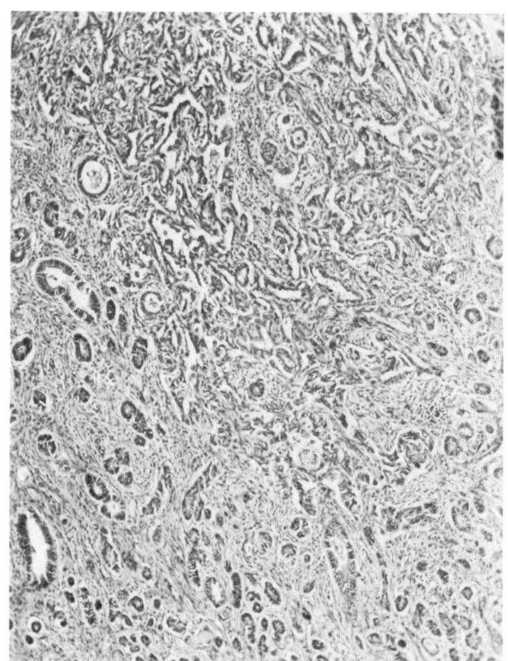

Fig 10–1.—High-power view showing focal severe glandular crowding and slight cytologic atypia. The bottom of the field contains small, evenly spaced mesonephric tubules. The top contains back-to-back oval or elongate tubules with focal papillary tufting. (Courtesy of Ferry JA, Scully RE: *Am J Surg Pathol* 14:1100–1111, 1990.)

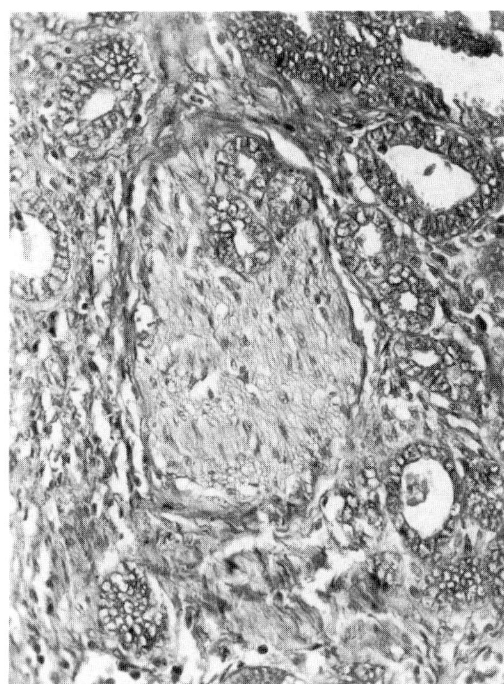

Fig 10–2.—Mesonephric carcinoma with perineural invasion. Well-differentiated tubules lined by cuboidal cells infiltrate a small nerve; in other areas, tubules were lined predominantly by stratified columnar cells. (Courtesy of Ferry JA, Scully RE: *Am J Surg Pathol* 14:1100–1111, 1990.)

imens obtained at surgery. One of 4 carcinomas in this series was initially misdiagnosed, emphasizing that physicians should be alert to the lesions.

Methods.—Forty-nine cervical specimens containing mesonephric remnants were found in a review of the consultation files dated 1964–1990. In 9 cases a periodic acid-Schiff stain was available for analysis.

Results.—The 45 patients with normal mesonephric remnants, lobular mesonephric hyperplasia, ductal hyperplasia, or diffuse mesonephric hyperplasia had a mean age of 37 years (range, 21–72 years). In 19 cases there was a description of the gross appearance of the cervix; it appeared normal in 15 patients, demonstrated Nabothian cysts in 2, and was "full" in another; a 10-mm cystic lesion was present in the left wall of the cervix in 1 instance. The 4 women with mesonephric carcinoma had a mean age of 49 years (range, 36–58 years). In these patients, 31 lesions were classified as lobular mesonephric hyperplasia. In 1 specimen with a focal endometrioid appearance, a superficially located 2-mm focus was observed (Fig 10–1). Among the 4 cases of mesonephric carcinoma, 1 focus of perineural invasion was seen (Fig 10–2). In another of these cases, 1 sample demonstrated a cytologically bland proliferation of widely separated tubules surrounding the tumor and extending into the vagina (Fig 10–3). Follow-up data for 31 of the patients with mesonephric remnants showed that all were disease free from 2 months to 24 years after diagnosis. All 4 patients with carcinoma died within approximately 2 years of diagnosis and treatment.

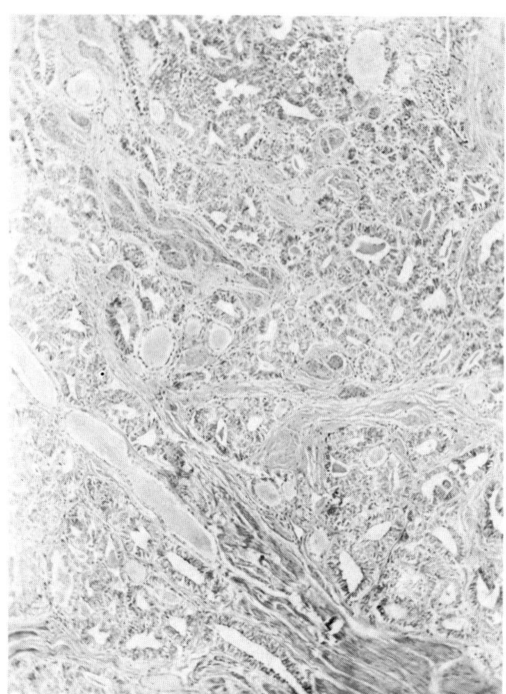

Fig 10–3.—Mesonephric carcinoma. Slightly less crowded tubules toward the periphery of the carcinoma. The neoplastic tubules are intermingled with mesonephric tubules with less cytologic atypia and lined by cuboidal epithelium. (Courtesy of Ferry JA, Scully RE: *Am J Surg Pathol* 14:1100–1111, 1990.)

Implications.—The correct diagnosis and classification of mesonephric lesions are necessary for proper patient management and therapy. In the absence of clearly malignant characteristics for mesonephric lesions, the following factors should be used to aid in the diagnosis: irregular, disorderly invasion; back-to-back glandular aggregation; nuclear atypicality; and focal loss of the basement membranes. These are important clues in the diagnosis of carcinoma.

▶ Cervical mesonephric remnants often represent problem findings in surgical pathology and are sometimes even misdiagnosed as minimum deviation cervical adenocarcinoma (1). The illustrations provided in this report should aid practicing pathologists in distinguishing between benign mesonephric remnants, mesonephric hyperplasia, and rare cases of mesonephric carcinoma.—R.M. Austin, M.D., Ph.D.

Reference

1. Ayroud Y, et al: *Int J Gynecol Pathol* 4:245, 1985.

Cystic Endocervical Tunnel Clusters: A Clinicopathologic Study of 29 Cases of So-Called Adenomatous Hyperplasia

Segal GH, Hart WR (Cleveland Clinic Found)

Am J Surg Pathol 14:895–903, 1990 10–5

Background.—Little is known about the clinical and histologic features of cystic endocervical tunnel clusters (CETCs). They may be mistaken for endocervical adenocarcinoma or interpreted as adenomatous hyperplasia. Twenty-nine patients with CETCs were studied to gain information to aid to recognizing this entity.

Patients.—Clusters were found in 19 of 322 consecutive hysterectomy patients and in 3 of 31 consecutive cervical conization specimens. Seven additional referral patients were also analyzed. The 29 patients ranged in age from 33 to 72, with a mean of 55 years, and all but 1 were multigravida, most having had at least 3 previous pregnancies. Hysterectomy patients with CETCs had significantly greater gravidity and age than those without CETCs. The lesions were generally discovered during routine cervical examination.

Findings.—The mean greatest dimension of the clusters was 2.4 mm. Multifocal clusters were seen in 82.8% of the patients (Fig 10–4). The

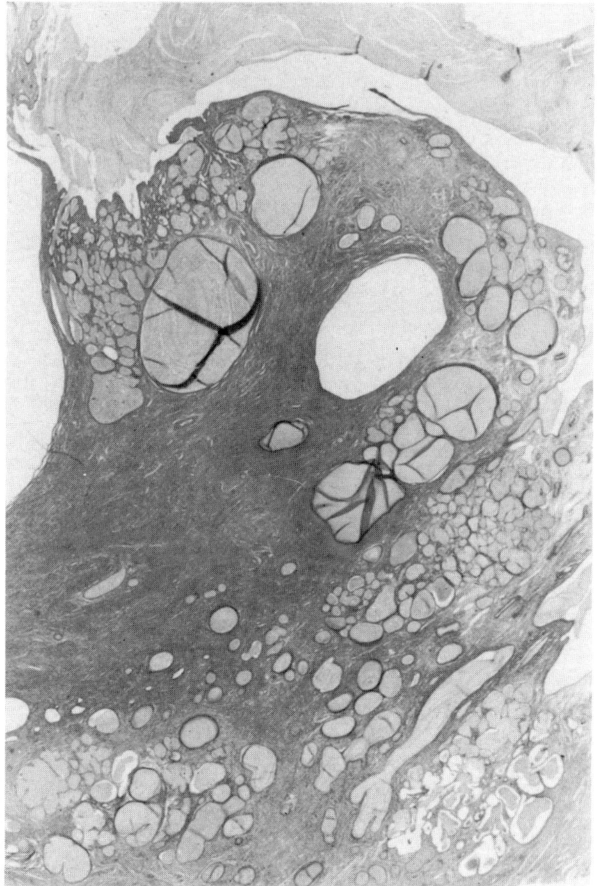

Fig 10–4.—Multiple lobules of cystic endocervical tunnel clusters with retention cysts of various sizes involving superficial endocervix. Each cluster has a relatively well circumscribed border. (Courtesy of Segal GH, Hart WR: *Am J Surg Pathol* 14:895–903, 1990.)

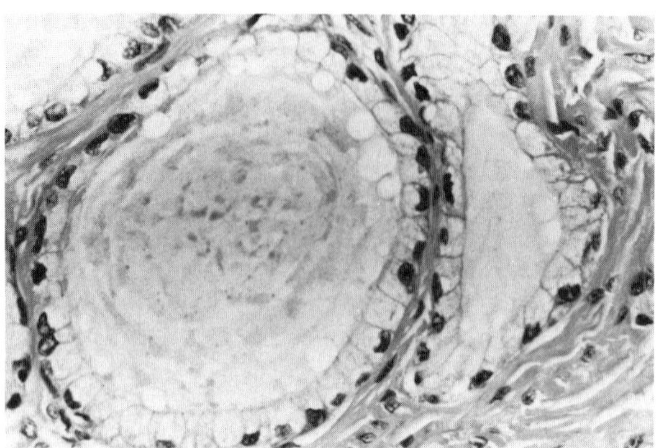

Fig 10–5.—Low columnar endocervical cells lining the tunnels have slightly enlarged, hyperchromatic nuclei. Such nuclear changes are usually inconspicuous and are of no clinical significance. (Courtesy of Segal GH, Hart WR: *Am J Surg Pathol* 14:895–903, 1990.)

clusters were made up of orderly, lobular aggregates of closely packed, dilated tubular endocervical glands in the superficial endocervix. Nine millimeters was the depth of the deepest clusters; they were often in association with multiple nabothian cysts that also penetrated deeply. One layer of flattened or cuboidal endocervical cells made up the lining epithelium, and there were no mitotic figures or significant cytologic atypia (Fig 10–5). Intracytoplasmic CEA immunoreactivity was not seen, but focal positive CEA staining along the luminal border of the endocervical cells was found in 52% of clusters.

Conclusions.—Cystic endocervical tunnel clusters are not related to cervical neoplasms and must be distinguished from other endocervical glandular lesions. They may arise from subinvolution of previous episodes of physiologic mucosal hyperplasia, most often caused by pregnancy.

▶ Cystic endocervical tunnel clusters are an important entity among a number of difficult pseudoneoplastic glandular lesions of the cervix. These processes include papillary endocervicitis, deep glands and deep nabothian cysts, microglandular hyperplasia, mesonephric hyperplasia, diffuse laminar endocervical glandular hyperplasia, glandular hyperplasia not otherwise specified, tubal metaplasia, intestinal metaplasia, endometriosis, Arias-Stella reaction, changes secondary to extravasation of mucin, and various infectious and reactive atypias (1).—R.M. Austin, M.D., Ph.D.

Reference

1. Young RH, Clements PB: *Semin Diagn Pathol* 8:234, 1991.

Autoimmune Oophoritis: A Clinicopathologic Assessment of 12 Cases

Bannatyne P, Russell P, Shearman RP (King George V Mem Hosp, Sydney, Australia; Royal Prince Alfred Hosp, Sydney; Sydney Univ)

Int J Gynecol Pathol 9:191–207, 1990 10–6

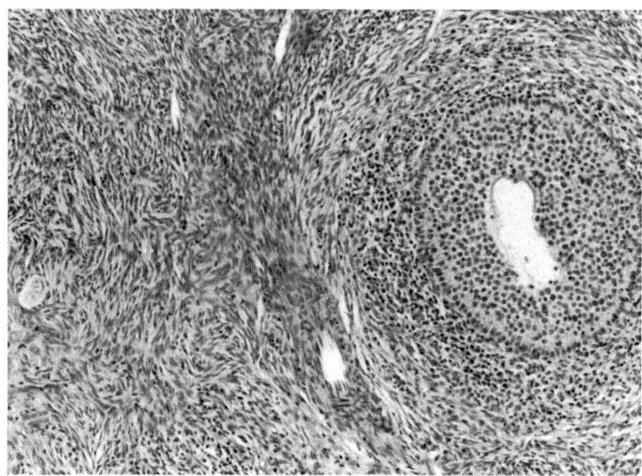

Fig 10–6.—A late primary or preantral follicle *(right)* with an obvious inflammatory infiltrate involving the theca but sparing the granulosa. The small primordial follicle *(far left)* is not affected. Hematoxylin and eosin; original magnification, ×100. (Courtesy of Bannatyne P, Russell P, Shearman RP: *Int J Gynecol Pathol* 9:191–207, 1990.)

Introduction.—Autoimmune oophoritis is not a well-established entity either clinically or pathologically. Perhaps because it is not identified in its early, active stages, it is not considered a potentially treatable cause of premature ovarian failure.

Patients.—Twelve patients with histologically verified autoimmune oophoritis, 8 found during a study of premature ovarian failure, were reviewed. The mean age at presentation was 32 years. Seven patients had secondary amenorrhea or oligomenorrhea; 4 of them also reported infertility. Three of the 12 patients had clinical evidence of other autoimmune disorders. Six patients had a range of circulating antibodies.

Outcome.—Two patients were actively but unsuccessfully treated to restore fertility. Two patients had menstrual-like episodes, and 1 of them is under consideration for immunosuppressive therapy.

Pathology.—Seven patients had enlarged ovaries. Primordial follicles were present in all patients (Fig 10–6). In 11 patients, there was a lymphoplasmacytic infiltrate involving early and late preovulatory follicles and corpora lutea but not involving primordial follicles. The remaining patient had granulomatous oophoritis with folliculotropic inflammation.

Recommendations.—Early biopsy is encouraged for women with premature ovarian failure. Autoimmune oophoritis is probably more common than the literature suggests. Prompt treatment might allow natural pregnancy in some patients. Studies for tissue antibodies can warn of developing Addison's disease or hypothyroidism.

▶ The authors describe 12 patients with "autoimmune" oophoritis, the majority of whom presented with premature ovarian failure. Of interest, 4 of these women also had other autoimmune diseases, specifically, Hashimoto's disease and Addison's disease. The illustrations (Fig 10–6) show relatively subtle findings that may be useful in the identification of this process as a cause of infertility or early ovarian failure.—G.F. Worsham, M.D.

Does Serum CA-125 Level Prior to Second-Look Laparotomy for Invasive Ovarian Adenocarcima Predict Size of Residual Disease?

Patsner B, Orr JW Jr, Taylor PT, Partridge E, Allmen T (Watson Clinic, Lakeland, Fla; State Univ of New York, Stony Brook; Univ of Virginia; Southern Gynecologic Oncology, Birmingham, Ala)

Gynecol Oncol 37:319–322, 1990 10–7

Introduction.—The presence of elevated CA-125 levels before planned second-look surgery is virtually pathognomonic of residual adenocarcinoma. It is not clear, however, whether this parameter can substitute for surgical exploration in patients who have completed chemotherapy and have no clinically evident disease. The extent of residual disease is critically important in predicting the outcome of invasive ovarian adenocarcinoma.

Patients.—Preoperative serum CA-125 levels were related to the extent of residual disease in 125 patients with invasive nonmucinous ovarian adenocarcinoma. The CA-125 levels in all patients were elevated at the time of initial cytoreductive surgery.

Findings.—The preoperative serum CA-125 level was elevated in 25% of 75 patients with positive laparotomy findings. Residual disease of less than 1 cm was nearly always associated with a normal CA-125 level. This was usually the case also for patients with disease of less than 2 cm. The serum CA-125 level was 93% specific but only 27% sensitive. Its positive and negative predictive values were 83% and 49%, respectively.

Conclusion.—Overlap of serum CA-125 levels makes it difficult to use this indication to precisely predict the extent of residual disease or to determine whether secondary debulking may be necessary.

▶ This important article demonstrates the high specificity but low sensitivity of CA-125 as a marker for ovarian carcinoma. Serum CA-125 levels should not replace second-look laparotomy for recurrent ovarian carcinoma at this time.—A.J. Garvin, M.D., Ph.D.

11 Breast

Borderline Epithelial Lesions of the Breast

Rosai J (Yale Univ)

Am J Surg Pathol 15:209–221, 1991 11–1

Background.—Controversy surrounds the idea of borderline epithelial lesions of the breast. Page and colleagues suggested that there is a continuum between hyperplasia and carcinoma in situ, with a correlation between the degree of proliferation and atypia and the development of invasive carcinoma. Subjectivity in making the diagnosis remains a problem.

Discussion.—To assess the problem of subjectivity among observers, 17 cases of proliferative ductal lesions or proliferative lobular lesions were submitted to 5 eminent pathologists for their diagnostic opinions. The reviewers did not agree unanimously on a diagnosis in any case, and 4 of 5 agreed in only 3 instances (table). It appears that the reviewers ei-

Results of Survey Carried Out With 10 Ductal and Screen Lobular Breast Lesions Among 5 Pathologists*

	Pathologist				
Lesion	A	B	C	D	E
D1	AH	AH	AH	H	H
D2	AH	AH	N	H	H
D3	CIS	CIS	AH	CIS	AH
D4	CIS	AH	CIS	H	AH‡
D5	AH	AH	H	H	H
D6	CIS	ALH	CIS	AH	H‡
D7	AH	H	AH	H	H
D8	AH	H	H	H	H†
D9	AH	AH	AH	AH	H‡
D10	CIS	AH	H	H	H‡
L1	CIS	AH	AH	AH	H[b]
L2	CIS	H	AH	AH	H[b]
L3	AH	H	H	AH	H
L4	CIS	AH	AH	AH	AH†
L5	CIS	CIS	CIS	AH	AH
L6	AH	H	AH	H	H
L7	CIS	H	AH	AH	H‡

*A through E identifies the 5 participating pathologists; D1 through D10 are the 10 ductal lesions; L1 through L7 are the 7 lobular lesions. The diagnoses listed are H, hyperplasia; AH, atypical hyperplasia; ALH, atypical lobular hyperplasia; CIS, carcinoma in situ; N, normal.

†Cases in which 4 of the 5 pathologists agreed on a given category.

‡Cases in which the disagreement spanned the range from hyperplasia (without atypia) to CIS.

(Courtesy of Rosai J: *Am J Surg Pathol* 15:209–221, 1991.)

ther did not use Page's criteria, or they used them differently than intended originally.

The use of ancillary techniques, including electron microscopy, immunohistochemistry, or morphological studies, to obtain more reproducible categories has not given the hoped-for results. Studies attempting to duplicate the correlation obtained by Page et al. are underway at 4 centers. Other investigators have suggested alternative criteria for atypical ductal hyperplasia: a lesion with cytologic findings of ductal carcinoma in situ (DCIS) but without its architectural growth pattern, or a lesion with both the cytologic and architectural features of DCIS but measuring less than 2 mm. The accuracy and reproducibility of these criteria remain to be proved.

Conclusions.—Given that the subjectivity of interpretation seems likely to persist, and that the terminology in current use suggests a sharper division in interpretation than currently exists, a term such as mammary intraepithelial endoplasia, ductal or lobular types is suggested. Alternatively, a 1- to 3-grade system from mild hyperplasia to carcinoma in situ could be adopted, following the prototype of the uterine cervix. Adoption of a new terminology would not solve the interpretive problems, but it might achieve other worthwhile goals.

▶ This article points out that unless specific criteria are agreed upon, the diagnosis of atypical hyperplasia in the breast is quite subjective. What it does not point out, however, is that although one is free to define his own criteria for atypical hyperplasia, the relative risk attributable to that diagnosis (4 times control populations) will not apply unless the criteria of Page et al. are utilized.— R.A. Jensen, M.D.

Metaplastic Carcinomas of the Breast. V. Metaplastic Carcinoma With Osteoclastic Giant Cells

Wargotz ES, Norris HJ (Maryland Med Lab at Doctor's Hosp, Lanham, Md; Armed Forces Inst of Pathology, Washington, DC)

Hum Pathol 21:1142–1150, 1990 11–2

Objective.—Osteoclastic giants cells (OGC) are a rare and unusual component of breast carcinoma. The clinical and pathologic features of 29 mammary metaplastic carcinomas with OGC in the stroma were reviewed and compared with other forms of metaplastic carcinoma with which it might be confused (table).

Pathology.—All 29 neoplasms were dominated by a bland-appearing spindle cell or sarcomatous component. Infiltrating duct carcinoma was present in 23 neoplasms and intraductal carcinoma in 6; all were admixed or contiguous with the osteoclastic stroma (Figs 11–1 and 11–2). In all neoplasms, OGC were present within cellular areas of stroma and were intimately associated with prominent thin-walled vessels. Hemorrhage and hemosiderin were prominent in most neoplasms. The stroma

Classification and Distribution of Cases of Metaplastic Carcinomas of the Breast

Type	No. of Cases
Matrix-producing carcinoma	26
Spindle cell carcinoma	100
Carcinosarcoma	70
Pure squamous cell carcinoma of ductal origin	22
Metaplastic carcinoma with osteoclastic giant cells	29
Total	247

(Courtesy of Wargotz ES, Norris HJ: *Hum Pathol* 21:1142–1150, 1990.)

contained osteoid, bone, or cartilage in 19 neoplasms, but these were prominent only in 5 neoplasms and OGC were not limited to these areas. The OGC were immunoreactive for vimentin and, to a lesser extent, actin. However, all neoplasms were uniformly negative for keratin and epithelial membrane antigen (EMA), confirming their mesenchymal nature. The stromal component was immunoreactive for keratin in 63%, for EMA in 34%, for S-100 protein in 54%, for actin in 84%, and for vimentin in 100% of neoplasms tested.

Outcome.—The cumulative disease-specific 5-year survival rate was 68%, similar to rates reported for other forms of metaplastic mammary carcinoma (e.g., matrix-producing carcinoma, spindle cell carcinoma, and pure squamous carcinoma of ductal origin), but it is higher than the survival rate for carcinosarcoma. Distant metastases developed in 11

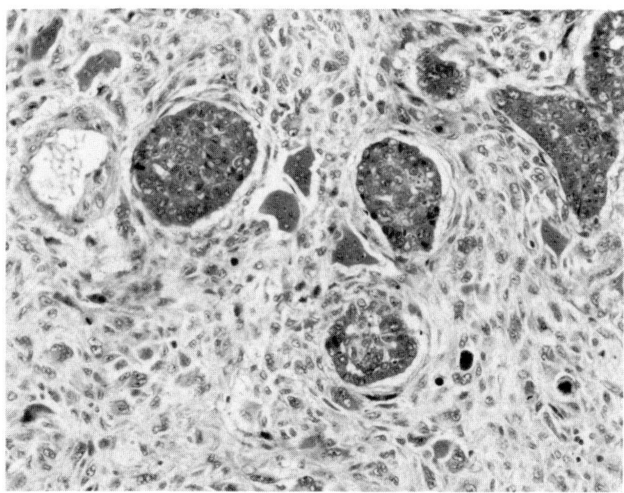

Fig 11–1.—Infiltrating carcinoma and osteoclastic giant cells within a high-grade polymorphous stroma. Original magnification, ×200. (Courtesy of Wargotz ES, Norris HJ: *Hum Pathol* 21:1142–1150, 1990.)

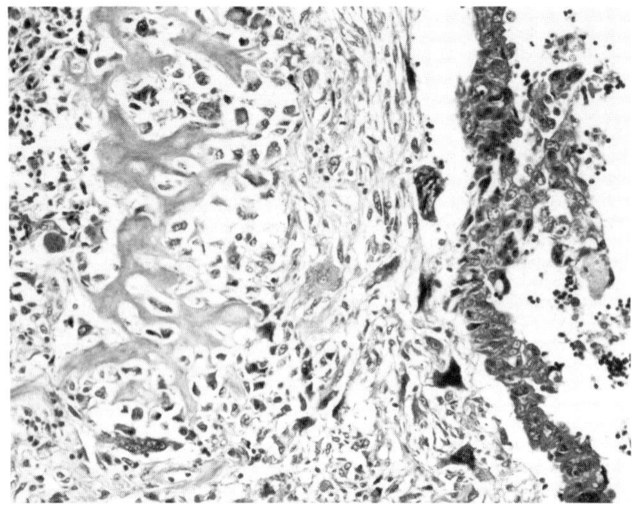

Fig 11–2.—Carcinoma, osteoclastic giant cells, and osteoid with a high-grade polymorphous stroma. Original magnification, ×200. (Courtesy of Wargotz ES, Norris HJ: *Hum Pathol* 21:1142–1150, 1990.)

women after initial therapy and all died of tumor. Metastastic potential was related to size and microscopic circumscription.

Conclusion.—Metaplastic carcinoma with OGC can be distinguished from other forms of metaplastic carcinoma, including matrix-producing carcinoma, by the presence of OGC. In addition, stromal hemorrhage, hemosiderin deposition, and prominent thin-walled vessels are features of metaplastic carcinoma with OGC.

▶ Osteoclastic giant cells are a rare feature of metaplastic carcinomas. Their presence does not alter prognosis.—R.A. Jensen, M.D.

Occult Breast Carcinoma Presenting With Axillary Lymph Node Metastases: A Follow-Up Study of 48 Patients

Rosen PP, Kimmel M (Mem Sloan-Kettering Cancer Ctr, New York)

Hum Pathol 21:518–523, 1990 11–3

Background.—An uncommon form of stage II breast cancer is carcinoma presenting with axillary metastases and no clinically apparent primary tumor. Published studies have described only small numbers of patients or limited follow-up information. Several authors have suggested that the prognosis is not exceptionally grave. A follow-up study was made of 48 patients—the largest series reported to date.

Findings.—Each patient was seen initially with an axillary mass that proved to be metastatic adenocarcinoma consistent with mammary origin when examined histologically. None of the patients had a palpable tumor. Mammography was negative in 76%, and suspicious or positive in 24%. Of 26 metastases, 35% were positive for estrogen (ER) and proges-

Follow-Up of Matched Patients With Occult and Palpable Breast Carcinomas

	Total		Number of Involved Lymph Nodes: 1-3		Number of Involved Lymph Nodes: 4 or More	
Patient Status	Occult (%)	Palpable (%)	Occult (%)	Palpable (%)	Occult (%)	Palpable (%)
NED	16 (73)	15 (36)	9 (75)	9 (38)	7 (70)	6 (33)
AWD	1 (5)	4 (10)	1 (8)	3 (13)	0 (0)	1 (6)
DOD	5 (23)	18 (43)	2 (17)	7 (29)	3 (30)	11 (61)
DOC	0 (0)	5 (12)	0 (0)	5 (21)	0 (0)	0 (0)
Total	22	42	12	24	10	18

(Courtesy of Rosen PP, Kimmel M: *Hum Pathol* 21:518–523, 1990.)

terone (PR) receptors; 38% were negative for both; and 27% were positive for ER and negative for PR. Primary treatment was mastectomy and axillary dissection in 38 patients; 21 received adjuvant chemotherapy. In 75% a primary tumor was found in the breast. Of 34 reviewed primary lesions, 79% were invasive and 21% were histologically noninvasive. They ranged in size from .1 to 6.5 cm. One to 65 lymph nodes were involved.

Outcome.—The patients were followed for a median of 5 years. Overall, 60% of the patients remained alive and free of disease. Of 15 patients who had recurrent carcinoma, 12 died of disease. Compared with a matched series of patients who had stage II disease with equivalent extent of disease and who presented with palpable breast tumors, patients with occult lesions had a better overall prognosis (table).

Conclusions.—Occult breast carcinoma with axillary lymph node metastases is uncommon. The results in this series are consistent with those of most other studies showing a prognosis similar to and possibly better than that of patients with stage II disease and a palpable breast mass. The actual pathologically determined TNM stage is probably a more important determinant of prognosis than apparent clinical stage on initial examination.

▶ This study represents the largest reported series for breast carcinoma presenting in axillary lymph nodes and confirms the importance of the TNM system in predicting prognosis for breast cancer patients.—R.A. Jensen, M.D.

Prognostic Importance of Occult Axillary Lymph Node Micrometastases From Breast Cancers

Bettelheim R, Price KN, Gelber RD, Davis BW, Castiglione M, Goldhirsch A, Neville AM, and the International (Ludwig) Breast Cancer Study Group (Bern, Switzerland)

Lancet 335:1565–1568, 1990 11–4

Background.—In 1981 the Ludwig Breast Cancer Study Group began an international trial of women aged 65 years and younger who had breast cancer, with or without ipsilateral axillary node disease. Micrometastases were sought by serial sectioning of ipsilateral axillary nodes in 921 patients after routine histologic study was negative.

Observations.—Node sectioning demonstrated occult micrometastases in 9% of the patients studied. Positive findings were more frequent in patients with larger tumors, those with peritumoral vascular involvement, and patients younger than age 50 years. Patients with micrometastases had a shorter survival than those with negative findings; the difference was most evident in postmenopausal women and in patients with invasive ductal carcinoma. Many patients with micrometastases had only a single positive node, in contrast to patients with involvement on routine node examination.

Discussion.—The detection of micrometastases in axillary lymph nodes may identify a high-risk group of patients. Sectioning probably should be part of the routine pathologic assessment. It might be best to divide each axillary node into 2-mm slices and stain them immunohistochemically.

▶ The need for serial sectioning of lymph nodes in mastectomy specimens is controversial. This study demonstrates that patients with micrometastases on serial sectioning have a slightly worse survival curve than those without.— R.A. Jensen, M.D.

Infiltrating Cribriform Carcinoma of the Breast: A Distinctive Clinicopathologic Entity

Venable JG, Schwartz AM, Silverberg SG (George Washington Univ)
Hum Pathol 21:333–338, 1990 11–5

Background.— Reportedly, the prognosis of infiltrating duct carcinoma (IDC) is improved if the cytologic features are those typically seen in cribriform carcinoma. Sixty-two cases of infiltrating cribriform carcinoma (ICC) were investigated to provide additional data for clinicopathologic correlation.

Methods.— Coded and available reports of primary breast carcinoma diagnosed from 1971 to 1975 and from 1981 to 1986 were reviewed to identify cases of pure and mixed ICC. The diagnosis of pure ICC required that all of the infiltrating components have a cribriform pattern and well- or moderately differentiated nuclei (Fig 11–3). Mixed tumors were classified as to having a cribriform component of more or less than 50%. On nuclear grading, grade 1 referred to highly differentiated nuclei and grade 3 to anaplastic nuclei (Fig 11–4).

Results.— The 62 at least focal ICC represented 6.2% of all infiltrating carcinomas in the first study period and 9% in the second study period;

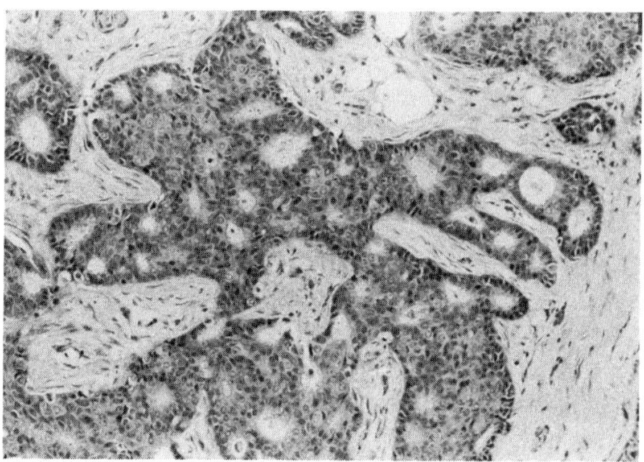

Fig 11–3.—Infiltrating cribriform carcinoma, showing angular nests of infiltrating tumor with surrounding and intervening scirrhous stromal response. The nests of well-differentiated carcinoma cells are punctuated by uniform punched-out spaces. (Hematoxylin-eosin; original magnification, ×200.) (Courtesy of Venable JG, Schwartz AM, Silverberg SG: *Hum Pathol* 21:333–338, 1990).

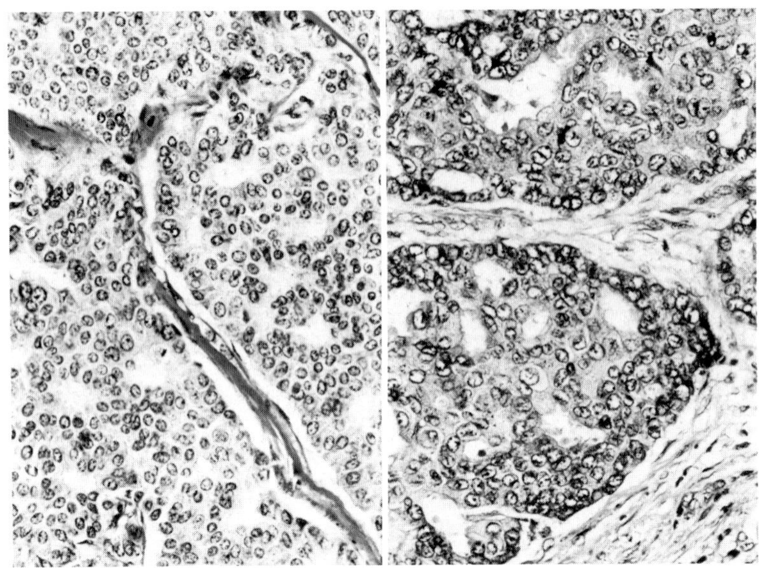

Fig 11–4.—Detail of infiltrating cribriform cases with *(left)* well-differentiated or grade 1 and *(right)* moderately differentiated or grade 2 nuclei. (Hematoxylin-eosin stain; original magnification, ×400.) (Courtesy of Venable JG, Schwartz AM, Silverberg SG: *Hum Pathol* 21:333–338, 1990).

the increase was not significant. The lesions tended to be seen in association with foci of tubular and intraductal carcinoma, often, but not always, of cribriform type, as reported previously. Pure ICC, tumors with mainly ICC and lesser amounts of infiltrating or other carcinomas, and any combination of ICC and tubular carcinoma commonly metastasized to the lymph nodes, but rarely to more than 3 nodes. Tumors composed of IDC not otherwise specified with less than 50% ICC and a control group of IDC more commonly involved 4 nodes or more. All ICC cases were estrogen-receptor positive, and 69% were progesterone-receptor positive. At 5 years the survival rates were 100% for patients with pure and 50% or more ICC, 88% for those with less than 50% ICC, and 78.3% for IDC controls.

Conclusions.—Infiltrating cribriform carcinoma was confirmed as a histologically distinct mammary carcinoma that is well differentiated and has a favorable clinical course. It must be distinguished from IDC and other tumors.

▶ This study emphasizes previous observations noting the importance of recognizing ICC because of its excellent prognosis.—R.A. Jensen, M.D.

Lymphomas of the Breast: A Clinicopathologic and Immunohistochemical Study of Primary and Secondary Cases

Cohen PL, Brooks JJ (Univ of Pennsylvania)

Cancer 67:1359–1369, 1991 11–6

TABLE 1.—Classification of Primary and Secondary Lymphoma of the Breast

	Primary	Secondary
Small cleaved	1	1
Follicular	0	0
Diffuse	1	0
Follicular and diffuse	0	1
Mixed small and large cell	5	2
Follicular	1	2
Diffuse	3	0
Follicular and diffuse	1	0
Large cell	10	14
Diffuse	10	14
Immunoblastic features	4	3
Lymphoblastic	0	1

(Courtesy of Cohen PL, Brooks JJ: *Cancer* 67:1359–1369, 1991.)

Introduction.—Primary lymphoma represents fewer than 1% of all malignant breast tumors and about 2% of extranodal lymphomas. Data were reviewed on 35 patients with lymphoid lesions of the breast.

Findings.—Eighteen lymphomas were secondary at presentation. Most primary lymphomas were of the diffuse large cell subtype (Table 1). The secondary lymphomas included 14 diffuse large cell lesions, 3 of which had immunoplastic features. All of the tumors were poorly circumscribed. Nine of the primary lymphomas were considered B cell lesions.

Outcome.—Excisional biopsy was the usual surgical approach to primary lymphoma of the breast (Table 2). Half of the patients with primary lymphoma had recurrent disease during a mean follow-up of 54 months. One patient died of metastatic disease. Survival is related to histologic features and stage of disease.

Discussion.—A large majority of breast lymphomas are of B cell origin. Some patients with primary lymphoma of the breast have done well after excisional biopsy alone. Survival appears to relate most closely to the stage of disease.

▶ Malignant lymphomas occurring in the breast are uncommon, but recognition of these neoplasms is important, as distinction from poorly differentiated carcinomas can be difficult. It is of interest that clinical, morphological, and immunologic features of some cases reported in this study are similar to recently described lymphomas of mucosa-associated lymphoid tissue (1).—J.B. Cousar, M.D.

Reference

1. Isaacson PG: *Histopathology* 16:617–619, 1990.

TABLE 2.—Clinical Characteristics of Primary Breast Lymphomas*

Patient no.	Age (yr)	Size (cm)	Site	Stage	Surgery	Histologic condition	Further treatment	Survival
1	35	4	R breast	I	Biopsy	D-LNC	3 cycles of CHOP, followed by RT	Recurrence in brain in 10 mos; AWD at 11 mo
2	53	1.5	R breast (mammographic lesion)	I	Biopsy	D-M SC + LC	None until recurrence; then RT and CHOP	Recurrence in brain in 18 mo; recurrence in R breast in 25 mo; recurrence in L breast in 41 mo; AWD at 41 mo
3	44	4	R breast	I	Biopsy	D-SCC	None	Alive NED 109 mo
4	67	1	R breast	I	Biopsy; mastectomy after recurrence	D-LNC	Chlorambucil	Recurrence in breast in 6 mo; lungs in <15 mo; DOD in 15 mo
5	49	2.2	R breast	I	Biopsy	D-LNC; IBL features	8 cycles of cytoxan, adriamycin, vincristine	Alive NED at 57 mo
6	44	NA	R breast	I	Biopsy	F-M SC + LC	None	Alive NED at 108 mo
7	47	1.5	R breast	I	Biopsy	F&D-M SC + LC	RT followed by 6 cycles of vincristine, alkeran and prednisone	Died of other causes at 48 mo; NED by autopsy
8	54	NA	R breast	II	Biopsy	D-LNC; IBL features	CHOP; may get RT	Alive NED at 10 mo

9	56	NA	L breast	I	Biopsy	D-M SC + LC	RT	Alive NED at 109 mo
10	35	NA	R breast	I	Biopsy	D-M SC + LC	8 cycles of CHOP	Recurrence in sub-Q at 44 mo; AWD at 48 mo
11	49	3.5	L breast	I	Radical mastectomy	D-LCC	None	Died of disseminated disease at 78 mo; was NED when lost to FU at 36 mo
12	50	2.5	R breast	I	Radical mastectomy	D-LCC	None	NED when lost to FU at 16 mo
13	61	1.2	L breast	I	Biopsy	D-LNC	CHOP	Recurrence in neck node at 39 mo; alive at 86 mo
14	74	3	L breast	I	Unknown	D-LNC; IBL features	Unknown	Recurrence in opposite breast and pelvic mass at 73 mo; AWD at 86 mo
15	88	20	L breast	II	Radical mastectomy	D-LNC; IBL features	None	Alive NED at 30 mo
16	83	NA	R breast	II	Biopsy	D-LNC	RT	Recurred in epitrochlear, axillary, and inguinal nodes at 6 mo; DOD at 13 mo

**Abbreviations: D-LCC*, diffuse large cleaved cell; *D-LNC*, diffuse large noncleaved cell; *D-SCC*, diffuse small cleave cell; *D-M SC + LC*, diffuse mixed small and large cell; *F-M SC + LC*, follicular mixed small and large cell; *F&D-M SC + LC*, follicular and diffuse mixed small cell and large cell; *IBL*, immunoblastic; *RT*, radiation therapy; *CHOP*, cyclophosphamide, hydroxydaunomycin, vincristine, and predisone; *FU*, follow-up; *NED*, no evidence of disease; *AWD*, alive with disease; *DOD*, dead of disease; *NA*, not available.

(Courtesy of Cohen PL, Brooks JJ: *Cancer* 67:1359–1369, 1991.)

Metastatic Tumors to the Female Breast: An Autopsy Study of 12 Cases

Di Bonito L, Luchi M, Giarelli L, Falconieri G, Viehl P (Univ of Trieste, Italy; Inst Curie, Paris)

Path Res Pract 187:482–486, 1991 11–7

Background.—Metastatic tumors to the female breast are rare. Prompt recognition of these tumors allows proper treatment to the primary tumor and thus avoids unnecessary mutilating breast surgery. The clinical and pathologic records of 12 women with metastatic tumors to the breast seen during a 19-year period were reviewed.

Findings.—The metastatic tumors of the breast were discovered incidentally at autopsy in 10 patients and diagnosed before death in 2; in 1 of the latter patients the tumor was misinterpreted as a primary. There were 4 malignant melanomas; 2 each of ovarian, renal, and gastric adenocarcinoma; and 1 each of pulmonary and pancreatic carcinoma. In both patients with gastric cancer, the breast was the only extra-abdominal site of metastases. One tumor showed a typical signet-ring cell pattern associated with massive gastric wall thickening and prominent perigastric lymph node, but not axillary node, involvement. The mean age of the patients was 58.5 years; those with melanoma were younger (mean age, 49.7 years). Half of the patients had bilateral breast metastases. The average interval between the diagnosis of primary tumor and occurrence of breast metastases was 2.5 years.

Conclusions.—Metastatic tumors to the breast are rare; an overall frequency ranging from 1.7% to 6.6% has been reported previously in necropsy studies. In addition to hematologic malignancy, melanoma and lung carcinoma are the most common metastatic tumors. Unfortunately, most of the suggested criteria that distinguish between primary and metastatic tumors to the breast are disputable. Pathologists should be wary when studying unusual histotypes in frozen or permanent paraffin-embedded sections. Further studies are warranted to define more sensitive diagnostic criteria.

12 Endocrine Disorders

The Pituitary Gland in Pregnancy: A Clinicopathologic and Immunohistochemical Study of 69 Cases

Scheithauer BW, Sano T, Kovacs KT, Young WF Jr, Ryan N, Randall RV (Mayo Clinic and Found, Rochester, Minn; St Michael's Hosp, Toronto)

Mayo Clin Proc 65:461–474, 1990 12–1

Introduction.—The pituitary gland enlarges during pregnancy; both the number and size of the chromophobic cells are increased. A detailed immunohistochemical study was made of the cellular components of the

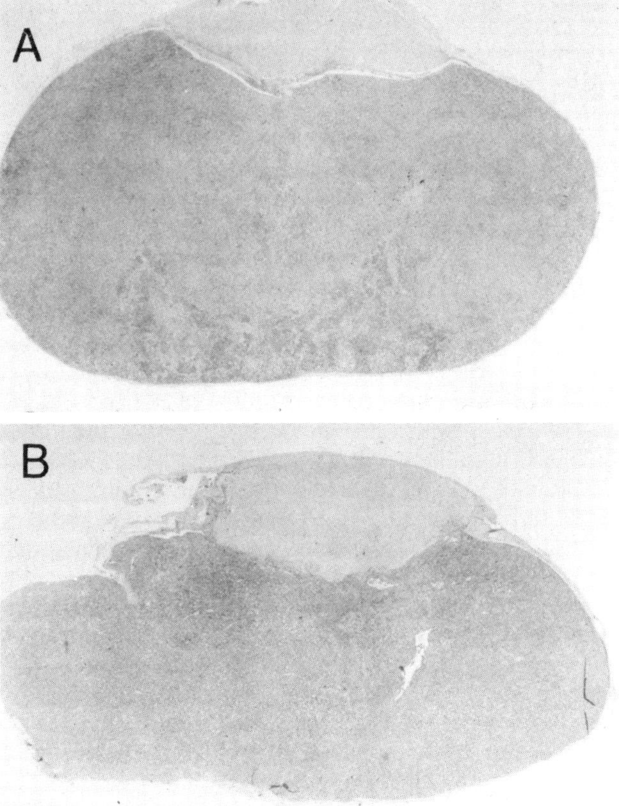

Fig 12–1.—Photographs of pituitary glands, showing hypertrophy in pregnancy. Pituitary from 32-year-old pregnant patient (gravida 10, para 9, abortion 1) at term, shown in horizontal section (**A**) dwarfs that of a nulliparous control (**B**). (Hematoxylin-eosin; original magnification, ×6.) (Courtesy of Scheithauer BW, Sano T, Kovacs KT, et al: *Mayo Clin Proc* 65:461–474, 1990.)

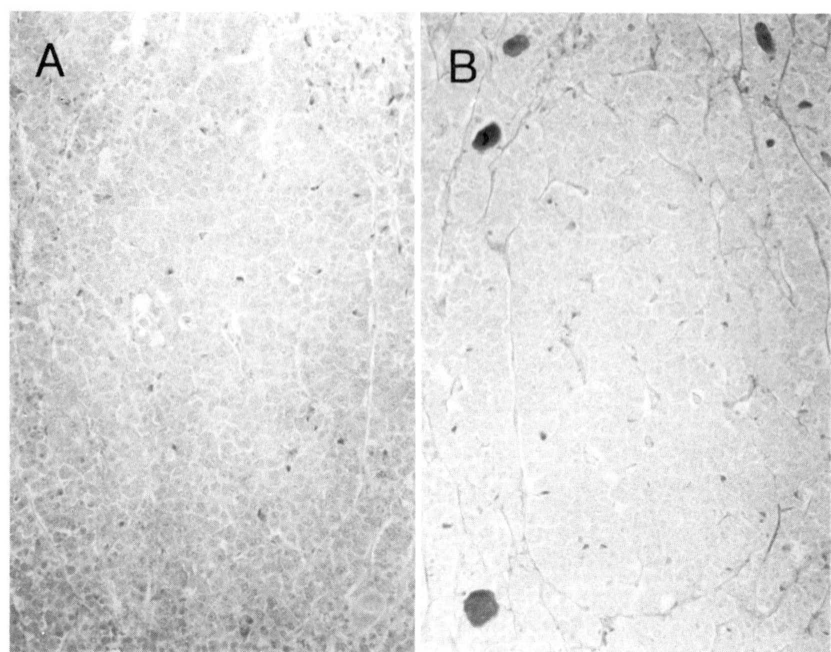

Fig 12–2.—Hyperplasia of prolactin cells, characterized by their relative abundance of chromophobic cytoplasm, causes not only a diffuse increase of such cells but also nodular aggregates (**A**), which result from expansions of the cord architecture (**B**). (Hematoxylin-eosin; original magnification, ×160.) (Courtesy of Scheithauer BW, Sano T, Kovacs KT, et al: *Mayo Clin Proc* 65:461–474, 1990.)

pituitary gland during all phases of pregnancy and the postpartum state. Glands were obtained at autopsy from 69 women who died during pregnancy, in the postpartum period, or after abortion. The mean age was 31 years.

Findings.—Pituitary enlargement was evident on gross inspection (Fig 12–1). Gland size incrased progressively during pregnancy and decreased in the postpartum period. The most conspicuous change was an increase in prolactin-secreting cells (Fig 12–2). Mitotic activity was readily apparent in prolactin-immunoreactive cells (Fig 12–3). Nonlactating patients generally exhibited less prolactin cell immunoreactivity at 1 month. Prolactin cell counts increased during pregnancy, whereas the number of growth hormone cells was relatively reduced. No significant changes in corticotrophic cells were noted. Gonadotropic cells were much less reactive during pregnancy. Thyrotropic cells were unchanged. Eight isolated adenomas were found in the study population.

Discussion.—Pituitary enlargement during pregnancy reflects a diffuse hyperplasia of prolactin cells, or so-called "pregnancy cells," which begins at 1 month and continues throughout gestation. Gonadotropic cells have a lowered hormone content during pregnancy. There is no evidence that pregnancy initiates the formation of pituitary adenomas or promotes their growth.

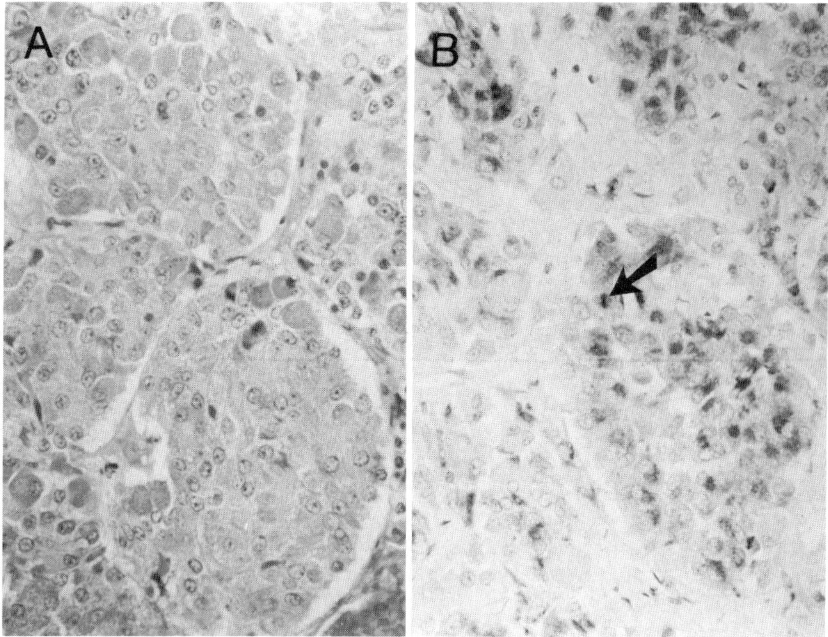

Fig 12–3.—Hyperplastic lactotrophs or "pregnancy cells" are large and chromophobic in appearance (**A**). On immunostain for prolactin, they show both a diffuse and Golgi pattern of reactivity (**B**). Because of their relative abundance, many cords appear to consist entirely of such cells. Mitotic activity (*arrow*), a highly unusual feature in otherwise normal pituitary glands, is a common finding in pregnancy. (×400.) (Courtesy of Scheithauer BW, Sano T, Kovacs KT, et al: *Mayo Clin Proc* 65:461–474, 1990.)

▶ Enlargement of the pituitary gland has long been recognized as part of normal pregnancy. After careful investigation, the authors of this article found that enlargement of the pituitary gland in this setting is caused by an increase in both size and number of chromophobic cells. The latter were immunoreactive for prolactin but not for other pituitary hormones. Routine histochemical studies and immunocytologic preparations show that the increase of chromophobic cells begins at 1 month and continues until delivery. The findings are very significant in the field of pituitary hormones in pregnancy, and further studies are warranted.—S.W. Wong, M.D.

Multiple Adenomas of the Human Pituitary: A Retrospective Autopsy Study With Clinical Implications

Kontogeorgos G, Kovacs K, Horvath E, Scheithauer BW (St Michael's Hosp, Toronto; Mayo Clinic and Found, Rochester, Minn)

J Neurosurg 74:243–247, 1991 12–2

Background.—Most pituitary adenomas grow at a slow rate, remain small, and produce no clinical symptoms. At least a fourth of all surgically removed pituitary adenomas are endocrinologically inactive. Although

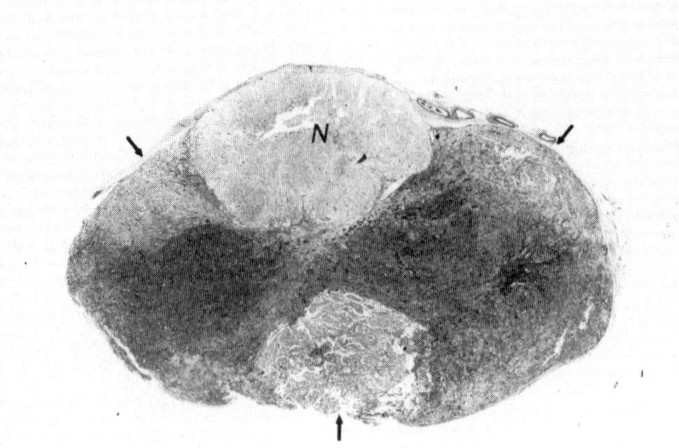

Fig 12–4.—Pituitary gland harboring 3 adenomas *(arrows)*, 2 in the lateral wing and 1 in the median wedge. *N*, neural lobe. Hematoxylin-phloxine-saffron; original magnification, ×5.4. (Courtesy of Kontogeorgos G, Kovacs K, Horvath E, et al: *J Neurosurg* 74:243–247, 1991.)

most pituitary adenomas are solitary tumors, sporadic cases of multiple adenomas have been reported. The autopsy material from 2 centers was reviewed to describe the clinicopathologic features of multiple adenomas.

Methods.—The combined study material consisted of 20 pituitary glands containing multiple adenomas obtained from 11 men and 9 women (mean age, 69 years at the time of death). All 20 patients had died of nonendocrine causes. The total number of tumors was 44. Sixteen pituitary glands contained 2 adenomas each, and the remaining 4 contained 3 adenomas each. Thirty-four adenomas were located in the lateral wings and 10 in the median wedge.

Analysis.—Thirty of the 44 tumors were measured for size; all were microadenomas measuring from 1 mm to 7 mm. Only 5 tumors were larger than 3 mm. The tumors were round or ovoid, and were demarcated from the surrounding pituitary parenchyma (Fig 12–4). Immunocytochemical analysis revealed that 11 adenomas contained prolactin, 3 contained adrenocorticotropic hormone, 1 contained growth hormone, and 1 contained α-subunit, follicle-stimulating hormone, and luteinizing hormone. Pituitary morphology did not correlate with clincical data, except in 1 patient who appeared to have had mild acromegaly. The frequency of adenomas found randomly at autopsy in pituitary glands was 10.4%. The frequency of multiple adenomas was .9%.

Conclusion.—Although multiple pituitary adenomas are uncommon, this phenomenon may underlie surgical failure in patients in whom 1 adenoma is removed and another is left behind.

▶ This article reminds us that pituitary adenomas, not unlike bad luck, may come in pairs or triplets. Multiple adenomas of the pituitary are not uncommon; therefore, surigcal failures may be expected from time to time when one is removed and the other is left behind.—S.W. Wong, M.D.

Nuclear Grooves: Valuable Diagnostic Feature in May-Grünwald-Giemsa-Stained Fine Needle Aspirates of Papillary Carcinoma of the Thyroid

Bhambhani S, Kashyap V, Das DK (Maulana Azad Med College, New Delhi)

Acta Cytol 34:809–812, 1990 12–3

Introduction.—Recent reports have suggested that the presence of nuclear grooves (clefts, notches) is helpful in diagnosing papillary thyroid carcinoma in fine-needle aspiration specimens. In most studies an alcohol-fixed material stained with either the Papanicolaou stain or hematoxylin-eosin was used.

Study Design.—Air-dried thyroid aspirates from 80 patients were stained by the May-Grünwald-Giemsa technique. The series included 25 papillary carcinomas, 15 follicular tumors, and 6 medullary carcinomas. There also were 15 cases each of chronic lymphocytic thyroiditis and colloid goiter and 4 cases of Hürthle cell adenoma.

Observations.—The grooves included thickened ridges passing between nuclei, ridges covering most of the nuclear diameter, and a notching or invagination covering about 25% of the nuclear diameter. Linear folding of the nuclear envelope along the longitudinal nuclear axis was noted in more than 75% of the cases. Nuclear grooves were seen in nearly 90% of the papillary thyroid cancers.

Conclusion.—Nuclear grooves are markers of possible papillary thyroid carcinoma in aspirates stained by the May-Grünwald-Giemsa method.

▶ Intranuclear cytoplasmic inclusions and nuclear grooves or clefts are well known clues to the diagnosis of papillary carcinoma in Papanicolaou-stained aspirates of the thyroid. These authors confirm that the latter finding may be seen in air-dried, May-Grünwald-Giemsa stained material. Many laboratories use air-dried methods alone or in combination with Papanicolaou-stained material in the thyroid because of the ability of the former to highlight colloid, an important finding in benign aspirates.—G.F. Worsham, M.D.

Anaplastic Carcinoma of the Thyroid: A Clinicopathologic Study of 121 Cases

Venkatesh YSS, Ordonez NG, Schultz PN, Hickey RC, Goepfert H, Samaan NA (Univ of Texas, Houston)

Cancer 66:321–330, 1990 12–4

Introduction.—Up to 14% of primary thyroid carcinomas are anaplastic. Anaplastic carcinoma is extremely aggressive, with a 5-year survival rate of only 7.1% and a mean survival period of 6.2 months. The data were reviewed on 121 cases of anaplastic carcinoma of the thyroid.

Classification.—Tumors were classified as either initial anaplastic or transformed anaplastic. The latter category included patients who had well-differentiated thyroid carcinoma at presentation but in whom anaplastic carcinoma developed subsequently. The stage of disease was categorized as "gland only," "gland and nodes," "gland, nodes, and neck," or "distant disease." Survival data were calculated from the time of tissue diagnosis. Immunohistochemical studies were performed on 30 tumors.

Pathology.— Patients ranged in age from 24 to 91 years (mean, 61.3 years); only 4 patients were younger than 40 years. The series included 54 men and 67 women. The most common presentation was a rapidly enlarging neck mass, with or without previous goiter. In addition to anaplastic carcinoma, 35% of the patients had areas of well-differentiated thyroid carcinoma elsewhere and 53% had metastases. Of the latter, 88% were to the lung and 15% to the bones. Tumors that consisted primarily of spindle cells had cells with a sarcomatoid appearance that were often arranged in fascicles resembling fibrosarcoma. Some tumors consisted primarily of large anaplastic cells containing single or multiple hyperpyknotic nuclei and eosinophilic cytoplasm that sometimes had a rhabdoid-like appearance. Of the 30 tumors analyzed, 24 stained for keratin, 28 stained for vimentin, and 10 stained for epithelial membrane antigen. Men and women had similar durations of survival. The mean survival was 7.2 months, but younger patients lived longer than older patients, and those whose disease was in an earlier stage at presentation responded better to treatment than those with metastatic disease. The duration of survival was not significantly increased by radical surgery. Ten of 12 long-term survivors received combined radiation therapy and chemotherapy after operation.

Conclusions.—Anaplastic carcinoma has a bleak prognosis, but multimodality therapy may offer the possibility of long-term survival. The outcome is most hopeful in younger patients who have less disease at the time of diagnosis.

▶ This large study of anaplastic carcinomas of the thyroid emphasizes features that have been recognized previously: association with well-differentiated thyroid carcinomas in a minority of patients and a poor prognosis (12% survival in initial anaplastic and 5% survival in transformed anaplastic cases). The immunochemical findings may prove useful in differentiating this neoplasm from soft tissue sarcomas and other anaplastic neoplasms in small biopsy material.— G.F. Worsham, M.D.

Needle Tract Implantation of Papillary Carcinoma of the Thyroid Following Aspiration Biopsy

Hales MS, Hsu FSF (Eden Hosp Med Ctr, Castro Valley, Calif)

Acta Cytol 34:801–804, 1990 12–5

Background.—Needle tract seeding of thyroid tumors resulting from fine-needle aspiration (FNA) is not commonly reported and usually involves high-grade malignancies. Cutaneous metastasis of a low-grade tumor of the thyroid resulted from FNA biopsy.

Case Report.—Woman, 36, underwent evaluation of a right thyroid mass that was present for 9 years. She had undergone 2 FNA biopsies 7 years and 5 years earlier in which 20- to 21-gauge needles were used; the third was done with a 25-gauge needle. This last specimen was composed mainly of histiocytes with intracytoplasmic pigmented material. Occasional groups of epithelial cells contained a single intranuclear inclusion. These findings suggested a papillary carcinoma arising in a benign nodule. The specimen from the biopsy performed 5 years earlier showed numerous phagocytic histiocytes and epithelial clusters with distinct cell borders and intranuclear cytoplasmic inclusions, also suggesting papillary carcinoma. A report of the first biopsy described "inclusion-like structures," and the pathologist had suggested surgical excision. The patient reported a .4-cm skin nodule over the right thyroid lobe several weeks later, at the site of the most recent biopsy. Right thyroid lobectomy, isthmectomy and excisional biopsy of the skin nodule were done. The surgical specimen was a 2-cm cyst partially rimmed by a papillary carcinoma. The thyroid parenchyma showed a separate .18-cm focus of papillary carcinoma and the dermis showed a .22-cm, partially cystic, focus of carcinoma embedded in a narrow rim of collagenous scar. The patient was well with no recurrence 1 year postoperatively.

Conclusions.—Cutaneous needle tract metastasis from a papillary thyroid carcinoma is unusual in that the implant arose from an indolent, slow-growing malignancy. The apparent rarity of this complication should not challenge the overall safety of FNA biopsy.

▶ This case report reviews the literature on tumor implantation along needle tracts after FNA biopsy using needles smaller than 18 gauge (1,2). It brings the number of reports of this rare complication to 21. Although the case history implies that the cutaneous implant was related to the 25-gauge FNA biopsy, the authors conclude that it was more likely to be related to one of the earlier biopsies done with a 20- or 21-gauge needle. This report emphasizes the rarity of this occurrence despite the widespread use of this procedure and is the first case to be reported involving relatively indolent papillary carcinoma of the thyroid.—G.F. Worsham, M.D.

References

1. Glasgow BJ, et al: *Am J Ophthalmol* 105:538, 1988.
2. Glaser KS, et al: *Lancet* 1:620, 1989.

Histogenesis of the Human Adrenal Medulla: An Evaluation of the Ontogeny of Chromaffin and Nonchromaffin Lineages

Cooper MJ, Hutchins GM, Israel MA (Natl Cancer Inst, Bethesda, Md; Johns Hopkins Med Insts)

Am J Pathol 137:605–615, 1990 12–6

Background.—Previous studies of the expression of chromaffin-related genes during development of the human adrenal medulla demonstrated both chromaffin and nonchromaffin adrenal neuroblasts. An attempt was made to better characterize the presumptive nonchromaffin progenitor cells by identifying the S-100 protein and HNK-1 immunoreactivity. The S-100 protein is expressed by sustentacular cells of the medulla and HNK-1 is an antibody that recognizes migratory neural crest cells.

Methods.—Paraffin-embedded blocks of 34 specimens of fetal and neonatal adrenal glands obtained from 42 days after conception to 5 years after birth were analyzed immunohistochemically for S-100 and HNK-1, as well as for chromogranin A (CGA), a major constituent of neurosecretory granules.

Findings.—In both chromaffin and nonchromaffin cells, HNK-1 immunoreactivity was present at different times during development. This marker identified the nonchromaffin lineage in midgestation and the chromaffin lineage neonatally. The S-100 protein was identified in some nonchromaffin neuroblasts; sustentacular cells were first seen at about 28 weeks' gestation.

Conclusions.—The nonchromaffin adrenal neuroblasts may include precursors of both sustentacular and ganglion cells. These lineages may be related more closely to one another developmentally than either lineage is to the chromaffin medullary lineage. It is possible that neuroblastomas can differentiate along several different lineages. Some tumors may arise in fetal life, perhaps in association with arrested phenotypic differentiation.

▶ The authors examine the cells of origin of the adrenal medulla. Using S-100 protein and HNK-1 antibodies to identify sustentacular and migrating neural crest cells, the authors' study of nonchromaffin adrenal neuroblasts indicated a possible development into sustentacular and ganglion cells. The possibility of maturation into chromaffin cells is also suggested. The authors relate this multipotential cell behavior to the multiple types of differentiation seen in neuroblastoma, a tumor arising in the adrenal medulla. They suggest that the biological behavior of these tumors may reflect the potentials of the early neuroblasts investigated in this paper.—A.J. Garvin, M.D., Ph.D.

Prognostic Value of Immunocytologic Detection of Bone Marrow Metastases in Neuroblastoma

Moss TJ, Reynolds CP, Sather HN, Romansky SG, Hammond GD, Seeger RC (Children's Cancer Study Group, Pasadena, Calif)

N Engl J Med 324:219–226, 1991 12–7

Introduction.—Conventional bone marrow examination has been a routine means of clinically staging neuroblastoma. Specific immunostaining of malignant cells using monoclonal antibodies should be a more sensitive procedure and might improve the detection of metastasis.

Methods.—Marrow aspirates obtained from 197 patients with neuroblastoma were analyzed. Immunoperoxidase staining employed monoclonal antibodies reacting strongly with neuroblastoma cells but not with normal marrow cells.

Findings.—Forty-six percent of patients had tumor cells in routine smears and trephine-biopsy specimens. In contrast, 67% were positive by immunocytologic analysis. The latter study detected marrow metastasis in 34% of the patients who were thought to have localized or regional disease. In cases of widespread disease, the immunocytologic study detected tumor cells that were not apparent on conventional study. Among patients with stage II or III disease diagnosed after age 1 year, those with occult marrow metastasis did poorly whereas those free of such disease did well. In patients with stage IV disease diagnosed before age 1 year, those with few or absent marrow metastases did relatively well.

Conclusion.—Immunocytologic study is a sensitive means of detecting marrow metastases of neuroblastoma and a good prognostic guide. The present findings illustrate the biological heterogeneity of neuroblastoma.

▶ The detection of occult metastasis in lymph nodes and bone marrow can be enhanced by the use of monoclonal antibodies. In this study of neuroblastoma patients, 34% of those thought to be marrow negative were in fact marrow positive. The ultimate prognosis, however, was also dependent on the patient's age and stage of the tumor. The use of mixtures of different monoclonal antibodies also was necessary to identify these occult metastases.—A.J. Garvin, M.D., Ph.D.

Clinical Relevance of Tumor Cell Ploidy and N-*myc* Gene Amplification in Childhood Neuroblastoma: A Pediatric Oncology Group Study

Look AT, Hayes FA, Shuster JJ, Douglass EC, Castleberry RP, Bowman LC, Smith EI, Brodeur GM (St Jude Children's Research Hosp, Memphis; Univ of Tennessee, Memphis; Univ of Florida; Univ of Alabama; Southwestern Med School, Dallas; et al)

J Clin Oncol 9:581–591, 1991 12–8

Background.—Neuroblastoma is a childhood tumor arising in the adrenal medulla and sympathetic nervous system. Tumor cell DNA content accurately discriminates between infants with disseminated neuroblastoma who will and will noat respond to cyclophosphamide and doxorubicin. The results of combined studies of DNA ploidy, karyotype, and N-*myc* copy number and their relationship to survival were examined in 298 children with neuroblastoma.

Findings.—Diploid tumor stem lines were identified in 34%, clonal hyperdiploid abnormalities in 65%, and hypodiploid stem lines in 1%. Ploidy had a highly age-dependent influence on prognosis in children with widely disseminated tumors at diagnosis. Among children younger than 12 months of age who were treated with cyclophosphamide-doxorubicin, hyperdiploidy was closely related to long-term disease-free survival, whereas diploidy predicted early treatment failures. In children aged 12–24 months treated with cisplatin-teniposide and cyclophosphamide-doxorubicin, diploidy consistently predicted early failure. Half of the children with hyperdiploidy, in contrast, attained long-term disease-free survival. In children older than 24 months with stage D tumors, there was no relationship between ploidy and treatment outcome. These children had a very low probability of long-term disease-free survival. N-*myc* gene amplification was found in 25% of the 147 tumors tested; the rest showed single-copy levels of the gene. N-*myc* gene amplification occurred more often in diploid than in hyperdiploid tumors and predicted a high likelihood of early treatment failure.

Conclusions.—These findings stress the importance of tumor stage and age at diagnosis in planning treatment and predicting outcomes in children with neuroblastoma. Among children younger than 24 months with disseminated disease, tumor cell ploidy and N-*myc* gene copy number provide complementary prognostic information that can distinguish children who can be cured with current regimens from those for whom new strategies are needed.

▶ Neuroblastoma is a childhood cancer associated with a survival rate of approximately 45%. Many attempts have been made to identify those patients who do not respond to routine therapy in order to provide a more aggressive chemotherapeutic regimen. Two characteristics of the tumor cells, the chromosome number (ploidy) and the number of copies of a proto-oncogene, N-*myc,* can be related to response to therapy. To measure those characteristics, fresh tissue from the tumor is required for flow cytometry/cytogenetics as well as Southern blots. This tissue should be obtained at the time of diagnosis and preserved for the optimal measurements of these properties.—A.J. Garvin, M.D., Ph.D.

Combined Analysis of DNA Ploidy Index and N-*myc* Genomic Content in Neuroblastoma

Bourhis J, DeVathaire F, Wilson GD, Hartmann O, Terrier-Lacombe MJ, Boccon-Gibod L, McNally NJ, Lemerle J, Riou G, Bénard J (Institut Gustave Roussy, Villejuif, France; Mt Vernon Hosp, Northwood, Middlesex, England; Hôpital Trousseau, Paris)

Cancer Res 51:33–36, 1991 12–9

Objective.—N-*myc* gene amplification and DNA ploidy index are reliable prognostic predictors in neuroblastoma. The prognostic effects of both N-*myc* amplification and DNA ploidy index were studied in a group of nonselected patients with neuroblastoma, taking into account potential confounding factors such as age and stage.

Methods.—The N-*myc* genomic content was analyzed by Southern blot hybridization, and the DNA ploidy index was analyzed by flow cytometry on neuroblastoma specimens obtained from 59 unselected patients. At diagnosis, 23 patients were younger than 1 year of age; 31 patients had stage IV disease, 10 had stage III, 5 had stage II, 8 had stage I, and 4 had stage IV-S.

Findings.—N-*myc* amplification was present in 9 tumors, including 1 stage IV-S, 2 stage III, and 6 stage IV tumors. Twenty-six neuroblastomas were diploid and 33 were aneuploid. Of the latter, 28 were near-triploid with DNA indexes between 1.25 and 1.68, 4 were near-diploid with DNA indexes up to 1.18, and 1 was hypotetraploid with DNA index of

1.85. There was a statistically significant correlation between the ploidy index and N-*myc* amplification; none of the 28 near-triploid neuoblastomas exhibited N-*myc* gene amplification, compared with 9 of 31 diploid, near-diploid, and hypotetraploid tumors. In addition, a significant proportion of near-triploid tumors occurred in patients younger than 1 year of age and those with stages I, II, and IV-S tumors.

Univariate analysis showed 4 factors that were significantly associated with a high risk of relapse: age, stage, DNA ploidy, and N-*myc* amplification. Multivariate analysis showed that only DNA index and N-*myc* amplification remained significantly associated with a high risk of relapse. The relative risk of relapse was threefold greater in tumors with N-*myc* amplification ≥3 copy number compared with <3 copy number, and ninefold greater among diploid or near-diploid tumors than near-triploid tumors.

Implications.—These findings suggest that the combined analysis of N-*myc* gene content and DNA index is a powerful indicator of tumor relapse in neuroblastomas. The combination of N-*myc* and DNA index should be included in routine management of neuroblastomas.

▶ This study demonstrates the importance of ancillary studies such as DNA index and N-*myc* amplification combined with the clinical information of age and stage for the routine managment of neuroblastomas. Of note is that each parameter does not always correlate with prognosis, but the combination gives the best profile for management.—A.J. Garvin, M.D., Ph.D.

Histopathology of Benign Versus Malignant Sympathoadrenal Paragangliomas: Clinicopathologic Study of 120 Cases Including Unusual Histologic Features

Linnoila RI, Keiser HR, Steinberg SM, Lack EE (Navy Hosp, Bethesda, Md; Natl Heart, Lung, and Blood Inst; Natl Cancer Inst, Bethesda, Md; Georgetown Univ)

Hum Pathol 21:1168–1180, 1990 12–10

Background.—Adrenal glands sometimes serve as the starting point for sympathoadrenal paragangliomas, rare tumors not often found in general practice. These tumors can also initiate in extra-adrenal sites (e.g., the pelvic floor). Logistic regression analysis was made of 16 nonhistologic and histologic parameters used to predict the biological behavior of these tumors.

Methods.—The medical records of the 120 patients (60 females, 60 males) with sympathoadrenal paragangliomas were examined. An average of 8 slides was available for analysis. Logistic regression analysis using PROC LOGIST of SAS was used to identify a predictive relationship between the clinicopathologic factors and the biologic behavior of the tumors.

Findings.—Clinical data were examined for 98 patients. The paragangliomas were clinically benign in 64 patients and malignant in 34. The

Histologic Features of Clinically Benign and Malignant Sympathoadrenal Paragangliomas

Histologic Features	Number of Tumors [n(%)] Malignant (n = 34)	Benign (n = 64)
Architectural pattern		
Alveolar (nesting, "zellballen")	15 (44)	19 (30)
Trabecular (anastomosing cords)	7 (21)	19 (30)
Mixed alveolar/trabecular	11 (33)	24 (38)
Diffuse/solid	0	2 (3)
Confluent tumor necrosis*	11 (32)	4 (6)
Mitotic rate (mean per 30 HPF, range)	3 (0-18)	1 (1-10)
Nuclear hyperchromasia/pleomorphism (mean in scale 1 to 3)	1.9	1.7
Extensive local invasion or vascular invasion*	11 (32)	7 (11)
Hyaline globules*	8 (32)	38 (59)
Features resembling ganglion cells	2 (6)	14 (22)
Proteinaceous material	4 (12)	16 (25)

*A statistically significant difference ($P_2 < .05$) between clinically malignant and benign tumors was found for the following: confluent tumor necrosis ($P_2 = .0023$), extensive local invasion ($P_2 = .022$), and hyaline globules ($P_2 = .0013$) by Fisher's exact test. The difference in features resembling ganglion cells (6% vs. 22%) was not statistically significant ($P_2 = .07$).

(Courtesy of Linnoila RI, Keiser HR, Steinberg SM, et al: *Hum Pathol* 21:1168–1180, 1990.)

average age of the patients with malignant tumors was 35.5 years. The malignant paragangliomas were significantly more often extra-adrenal than were the benign lesions. The pheochromocytomas of multiple endocrine neoplasia syndrome type 2 were bilateral in 8 of 17 patients, with a distinctive gross appearance. The table presents the histologic results from both the benign and the malignant paragangliomas. These were not different from each other with regard to overall architectural patterns or degree of nuclear hyperchromasia or pleomorphism. Mitotic shapes appeared in 45% of the benign lesions and in 65% of the malignant tumors. Regression analysis demonstrated that the most accurate parameters for predicting malignant tumors included extra-adrenal location, coarse tumor nodularity or multinodularity, confluent tumor necrosis, and lack of intracytoplasmic hyaline globules.

Conclusions.—Clinically benign and malignant sympathoadrenal paragangliomas have some different nonhistologic and histologic characteristics. Long-term clinical follow-up is required, however, to verify the overall usefulness of these factors in diagnosis.

▶ Neither gross nor microscopic features reliably predictive of malignant behavior have been identified for sympathoadrenal paragangliomas. However, this large series suggests that certain characteristics may be of value. The features outlined here (i.e., extra-adrenal location, coarse tumor nodularity, confluent tumor necrosis, and absence of hyaline globules), when present in the aggregate, appear to portend malignant behavior. Conceivably, recognition of these features and other molecular changes conferring abnormal growth regulation, invasiveness, and loss of cellular differentiation (i.e, reduced neuropetide synthesis) may afford early identification of malignant potential.—M. Johnson, M.D., Ph.D.

Extraadrenal Retroperitoneal Paragangliomas: Natural History and Response to Treatment

Sclafani LM, Woodruff JM, Brennan MF (Mem Sloan-Kettering Cancer Ctr, New York)

Surgery 108:1124–1130, 1990 12–11

Background.—Because extra-adrenal retroperitoneal paragangliomas are uncommon tumors, there is little information about their natural history and response to treatment. Data were reviewed on a relatively large series of patients with these tumors, treated at a single institution.

Patients.—Twelve men and 10 women (mean age, 42 years) with retroperitoneal paragangliomas were treated during a 41-year period. The mean follow-up time was 62 months for survivors and 75 months for those who died. Functional tumors were present in 8 patients. Ten patients were admitted with pain and 4 with a mass. The duration of symptoms, tumor size, and survival were similar whether tumors were functional or nonfunctional.

Outcome.—Fifty percent of the paragangliomas were classified as malignant because of metastasis. The 5-year disease-free survival rates were 19% for patients with nonresected tumors and 75% for those with completely resected tumors. The 10-year disease-free survival rates were 19% and 45%, respectively. The 5-year survival rate was 36% for metastatic tumors, the longest survival in this group being 76 months. Complete tumor resection was a predictor of survival, but tumor size and functional status were not. A clinical response was seen in some patients who received chemotherapy or radiotherapy, but there was no survival benefit.

Conclusions.—Aggressive surgery is indicated for retroperitoneal paragangliomas because of their high rate of malignant behavior. Patients must be followed for a long time because late metastasis may occur. Survival may be prolonged even after metastasis has occurred.

▶ This series documents the natural history of retroperitoneal paragangliomas. Half of the tumors were classified as malignant on the basis of metastasis. Complete surgical resection of the malignant tumors was an important predictor in survival.—A.J. Garvin, M.D., Ph.D.

13 Musculoskeletal System and Soft Tissue

Histopathology of Metastatic Temporal Bone Tumors

Nelson EG, Hinojosa R (Univ of Chicago)

Arch Otolaryngol Head Neck Surg 117:189–193, 1991 13–1

Introduction.—Temporal bone metastases are being reported at an increasing rate. Data were reviewed on a series of 60 temporal bones from 33 patients with metastatic malignancy; cases of lymphoma and leukemia were excluded. The specimens were collected over more than 50 years. Nineteen different primary malignancies were represented, with breast cancer being most frequent.

Findings.—Metastases were bilateral in 27 cases. Metastases secondary to hematogenous spread were present in the petrous apex. Tumors that metastasized to the meninges and involved the temporal bone secondarily were found in the internal auditory canal. Head-neck tumors extending directly to the temporal bone most often involved the petrous apex and foramen lacerum. Only 10 patients had a history of otologic symptoms, usually hearing loss. Diffuse metastases were present throughout the body in all cases of hematogenous or meningeal spread. In 1 case of hematogenous metastases a vascular otosclerotic focus was involved by metastatic tumor.

Discussion.—The findings in these cases represent an end-stage process. Temporal bone metastases often do not produce symptoms, even in patients with advanced disease.

▶ Utilizing the unusual resource of a collection of more than 1,200 temporal bones acquired in a 53-year autopsy experience, the authors performed a very detailed study of metastatic cancer in the temporal bones from 33 patients. All of the patients also had metastases elsewhere in the body, but only a third of the temporal bone metastases resulted in symptoms. In only 2 cases did the symptoms lead to the diagnosis of the primary tumor or metastatic disease. The authors also include a review of 148 cases of temporal bone metastases from the literature. This unique study sheds an interesting light on the patterns of involvement of the temporal bone by metastatic cancer.—J.A. Tucker, M.D.

Prognostic Value of Histopathology in Ewing's Sarcoma: Long-Term Follow-Up of Distal Extremity Primary Tumors

Hartman KR, Triche TJ, Kinsella TJ, Miser JS (Walter Reed Army Med Ctr, Washington, DC; Childrens Hosp Los Angeles/Univ of Southern California; Univ of Wisconsin Clinical Cancer Ctr, Madison; Mayo Clinic and Found, Rochester, Minn)

Cancer 67:163–171, 1991 13–2

Background.—Unlike most common childhood tumors, Ewing's sarcoma has no generally accepted, prognostically useful histopathologic criteria. The histopathologic findings and clinical course in a series of Ewing's sarcoma patients were reviewed.

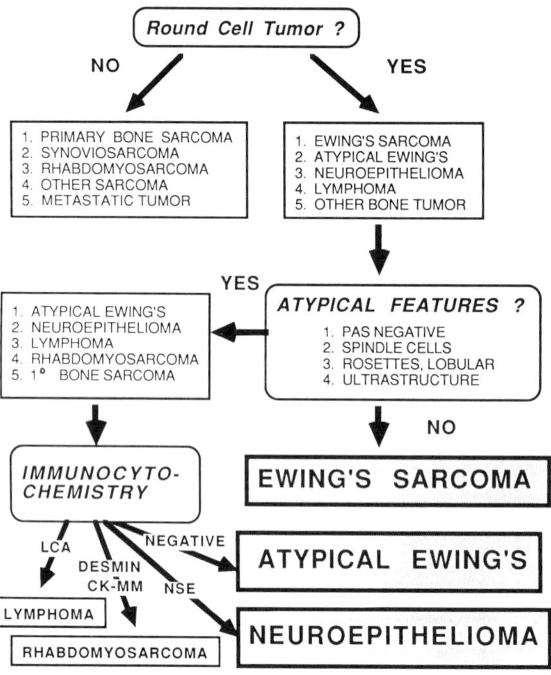

Fig 13–1.—Diagnosis of Ewing's sarcoma. This flow chart illustrates the sequence of decisions made in the process of arriving at a diagnosis of Ewing's sarcoma or related tumors (atypical Ewing's, peripheral neuroepithelioma, or other) in the present study. First, all non–round cell tumors were excluded *(first rounded box)*. Second, any atypical features *(second rounded box)* resulted in exclusion from the typical Ewing's sarcoma category *(first shaded box)*. Third, cases categorized as atypical were subjected to diagnostic immunocytochemistry (in parallel with matched typical cases); cases negative for all markers were simply categorized as atypical *(second shaded box)*. Positive results with NSE (and negativity for the muscle markers desmin and CK-MM) resulted in a diagnosis of peripheral neuroepithelioma *(third shaded box)*. Positive muscle markers or panhematopoietic markers resulted in diagnosis of rhabdomyosarcoma and lymphoma, respectively. The single primary sarcoma of bone was a round cell tumor categorized as atypical, and osteoblastic in particular, based on ultrastructural findings. (Courtesy of Hartman KR, Triche TJ, Kinsella TJ, et al: *Cancer* 67:163–171, 1991.)

Methods.—The series included 56 children with primary tumors of the distal extremities enrolled in Ewing's sarcoma study protocols during a 16-year period. Diagnostic material was obtained and reviewed in blinded fashion. Tumors were categorized histologically into 3 diagnostic groups, based on recent pathologic criteria; typical Ewing's sarcoma, atypical Ewing's sarcoma, and other (mainly peripheral neuroepithelioma) (Fig 13–1). The patients' records were reviewed for clinical data, and survival analyses were done.

Results.—Typical Ewing's sarcoma was present in 57% of the patients and atypical Ewing's sarcoma in 23%; 20% of the patients comprised the "other" category. Thirteen percent had peripheral neuroepithelioma; there were 2 cases of primitive rhabdomyosarcoma and 1 each of primitive bone sarcoma and synovial sarcoma. At diagnosis, disease was localized in 45 patients and metastatic in 11. Metastasis was present in only 2 of 32 patients with typical Ewing's sarcoma, compared with 9 of the remaining 24 patients. Of the latter group, 5 had lymph node metastases and 2 had brain metastases. The histologic grouping was independently prognostic of clinical outcome in patients with localized disease, although metastatic disease was a strongly negative prognostic factor. Overall survival was improved in patients with typical osseous Ewing's sarcoma, whereas disease-free survival was poorer in patients in the other 2 groups.

Conclusions.—In Ewing's sarcoma, any atypical appearance, neuroectodermal or otherwise, is associated with a poorer prognosis. This finding is particularly important because there are no generally accepted histopathologic prognostic criteria for this tumor. These findings must be confirmed in larger retrospective series and in prospective studies.

▶ Ewing's sarcoma is one of the common round cell tumors of childhood. In this report, the authors define the histologic and histochemical criteria for a diagnosis of "atypical" Ewing's sarcoma. The atypical features are defined in the flow diagram of Figure 13–1 and the criteria for the diagnosis of other tumors are presented. The histologic features as first described by James Ewing plus the requirement for diastase-sensitive, glycogen-containing tumors were used to define the typical cases. Based on these criteria, the authors found that survival was improved in the group with typical compared to the group with atypical Ewing's and other round cell tumors.

Although the number of cases in the "atypical" group (13) and in the "other" diagnoses group (11) was small, this study suggests that these histologic criteria may predict survival in patients with Ewing's sarcoma. Additional studies need to be performed with the additional criterion of the presence of a known 11:22 chromosomal translocation.—A.J. Garvin, M.D., Ph.D.

Chondrosarcomas of the Synovium

Bertoni F, Unni KK, Beabout JW, Sim FH (Mayo Clinic and Found, Rochester, Minn)

Cancer 67:155–162, 1991 13–3

Background.—No clear radiographic or histologic criteria exist to distinguish chondrosarcoma from synovial chondromatosis in the clinical setting. Data were reviewed on 10 patients with synovial chondromatosis in an attempt to define features that characterize the 2 conditions.

Patients.—The clinical charts, radiographs, and microscopic slides of 6 women and 4 men aged 30–70 years were studied. Five lesions were located in the knee, 3 in the hip, and 1 each in the elbow and the ankle.

Findings.—Radiographs, available for 9 of the 10 patients, all had evidence of a soft tissue mass at the involved joint. Four patients had calcifications in the soft tissue, and 3 had marginal erosion of bone at

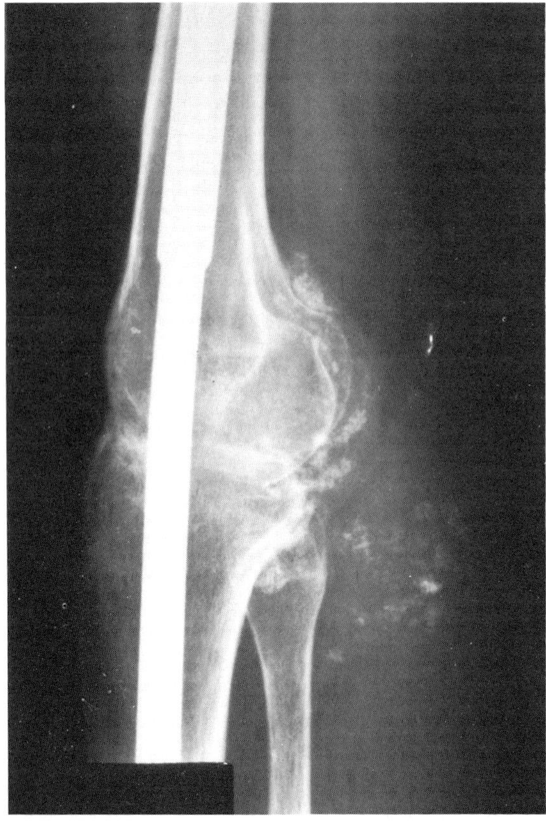

Fig 13–2.—Lateral view. Postoperative recurrence of soft tissue mass in knee. Mass contains clumps of calcification that suggest diagnosis of synovial chondromatosis. (Courtesy of Bertoni F, Unni KK, Beabout JW, et al: *Cancer* 67:155–162, 1991.)

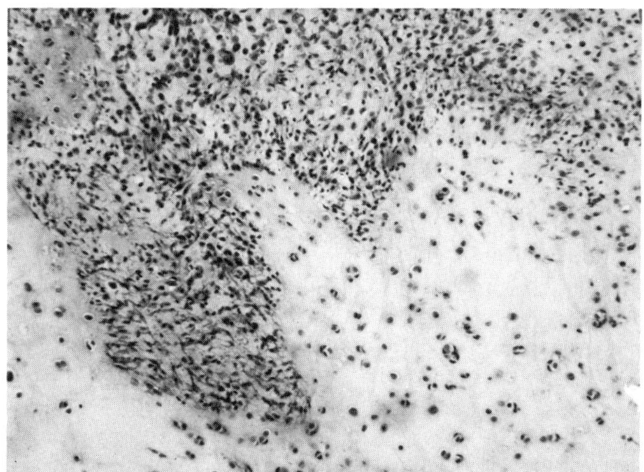

Fig 13–3.—Areas of synovial chondromatosis associated with areas in which cells lose clustering effect and have a sheetlike arrangement. Hypercellularity with small undifferentiated and spindle cells, features of grade 2 chondrosarcoma associated with synovial chondromatosis (hematoxylin-eosin; ×110). (Courtesy of Bertoni F, Unni KK, Beabout JW, et al: *Cancer* 67:155–162, 1991.)

the involved joint. For those patients with tumor calcification, synovial chondromatosis was the most likely diagnosis (Fig 13–2). In patients with uncalcified tissue, the suggested diagnoses included chronic synovitis, pigmented villonodular synovitis, and synovial chondromatosis. Five patients had histologic evidence of synovial chondromatosis, and in 3 of these 5 both synovial chondromatosis and chondrosarcoma were present at diagnosis (Fig 13–3). Synovial chondromatosis was characterized by nodules of metaplastic cartilage in the synovium, with chondrocytes arranged in groups surrounded by abundant intervening matrix. Chondrosarcoma was distinguished by a nodular lesion with an extending or permeative edge, with chondrocytes lined up in sheets without a clustering pattern. Myxoid change of the matrix with formation of microcysts was present in 6 cases, with focal necrosis in 4. One patient was lost to follow-up. All of the other 9 patients had a recurrence within 2–26 months after surgery. Although wide excision margins and aggressive operative techniques were used, 5 patients had metastatic disease.

Conclusions.—The clinical features and radiographic evidence did not help to distinguish synovial chondromatosis from chondrosarcoma. The characteristics most useful for diagnosis include qualitative differences in the cartilage in the various areas of the tumor, the myxoid change in matrix, hypercellularity with crowding and spindling of nuclei at the edge (a sign of malignancy), and necrosis, which indicates malignancy.

▶ The article delineates clearly the morphological distinction between chondrosarcoma and synovial chondromatosis in contrast to the inability of radiologic and clinical features to do so.—A.J. Garvin, M.D., Ph.D.

Histopathological Grading of Soft Tissue Tumours: Prognostic Significance in a Prospective Study of 278 Consecutive Cases

Jensen OM, Høgh J, Østgaard SE, Nordentoft AM, Sneppen O (Univ of Aarhus, Denmark)

J Pathol 163:19–24, 1991 13–4

Background.—A system of grading soft tissue tumors, described in 1983, is based on the histogenetic type and subtype of tumor, the number of mitoses, the degree of cellularity, anaplasia, and necrosis. The system was applied to 278 soft tissue sarcomas assessed prospectively between 1979 and 1988.

Methods.—Specimens were fixed in formalin and embedded in paraffin; subsequent sections were stained with hematoxylin and eosin. Certain tumors (e.g., embryonal and alveolar rhabdomyosarcomas, synovial sarcomas, and osteosarcomas and chondrosarcomas) were classified *a priori* as high-grade lesions. Liposarcomas were graded by subtype; those that were well differentiated were considered low grade, whereas myxoid lesions were intermediate and pleomorphic ones were high-grade tumors. Other tumors were designated grade 1 if there was less than 1 mitosis in 10 high-power fields of viable areas of tumor, grade 2 if there were 1–5 mitoses, and grade 3 when more than 5 mitoses were observed.

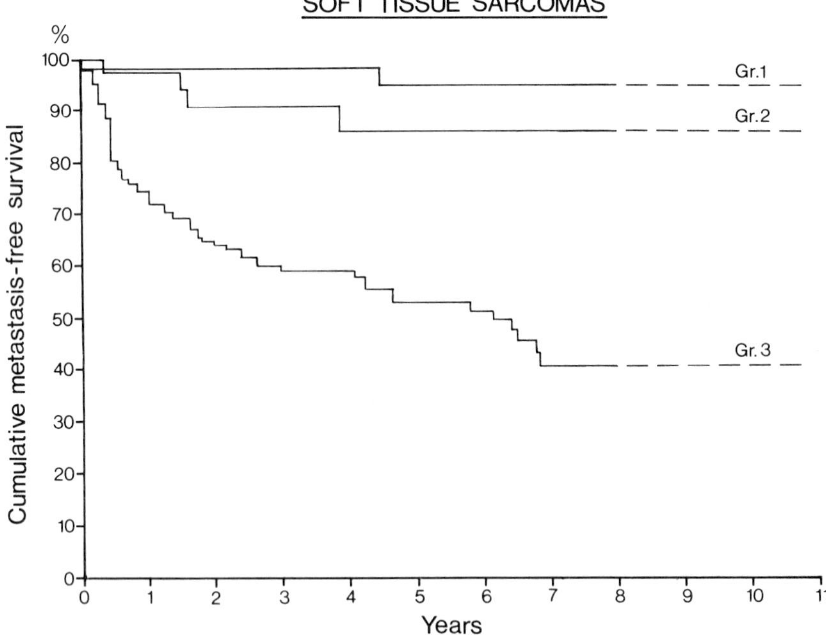

Fig 13–4.—Metastasis-free survival (disease-free survival) in relation to histopathologic grade of malignancy in 248 patients with soft tissue sarcomas (30 patients with metastasis at referral are excluded). The difference between survival in grades 1 + 2 and grade 3 is highly significant ($p < .0001$). (Courtesy of Jensen OM, Høgh J, Østgaard SE, et al: *J Pathol* 163:19–24, 1991.)

Soft Tissue Sarcomas (1979-1988): Distribution of Histologic Types and Grades

Type	Number (%)	Grade 1	Grade 2	Grade 3A	Grade 3B	Grade 3NOS
Malignant fibrous histiocytoma	75 (30·0)	12	7	33	18	5
Liposarcoma	41 (14·7)	11	13	5	9	3
Fibrosarcoma	38 (13·7)	22	4	7	4	1
Leiomyosarcoma	27 (9·7)	2	4	12	7	2
Malignant schwannoma	19 (6·8)	1	6	6	5	1
Synovial sarcoma	16 (5·8)	0	0	4	11	1
Dermatofibrosarcoma protuberans	13 (4·7)	6	6	1	0	0
Osteo- and chondrosarcomas, extraoss.	12 (4·3)	0	0	4	8	0
Rhabdomyosarcoma	11 (4·0)	0	0	2	9	0
Vasc. sarcomas	10 (3·6)	1	2	4	2	1
Others	7 (2·5)	1	1	1	1	3
Unclassified	9 (3·2)	1	0	1	4	3
Total	278	57	43	80	78	20
(%)	(100)	(20·5)	(15·5)	(28·8)	(28·1)	(7·2)

(Courtesy of Jensen OM, Høgh J, Østgaard SE, et al: *J Pathol* 163:19–24, 1991.)

Clinical Data.—Patients had a mean age of 54 years. More than one third of the tumors were at superficial sites, and more than half were larger than 5 cm in diameter. The most common types were malignant fibrous histiocytomas, liposarcoma, and fibrosarcoma (table).

Prognostic Factors.—Low-grade tumors were seen in 20.5% of patients, intermediate-grade tumors in 15.5%, and high-grade tumors in 64%. Among all prognostic factors, grade had the most predictive value. Five-year survival rates in low- and intermediate-grade cases were 95% and 86%, respectively, compared with 50% for high-grade cases (Fig 13–4). Other adverse prognostic factors included age older than 65 years, deep-seated tumor, and local recurrence at the time of referral.

▶ A widely accepted single grading system of soft tissue sarcomas has been the goal of a number of articles. Such a system would permit clinical classification of this uncommon and complex group of tumors so that clinicians may more easily categorize, and thereby select therapy for patients. This paper represents a follow-up study of their original work (1) in which they reported on 261 retrospectively reviewed patients with soft tissue sarcomas. These authors thus have the largest published experience using a single grading system for these lesions. The scheme uses parameters familiar to all pathologists and recognizes certain poor prognostic subtypes regardless of other features. This idea is useful in the evaluation of incisional biopsy that may not include areas of tumor necrosis, required by some classifications for the high-grade designation (2). Ongoing publication of large series with well-articulated criteria and complete follow-up will continue to improve pathologic classification and could potentially improve comparison in interinstitutional clinical trials.—G.F. Worsham, M.D.

References

1. Myhre Jensen O, et al: *Acta Pathol Microbiol Immunol Scand [A]* 91:145, 1983.
2. Costa J, et al: *Cancer* 53:530, 1984.

Angiomatoid Malignant Fibrous Histiocytoma: A Follow-Up Study of 108 Cases With Evaluation of Possible Histologic Predictors of Outcome

Costa MJ, Weiss SW (Emory Univ; Univ of Michigan)

Am J Surg Pathol 14:1126–1132, 1990 13–5

Background.—Angiomatoid malignant fibrous histiocytoma (MFH) is a distinctive tumor seen in adolescents and young adults. It is characterized by sheets of round or spindled cells separated by areas of cystic hemorrhage. Experience with about 40 cases has suggested a low-grade malignancy. Findings were reviewed in 108 new cases of angiomatoid MFH; follow-up data were available for 87% of cases.

Clinical Findings.—The mean age at surgery was 17 years. Two thirds of the tumors were on the extremities, and most of the others were on the trunk. The mean duration of known tumor was 1 year; the usual clinical diagnosis was benign cyst. Nine of 11 patients with local recurrences were cured after wide local excision. Another patient was lost to follow-up; 1 patient had local metastasis but was well after further excision.

Pathologic Findings.—Most of the tumors were cystic and filled with hemorrhagic fluid or blood. Twenty-one lesions were considered more pleomorphic than usual. Mitotic figures were frequent in 7% of cases. A large majority of tumors involved the subcutaneous tissue.

Clinicopathologic Correlation.—Local recurrences were associated with an irregular tumor border and the presence of tumor in the head and neck region. Local and distant metastasis (seen in 5 patients) correlated with invasion of deep fascia or muscle, but not with mitotic rate and pleomorphism.

Conclusions.—Angiomatoid MFH appears to be a low-grade tumor. One patient in this series died of disease. These tumors contrast with conventional MFHs, the majority of which are high-grade sarcomas.

▶ Since its original description (1), this rate variant of MFH has been considered of low-grade malignancy in contrast to its more common relatives. This paper does not address the issue of histogenesis, which continues to be uncertain, although the authors quote previous studies linking it to a histiocytic or endothelial origin. The study does confirm the previous impression of a relatively low-grade sarcoma. A number of histopathologic parameters, including mitotic activity, pleomorphism, tumor size, and inflammatory response, did not correlate well with clinical course. As might be expected, the best correlates with local recurrence were deep location, origin in the head and neck, and infiltrative margins. In this initial report, a number of cases had peculiar symptoms, including severe anemia, fever, and weight loss; however, in the current series, these clinical features were less prominent, attributed by the authors to earlier diagnosis and prompt therapy.—G.F. Worsham, M.D.

Reference

1. Enzinger FM: *Cancer* 44:2146, 1979.

Intra-Abdominal Desmoplastic Small Round-Cell Tumor: Report of 19 Cases of a Distinctive Type of High-Grade Polyphenotypic Malignancy Affecting Young Individuals

Gerald WL, Miller HK, Battifora H, Miettinen M, Silva EG, Rosai J (Yale Univ; City of Hope Natl Med Ctr, Duarte, Calif; Thomas Jefferson Univ; Univ of Texas, Houston)

Am J Surg Pathol 15:499–513, 1991 13–6

Introduction.—Small round cell tumors (SRCT) comprise a continuously evolving family of neoplasms of infancy and childhood. The latter are characterized by high cellularity, a small cell size, an overall blue appearance in hematoxylin-eosin–stained specimens, and a diffuse growth pattern. Nineteen malignant small cell tumors that appear distinct from the well-recognized members of SRCT were studied.

Clinical Features.—The mean age of the patients at diagnosis was 18.6 years. The male-to-female ratio was more than 5:1. The tumors displayed extremely aggressive behavior, 15 patients dying within 6 months to 4 years after diagnosis.

Pathologic Features.—The tumors were predominantly located intra-abdominally, with only inconstant and secondary organ involvement. The tumors were found as multiple firm or hard nodules attached to the peritoneal surface. The cut surface was gray-white, sometimes myxoid, with sharply outlined necrotic foci (Fig 13–5). Microscopically, they appeared as sharply outlined clusters of tumor cells varying in size and shape separated by a cellular (desmoplastic) stroma (Fig 13–6). Focal

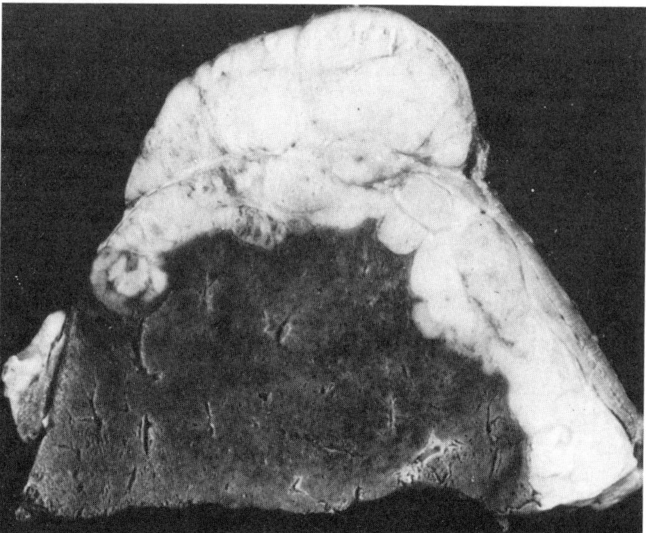

Fig 13–5.—Gross appearance of cut surface of the tumor, which involved the peritoneal surface and extended into the liver. The neoplasm has a solid white appearance and a nodular quality, and it exhibits several foci of necrosis. (Courtesy of Gerald WL, Miller HK, Battifora H, et al: *Am J Surg Pathol* 15:499–513, 1991.)

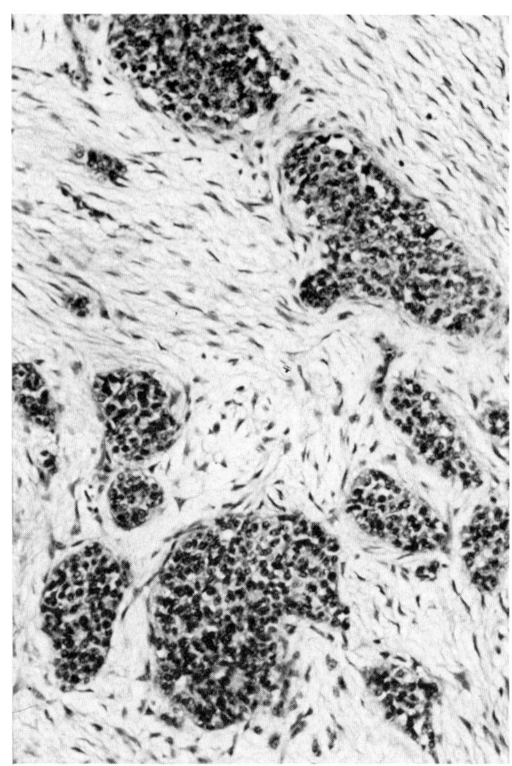

Fig 13–6.—Photomicrograph illustrating typical appearance of the tumor. Well-defined neoplastic nests of varying size and shape are separated by abundant stroma containing numerous mesenchymal spindle cells. (Courtesy of Gerald WL, Miller HK, Battifora H, et al: *Am J Surg Pathol* 15:499–513, 1991.)

rhabdoid features and central necrosis were common. Immunohistochemical studies revealed positivity for keratin, epithelial membrane antigen, neuron-specific enolase, vimentin, and desmin. In particular, the extensive coexpression of keratins and desmin appeared to be unique, as did the reactivity for desmin without expression of muscle-specific actin.

Discussion.—These tumors may represent another SRCT of infancy and childhood with distinctive topographic, morphological, and immunohistochemical features and a capacity for simultaneous multidirectional phenotypic expression.

▶ The authors present good evidence for considering these neoplasms as a distinctive type of SRCT that expresses epithelial as well as muscle-associated and neural markers. Features of these neoplasms include male predilection, intra-abdominal location, desmoplastic response, vascular proliferation, coexpression of keratin and desmin (in the absence of expression of muscle specific actin), expression of neuron-specific enolase (and, in 2 cases, apparent neuroendocrine granules ultrastructurally), and an aggressive clinical course. Trying to classify one of these lesions on the basis of previously recognized neoplastic categories would be difficult, and this new category appears useful both for providing prognostic information and for accruing additional cases that may ultimately provide a better understanding of this unusual entity. In addition to the description of the intra-abdominal desmoplastic SRCT, the authors provide a useful, brief review of SRCTs, including information such as the recent recognition of keratin expression in Ewing's sarcoma and rhabdomyosarcoma.—J.A. Tucker, M.D.

Keratin Subsets in Spindle Cell Sarcomas: Keratins Are Widespread But Synovial Sarcoma Contains a Distinctive Keratin Polypeptide Pattern and Desmoplakins

Miettinen M (Thomas Jefferson Univ)

Am J Pathol 138:505–513, 1991 13–7

Background.—Contrary to original teachings, recent studies indicate that keratins are not phenotypically restricted to epithelial cells, and have been expressed in mesenchymal cells, smooth cells and their neoplasms, and certain fetal striated muscle cells. The recognition of 20 (cyto)keratins facilitated attempts in carcinoma subclassification by keratin typing.

Methods.—The presence of individual keratin polypeptides and desmoplakins was analyzed immunohistochemically in 25 spindle cell sarcomas.

Findings.—Keratins 8 and 18 were present in all 9 synovial sarcomas, 5 of 7 leiomyosarcomas, all 5 malignant schwannomas, and 1 of 4 undifferentiated spindle cell sarcomas. In addition, the glandular epithelial cells in synovial sarcoma exhibited prominent reactivity with antibodies to keratins 7 and 19, and showed desmoplakin immunoreactivity in a typical luminal distribution. Keratin 13 also was evident in 4 of 9 synovial sarcomas. In contrast, keratins 7, 13, and 19 were not evident in leiomyosarcomas, malignant schwannomas, or undifferentiated spindle cell sarcomas, and none showed desmoplakin immunostaining.

Conclusion.—This study shows the widespread presence of keratins in various spindle cell sarcomas. However, synovial sarcomas have a more complex keratin pattern and contain desmoplakins, compared with the other spindle cell sarcomas. The presence of keratins 7 and 19 and desmoplakins in synovial sarcomas coincides with morphologically observed epithelial differentiation restricted to synovial sarcomas among spindle cell sarcomas.

▶ Spindle cell sarcomas have been shown to express keratins primarily of the 8 and 18 types. Synovial sarcomas with an epithelial component also express keratins 7 and 19, which are more characteristic of epithelial cells, as well as desmoplakins.

A.J. Garvin, M.D., Ph.D.

Is Fetal Cellular Rhabdomyoma an Entity or a Differentiated Rhabdomyosarcoma? A Study of Patients With Rhabdomyoma of the Tongue and Sarcoma of the Tongue Enrolled in the Intergroup Rhabdomyosarcoma Studies I, II, and III

Kodet R, Fajstavr J, Kabelka Z, Koutecky J, Eckschlager T, Newton WA Jr (Charles Univ, Prague, Czechoslovakia; Intergroup Rhabdomyosarcoma Study, Childrens' Hosp, Columbus, Oh)

Cancer 67:2907–2913, 1991 13–8

Background.—It generally has been considered necessary to distinguish rhabdomyoma from rhabdomyosarcoma, to avoid unnecessary treatment. An exception to this distinction is suggested by a patient having a highly differentiated striated muscle tumor consistent with fetal cellular rhabdomyoma, which recurred and transformed to a mixed embryonal/alveolar rhabdomyosarcoma during a period of 22 months.

Case Report.—Infant, 18 months, had a tumor of the tongue that recurred 10 months after initial excision and again at 40 months. Examination of the first recurrence showed increased nuclear irregularity and more evident mitotic activity. The second recurrence was rhabdomyosarcoma.

For comparison, data were reviewed on 8 children and adolescents with primary sarcomas of the tongue. Five had embryonal rhabdomyosarcomas and 1 patient each had an alveolar, mixed embryonal/alveolar, and undifferentiated myxoid sarcomatous lesion. Five tumors were poorly differentiated, whereas 2 exhibited moderate myogenesis. Two patients died of their disease.

Discussion.—The concept of cellular rhabdomyoma as always being benign may be questioned. Two possibilities exist: that malignant change may occur in a rhabdomyoma, and that a highly differentiated rhabdomyosarcoma may be difficult to distinguish from a rhabdomyoma.

▶ The authors describe the transformation of a fetal cellular rhabdomyoma to a rhabdomyosarcoma with recurrence. The concept of a cellular rhabdomyoma should be reviewed in light of recent descriptions of a spindle cell (leiomyomatous) rhabdomyosarcoma with low malignant potential (1).—A.J. Garvin, M.D., Ph.D.

Reference

1. Carazzana AO, et al: *Proceedings, Symposium on Childhood Rhabdomyosarcoma,* Columbus, Oh, 1989.

Dermatofibroma Extending Into the Subcutaneous Tissue: Differential Diagnosis From Dermatofibrosarcoma Protuberans

Kamino H, Jacobson M (New York Univ)

Am J Surg Pathol 14:1156–1164, 1990 13–9

Histologic Criteria

Dermatofibroma (fibrous variant)	Dermatofibrosarcoma protuberans
1. Plump fibroblasts in a haphazard array	1. Slender cells frequently in a storiform pattern
2. Polarizable (birefringent, doubly refractile) collagen bundles	2. Nonpolarizable thin delicate collagen fibers
3. Preexisting collagen bundles: thick and straight[a]	3. Preexisting collagen: wavy and infiltrated by spindle cells[a]
4. Perivascular inflammatory infiltrate of lymphocytes and usually plasma cells at the periphery	4. Infrequent inflammatory infiltrate
5. Occasional foamy histiocytes	5. Rare foamy histiocytes
6. Occasional multinucleated histiocytes	6. Rare multinucleated cells
7. Frequent hemosiderin deposits	7. Rare hemosiderin deposits
8. Scant stromal mucin	8. Variable amounts of stromal mucin
9. Fat cells at the interface between the lesion and the subcutaneous fat or in preexisting areas around adnexa[a]	9. Fat cells scattered throughout the lesion[a]
10. Frequent epidermal hyperplasia with hyperpigmentation of basal layer	10. Epidermis usually thin

(Courtesy of Kamino H, Jacobson M: *Am J Surg Pathol* 14:1156–1164, 1990.)

Background.—Dermatofibromas usually are well defined histologically when they are found confined to the dermis. However, the fibrous variety of dermatofibroma can extend into the subcutaneous tissue, making diagnosis difficult. The appearance of specimens of fibrous dermatofibroma with extension into the subcutaneous tissue was ana-

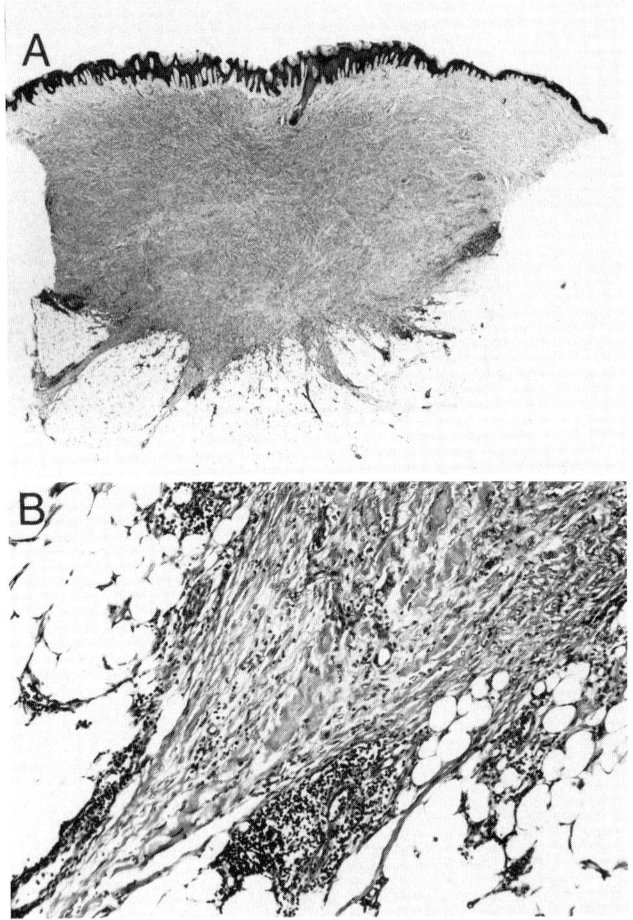

Fig 13–7.—**A,** dermatofibroma with radial pattern of extension into the subcutaneous tissue. **B,** a wedge-shaped extension along the septum with fibroblasts and thick collagen bundles. At the periphery is an inflammatory cell infiltrate. (Courtesy of Kamino H, Jacobson M: *Am J Surg Pathol* 14:1156–1164, 1990.)

lyzed and compared with that of specimens of dermatofibrosarcoma protuberans.

Methods.—A retrospective review was made of 185 specimens of excised fibrous dermatofibroma and 40 specimens of excisional or incisional biopsy specimens of dermatofibrosarcoma protuberans. The criteria for sample analysis are shown in the table.

Findings.—The dermatofibromas appeared to have 2 main patterns of extension into the subcutaneous tissue: 133 of 185 specimens demonstrated an irregular vertical or radial extension producing a wedge-like appearance, whereas 52 specimens exhibited a smooth, well-demarcated, deep margin bulge into the subcutaneous tissue (Figs 13–7 and 13–8).

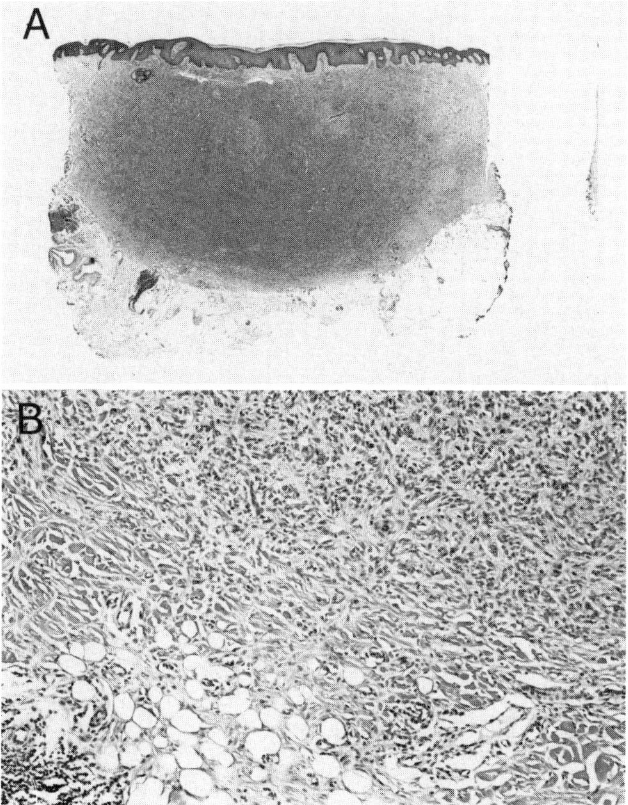

Fig 13–8.—**A,** dermatifibroma with a smooth and well-demarcated deep margin that bulges into the subcutaneous tissue. **B,** fat cells intermingled with fibroblasts and collagen bundles at the interface between the lesion and the subcutaneous tissue. (Courtesy of Kamino H, Jacobson M: *Am J Surg Pathol* 14:1156–1164, 1990.)

Fat cells mixed with collagen bundles in both patterns only at the interface between the lesion and the subcutaneous tissue. All dermatofibromas had large fibroblasts arranged as interlacing fascicles, keloidal collagen bundles, and patchy inflammatory infiltrates. These characteristics were seen both in dermatofibromas found in the dermis and in those extending into the subcutaneous tissue. The dermatofibrosarcoma protuberans specimens had 2 infiltration patterns: a honeycomb or lacelike arrangement with spindle-shaped cells found along the septa, and a multilayer arrangement of spindle-like cells bundled and parallel to the surface of the skin. Other features of the dermatofibrosarcoma protuberans were infiltration of the hair muscles, blood vessel walls, and eccrine glands.

Conclusions.—These findings indicate that the histologic patterns of extension of dermatofibromas into the subcutaneous tissue vary distinctively from those of dermatofibrosarcoma protuberans. Knowledge of the differences in these extension patterns can aid in the differential diagnosis of these 2 conditions and can prevent overtreatment of the benign dermatofibroma and underdiagnosis of the more serious tumor.

▶ Dermatofibromas are usually diagnosed easily and recur uncommonly even when incompletely excised. Dermatofibrosarcoma protuberans is much less frequently encountered in practice and can be difficult to distinguish from both dermatofibromas and, occasionally, neurofibromas. These authors describe 2 patterns of infiltration of the adjacent subcutaneous fat that should be useful to dermatopathologists and general surgical pathologists in making this distinction. Other features emphasized in the table may be helpful in distinguishing these 2 entities in biopsy specimens that do not include the interface between the dermis and the subcutis.—G.F. Worsham, M.D.

Myolipoma of Soft Tissue

Meis JM, Enzinger FM (Armed Forces Inst of Pathology, Washington, DC)

Am J Surg Pathol 15:121–125, 1991 13–10

Introduction.—Nine cases of soft tissue myolipoma—a presumably benign but previously undescribed entity—were found in a search of the Armed Forces Institute of Pathology database for 1980–1990.

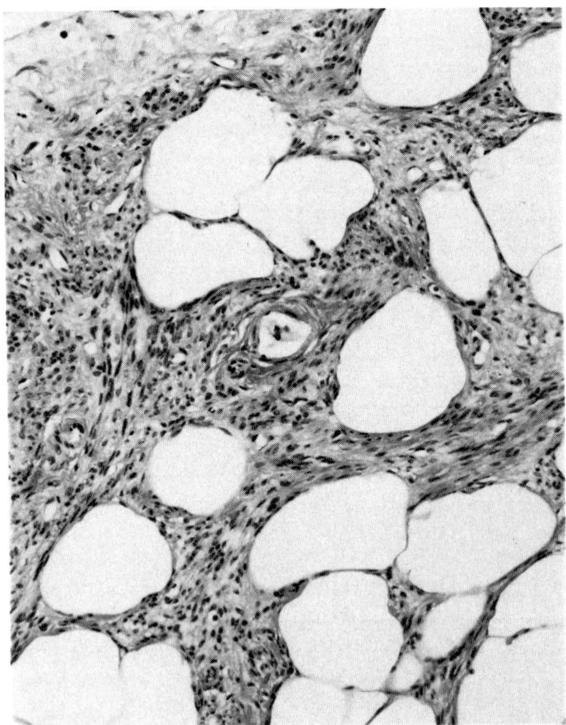

Fig 13–9.—The smooth muscle component is cytologically bland. There is no atypia of the adipocytes. (Courtesy of Meis JM, Enzinger FM: *Am J Surg Pathol* 15:121–125, 1991.)

Clinical.—The patients (aged 28–73 years) had glistening, tan-yellow to pink, myxoid-appearing tumors. Tumor sites were varied and included the anterior abdominal wall, abdominal cavity, retroperitoneum, and subcutaneous fat. The tumors averaged 16 cm in greatest dimension. Seven tumors were clinically palpable. No recurrences developed in 5 patients followed for up to 10 years.

Pathologic Features.—The tumors consisted of varying amounts of benign smooth muscle and mature fat tissue (Fig 13–9). Five were at least partly encapsulated. A nonlipomatous component was grossly apparent in 3 cases. Fuchsinophilic staining of myofibrils with trichrome stain confirmed the impression of myogenic differentiation.

Discussion.—Soft tissue myolipoma is a distinctive lesion usually considered benign. Its recognition will prevent confusion with more aggressive smooth muscle and lipomatous tumors of the abdomen and retroperitoneum.

▶ Continuing the tradition of identifying unusual soft tissue tumors within the material at the Armed Forces Institute of Pathology, Dr. Meis, the new Chairman of the Department of Soft Tissue Pathology, and Dr. Enzinger describe 9 cases of a unique benign tumor with both smooth muscle and adipose tissue components, all of which occurred outside of the kidney. None of their patients had tuberous sclerosis. Also reported during this period, and noted by the above authors in proof, was an additional series (1). The mesenchymal tumors in this second series had atypia within the fat cells and 2 of the 3 cases recurred. One of these patients had multiple recurrences and eventually died of tumor, which in its later manifestations resembled dedifferentiated liposarcoma. These 2 reports suggest that these rare mesenchymal tumors with biphasic differentiation have a range of morphological expression that reflects their biological potential.—G.F. Worsham, M.D.

Reference

1. Evans HL, *Am J Surg Pathol* 14:714, 1990.

14 Dermatopathology

Histopathologic Diagnosis of Dysplastic Nevi: Concordance Among Pathologists Convened by the World Health Organization Melanoma Programme

Clemente C, Cochran AJ, Elder DE, Levene A, MacKie RM, Mihm MC Jr, Rilke F, Cascinelli N, Fitzpatrick TB, Sober AJ (Natl Tumor Inst, Milan, Italy; Univ of California; Hosp of Univ of Pennsylvania; Humana Hosp Wellington, London; Univ of Glasgow, et al)

Hum Pathol 22:313–319, 1991 14–1

Introduction.—Dysplastic nevi are a useful indicator of the risk of cutaneous malignant melanoma, but diagnostic precision has been lacking.

Study Design.—A panel of 6 dermatopathologists reviewed various criteria for diagnosing dysplastic nevus and agreed on a set of diagnostic measures. The set of criteria then was applied to 114 cases of acquired nevus, dysplastic nevus, and early (radial-growth phase) melanoma.

Criteria.—The major diagnostic criteria are basilar proliferation of atypical nevomelanocytes (extending at least 3 rete ridges or pegs beyond any dermal nevocellular component) and proliferation in a lentiginous or epithelioid-cell pattern. Minor criteria include lamellar fibrosis or concentric eosinophilic fibrosis, neovascularization, inflammation, and fusion of rete ridges. Both major criteria and at least 2 minor signs are needed for diagnosis.

Observations.—The mean degree of diagnostic concordance for the 114 cases exceeded 92%. Concordance values for benign acquired nevi, dysplastic nevi, and early melanoma were 95%, 88%, and 95%, respectively. Concordance with the original histopathologic diagnosis was 82%.

Conclusion.—Agreement exceeding 90% now can be expected when a set of histopathologic criteria are applied to benign and dysplastic nevi and early melanomas.

▶ This paper describes a study in which 114 melanocytic neoplasms were subjected to a set of diagnostic criteria that had been agreed on by a panel of 6 dermatopathologists. Using these criteria, the neoplasms were characterized as being common acquired nevi, dysplastic nevi, or early melanoma. Concurrence between members of the panel was said to exceed 90%. This study demonstrates that once morphologic criteria are established, it is possible for dermatopathologists to apply them and reach agreement about diagnosis in about 90% of cases. However, the validity of the criteria used in this study was not established.—J.S. Metcalf, M.D.

Multiple Rhabdomyomatous Mesenchymal Hamartomas of Skin

Sahn EE, Garen PD, Pai GS, Levkoff AH, Hagerty RC, Maize JC (Med Univ of South Carolina)

Am J Dermatopathol 12:485–491, 1990 14–2

Background.—Solitary rhabdomyomatous mesenchymal hamartoma of the skin in an infant has only recently been reported in the literature. This particular case was characterized by an abnormal arrangement of dermal mesenchymal elements dominated by the presence of skeletal muscle, with striated muscle and admixed mature adipose tissue located entirely within the dermis. Multiple rhabdomyomatous mesenchymal hamartomas of the skin was observed in a neonate.

Case Report.—Neonate, born after uncomplicated gestation and delivery, had many fleshy polyps and soft nodules over the periorbital and periauricular areas of the face (Fig 14–1). These nodules ranged in size from a few millimeters to a few centimeters in length. The infant had bilateral preauricular sinuses, not observed in either parent. The child's ears were low-set and he had bilateral diffuse sclerocorneas with probable retinal dysplasia or an orbital cyst seen on ultrasonograms. The 32-year-old mother denied use of alcohol, cigarettes, or illicit drugs during the pregnancy. Chromosome analysis showed a normal male karyotype. The infant fed and behaved well. The lesions were successfully excised under general anesthesia on the tenth day of life.

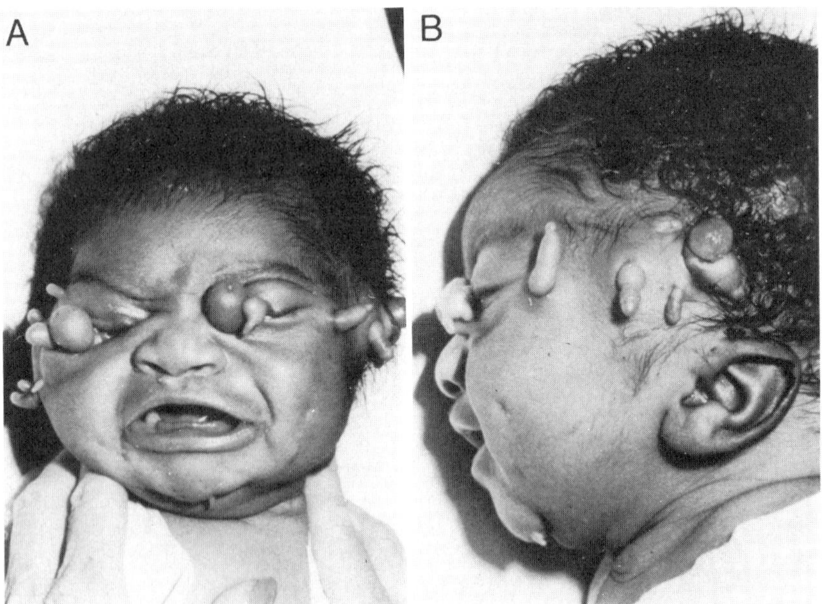

Fig 14–1.—Multiple elongate and globular polyps on the face of a 2-day-old infant. Note constrictions near tips of elongate polyps and dimples on globular polyps. Note also low-set ears in **B.** (Courtesy of Sahn EE, Garen PD, Pai GS, et al: *Am J Dermatopathol* 12:485–491, 1990.)

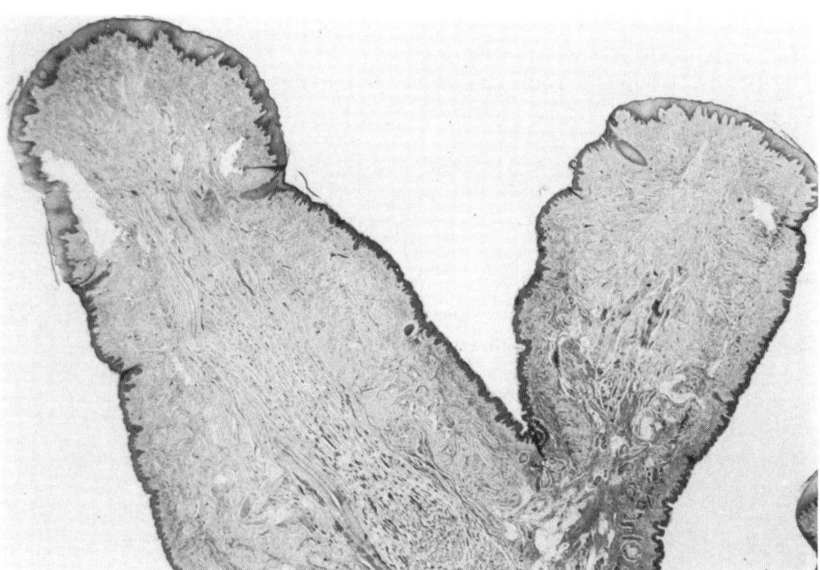

Fig 14–2.—Bifid polyp with central core of skeletal muscle fibers (hematoxylin-eosin; ×10). (Courtesy of Sahn EE, Garen PD, Pai GS, et al: *Am J Dermatopathol* 12:485–491, 1990.)

Findings.—The histopathologic tests showed polyps covered by squamous epithelium and possessing normal follicular units (Fig 14–2). The bundles of skeletal muscle contained regular cross-striations in the muscle fibers. Skeletal muscle histochemical staining of lesion tissue demonstrated the presence of types 1 and 2 muscle fibers, and electron microscopy showed a normal skeletal banding pattern. Several lesions had spontaneous movement, which showed functional skeletal muscle involvement.

▶ This paper is a case report of an infant with multiple congenital cutaneous hamartomas, which appeared clinically as polyps and nodules located in the periorbital and periauricular areas. These cutaneous lesions are described in detail clinically, histopathologically, and ultrastructurally; the histologic features are distinguished from fetal rhabdomyoma, nevus lipomatosis cutaneous superficialis, fibrous hamartoma of infancy, and benign Triton tumors.—J.S. Metcalf, M.D.

Benign Cutaneous Adnexal Tumors in Childhood and Young Adults, Excluding Pilomatrixoma: Review of 28 Cases and Literature

Marrogi AJ, Wick MR, Dehner LP (Washington Univ)

J Cutan Pathol 18:20–27, 1991 14–3

Introduction.—In children, dermal neoplasms arising from the cutaneous appendages are not common. Some of these tumors are easily recognized, but others may be difficult to classify.

Pathology.—All eccrine tumors, trichogenic lesions, and apocrine neoplasms identified for a review of surgical pathology files were considered for evaluation of hematoxylin-eosin–stained slides. Each patient's clinical records were also examined.

Observations.—The patients were 23 females and 5 males, mean age 15 years. There were 12 benign hair follicular tumors and 15 benign sweat gland tumors. Lesions were most commonly described as papules, and they were located on the face, scalp, and neck in 75% of cases. Trichoepithelioma, including desmoplastic variants, and syringoma made up 56% of all neoplasms. A family history of trichoepitheliomas was seen in 1 case. All lesions were locally excised, and only 1 eccrine acrospiroma recurred.

Conclusion.—A series of cutaneous adnexal neoplasms in young persons is evaluated. These tumors probably occur as sporadic growths rather than as manifestations of heredofamilial disorders or hamartoma. Tumors are typically underdiagnosed until the second decade of life.

▶ The authors describe a study of benign cutaneous adnexal tumors in young patients. Of these, 12 were thought to be of trichogenic origin, including trichoepitheliomas (both typical and desmoplastic), trichofolliculoma, trichoblastoma, and steatocystoma. Also described were eccrine and apocrine tumors, including acrospiromas, hidrocytomas, syringomas, and syringocystadenomas papilliferum. In the majority of the group of 28 patients, the adnexal tumors were thought to have developed sporadically, although 1 of the patients with trichoepithelioma had a family history of multiple trichoepitheliomas. There is marked female predominance.—J.S. Metcalf, M.D.

Folliculocentric Basaloid Proliferation: The Bulge *(der Wulst)* Revisited

Leshin B, White WL (Bowman Gray School of Medicine of Wake Forest Univ)

Arch Dermatol 126:900–906, 1990 14–4

Introduction.—Standard frozen sections obtained from 22 patients undergoing Mohs' micrographic surgery for nasal or perinatal basal cell carcinoma demonstrated folliculocentric basaloid proliferation (FBP). The patients, all women, were aged 58–86 years. Folliculocentric basaloid proliferation has occurred in 5.7% of all patients found to have nasal or perinasal basal cell carcinoma at micrographic surgery.

Observations.—Folliculocentric basaloid proliferation shares many histologic features with basal cell carcinoma, but several criteria are available for distinguishing between these lesions. On scanning magnification, FBP has an overall vertical orientation and a flasklike configuration, whereas basal cell carcinoma usually is oriented horizontally. Folliculocentric basaloid proliferation never occurs deep in skeletal muscle or subcutaneous fat. Single cell necrosis and mitotic figures are rare in FBP but are seen frequently in basal cell carcinoma. Another feature distinguishing FBP is the presence of a prominent hyaline basement membrane at the periphery of many basaloid aggregates.

Conclusion.—Follicular basaloid proliferation probably represents a proliferative epiphenomenon to basal cell carcinoma. Follow-up studies to date have confirmed the absence of tumor.

▶ One of the difficulties frequently encountered by the dermatopathologist is the assessment of margins of basal cell carcinoma. Resection of basal cell carcinomas from the central face are particularly problematic because of the prominence of sebaceous glands and their associated follicles. Benign basaloid proliferations, associated with hair follicles, particularly when sectioned obliquely or tangentially, are easily misinterpreted as extensions of basal cell carcinoma. These occur in the region of "the bulge" where follicular stem cells are thought to be located.

This paper is useful in that it delineates the morphologic features that distinguish benign, follicular-associated basal cell proliferations (folliculocentric basaloid proliferations) from basal cell carcinoma. Several of these criteria, such as the absence of single-cell necrosis and mitoses in these benign proliferations and the presence of prominent hyaline basement membrane material, can be applied even when the relationship of the proliferation to a hair follicle is not immediately evident.—J.S. Metcalf, M.D.

Collagenous Spherulosis in Chondroid Syringomas

Argenyi ZB, Balogh K (Univ of Iowa; New England Deaconess Hosp, Boston)

Am J Dermatopathol 13:115–121, 1991 14–5

Background.—Collagenous spherulosis (CS) was recognized as a separate entity in 1987, when the presence of intraluminal eosinophilic globules was found in benign breast lesions. The eosinophilic globules of CS had characteristic concentric or radiating fibrillary structures that stained for collagen and reticulin fibers, acidic mucin, and PAS-positive, basal

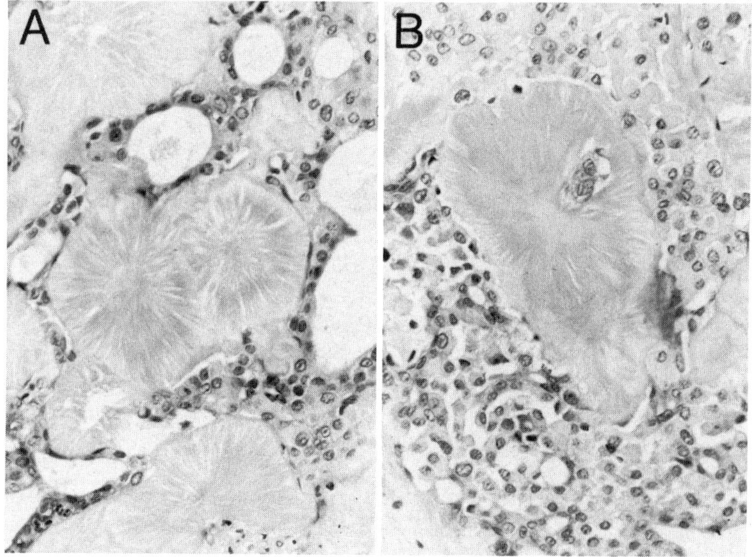

Fig 14–3.—A, higher magnification of the spherules shows a radiating fibrillary architecture associated with fenestrated epithelial structures. **B,** occasional solitary spherules are embedded in loose nests of hyaline cells. (Courtesy of Argenyi ZB, Balogh K: *Am J Dermatopathol* 13:115–121, 1991.)

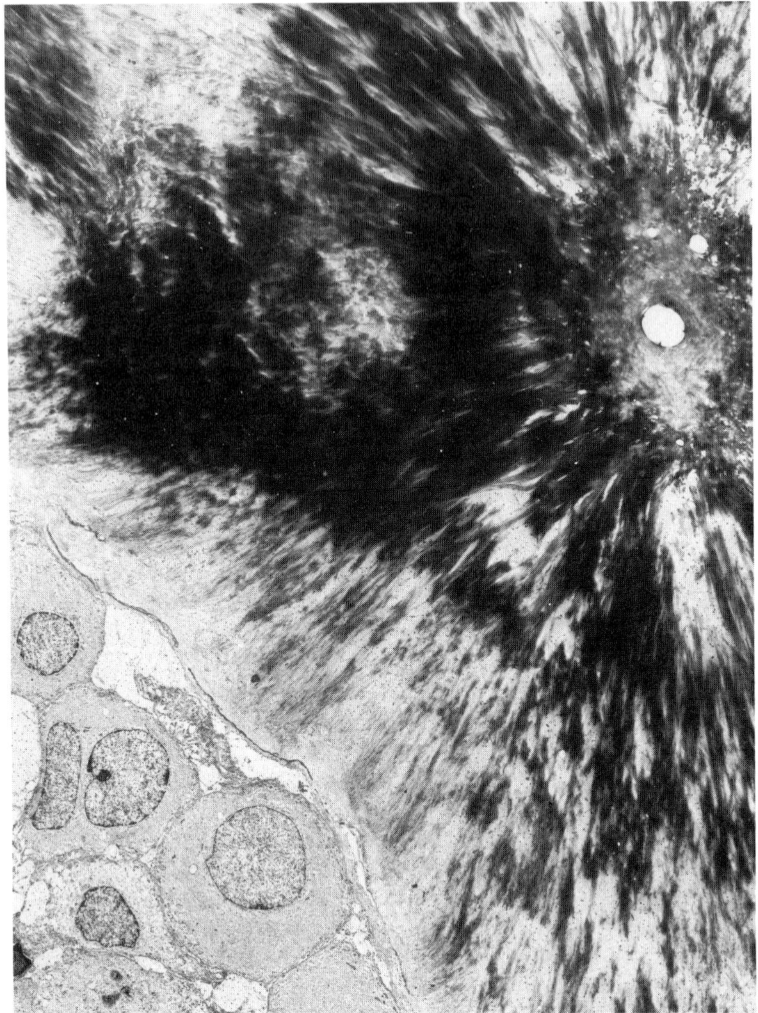

Fig 14–4.—Low-magnification electron micrograph of a spherule shows radiating fibers and adjacent hyaline cells (×1,400); shown here at 80%. (Courtesy of Argenyi ZB, Balogh K: *Am J Dermatopathol* 13:115–121, 1991.)

lamina-like material. To date, CS has been considered a distinct lesion of the breast. A case of similar structures in a chondroid syringoma of the skin was described.

Case Report.—Man, 75, had a .5-cm skin-colored papule on his face. He had no history of injury or treatment to the area. The lesion was excised and studied by routine light microscopy, special stains, immunohistochemical techniques, x-ray spectrophotometry, and electron microscopy. On light microscopy, there were solitary and confluent eosinophilic globules with radiating fibrillary structures in and around the lumina of the tubuloglandular components of CS. The fibrillary structures stained intensely for collagen and reticulum. Staining was less intense for acidic mucopolysaccharides. Immunohistochemical study showed that the globules were focally positive only for collagen type IV. On electron microscopy, radiating collagen fibers surrounded by basal lamina-like material were seen (Figs 14–3 and 14–4).

Conclusions.—Collagenous spherulosis is not specific to breast. It also occurs in chondroid syringomas. The term "collagenous spherulosis" is appropriate because, in this case, collagen fibers were found histochemically and ultrastructurally in the spherules. Apparently, CS is associated with tubular epithelial structures. In the case studied, there were no immunohistochemical signs of myoepithelial differentiation.

▶ This case report describes chondroid syringoma containing eosinophilic globules with light microscopic and ultrastructural features of collagenous spherulosis, structures that have been described previously in the breast. The figures show the radiating fibrillary architecture of these peculiar structures and their location within the chondroid syringoma.

It is not too surprising that there should be similarities between certain lesions of eccrine sweat glands and lesions of the breast. Topographical and immunohistochemical differences between the 2 sites are described by the authors.—J.S. Metcalf, M.D.

15 Neuropathology

Mixed Glioblastoma Multiforme and Sarcoma: A Clinicopathologic Study of 26 Radiation Therapy Oncology Group Cases

Meis JM, Martz KL, Nelson JS (Armed Forces Inst of Pathology, Bethesda, Md; RTOG Statistical Unit, Philadelphia)
Cancer 67:2342–2349, 1991 15–1

Background.—Mixed glioblastoma multiforme (GBM) and sarcoma, or gliosarcoma (GS), is a primary CNS tumor consisting of malignant glial and mesenchymal cell populations. All clinicopathologic views of GS come from a single comparative study with GBM.

Methods.—Twenty-six cases of GS were drawn from a series of 1,479 GBM that were part of 5 consecutive randomized phase II or III malignant glioma protocols begun in a 9-year period. Frequency of GS was only 1.8%. The classification of GS required 2 distinct malignant populations, 1 of them astrocytic in origin. The glial nature of the spindled malignant cells was often identified by reticulin stains and immunostaining for glial fibrillary protein. At least 1 confluent sarcomatous area filling 1 medium-power field was also required; 25 of the cases had large confluent sarcomatous growths. The patients received photon radiation alone, combined photon and neutron radiation, or combined photon radiation and chemotherapy.

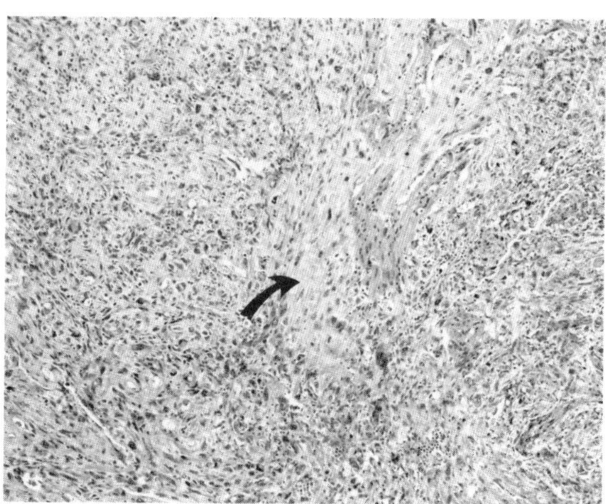

Fig 15–1.—Gliosarcoma in which the malignant glial component *(arrow)* is somewhat obscured by the sarcomatous component, which in this case was a malignant fibrous histiocytoma (hematoxylin-eosin; original magnification, ×75). (Courtesy of Meis JM, Martz KL, Nelson JS: *Cancer* 67:2342–2349, 1991.)

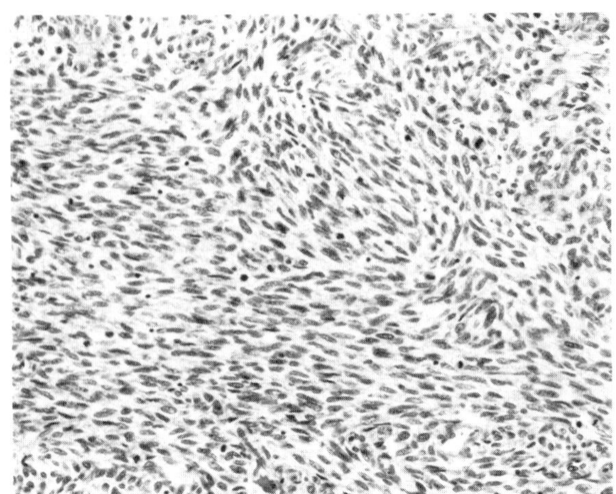

Fig 15–2.—Fibrosarcomatous component in a gliosarcoma. The cells are uniform and arranged in a herringbone pattern (hematoxylin-eosin; original magnification ×200). (Courtesy of Meis JM, Martz KL, Nelson JS: *Cancer* 67:2342–2349, 1991.)

Results.—Twenty patients were classified as having malignant fibrous histiocytoma based on the presence of malignant spindled mesenchymal cells, at least mildly pleomorphic, and arranged in a storiform or haphazard pattern (Fig 15–1). Five cases of fibrosarcoma showed a uniform malignant spindle cell proliferation comprising most of the mesenchymal part of the tumor (Fig 15–2). Gliosarcoma patients did not differ significantly from patients with GBM in terms of age, sex, pretreatment Karnofsky performance status, tumor location, size, or actuarial survival. Median survivals were 8.3 months for patients with GS and 9.6 months for patients with GBM. No treatment improved the survival of patients with GS over those with GBM. The temporal lobe was not selectively involved in GS.

Conclusions.—Using stringent diagnostic criteria, GS does not occur as frequently as previously reported and it does not selectively involve the temporal lobes. Affected patients are usually over age 60 years. The behavior of the tumor is similar to that of GBM, regardless of treatment. Gliosarcoma is not noted to metastasize more often than GBM.

▶ Surprisingly, few clinicopathologic studies are available to aid surgical pathologists in their recognition of gliosarcomas and the prognostic significance of this diagnosis. This study presents minimal criteria to facilitate differentiation of these lesions from more common glioblastomas. Requiring the presence of reticulin-positive, glial fibrillary protein-negative sarcoma that span at least 1 medium power field should reduce the number of mislabeled glioblastomas. Moreover, this relatively large series challenges previous observations that gliosarcomas are more common in the temporal lobe and metastasize more frequently than glioblastomas. The study reaffirms the dismal prognosis of these neoplasms.—M. Johnson, M.D., Ph.D.

Cellular Schwannoma: A Clinicopathologic Study of 57 Patients and 58 Tumors

White W, Shiu MH, Rosenblum MK, Erlandson RA, Woodruff JM (Mem Sloan-Kettering Cancer Ctr, New York)

Cancer 66:1266–1275, 1990 15–2

Introduction.—Cellular schwannoma, a variety of schwannoma with predominant cell growth without Verocay bodies, is often considered malignant. In 1981, 14 cases of a type of schwannoma considered benign were examined. The clinical and pathologic characteristics of 57 patients with this disorder were studied.

Methods.—Between 1974 and 1989, the records of 57 patients with 58 tumors were reviewed. Fifteen of these cases had been reported previously. All removed tumors had been preserved in formalin and stained with hematoxylin-eosin. Thirteen cases were assessed by transmission electron microscopy.

Results.—The 56 patients had a mean age of 44 years (range, 15 months–81 years) and 35 (63%) were female. Tumors most often occurred in the retroperitoneum, the mediastinum, the head and neck, and in an extremity. Bone erosion was verified by roentgenogram or on CT in 11 patients (19%). Surgical excision was the primary treatment for these

Data on 75 Patients With Cellular Schwannoma

No. tumors	76
Sex	60% female, 40% male
Age	Range, 15 months to 81 years; mean age, 44 years
VRN	4%
Associated nerve	46%
Sites	Widely distributed including cranial nerves and extremities, but most commonly in the posterior mediastinum and retroperitoneum
Mean size	6.2 cm
Bone erosion	15%
Histologic malignant diagnosis	28%
Treatment	Usually only surgical resection; incomplete resection in 9%
Follow-up	Available for 65% (49) of the patients
	1–2 years 10%
	2–5 years 29%
	5–10 years 29%
	10–20 years 18%
	20–32 years 14%
Outcome	Persistent local tumor, 9%; locally recurrent tumor, 5%; NED, 86%

**Abbreviations: VRN,* von Recklinghausen's neurofibromatosis; *NED,* no evidence of disease.

†Current data combined with those of Fletcher et al.

(Courtesy of White W, Shiu MH, Rosenblum MK, et al: *Cancer* 66:1266–1275, 1990.)

tumors. Incomplete excision occurred in 7 patients who then received radiotherapy and/or chemotherapy. Some 61% of the cases were available for follow-up 1 year after the initial surgery, and none of these patients had metastatic schwannoma or had died of the tumor. Pathologic findings showed that the tumors were usually spheric or ovoid and firm or rubbery, more cellular than a classic schwannoma, and did not have well-defined Verocay bodies. Twenty-eight percent of the tumors were cellulary uniform, but the other 72% were biphasic. Immunohistochemical analysis showed that 96% of the 23 samples reacted to S-100 protein. Ultrastructure determination showed tumors consisting of plump spindly cells with long bipolar cytoplasmic processes. These data correspond with previous reports (table).

Implications.—Surgeons should be aware that these tumors do exist to avoid unnecessary excision of functionally important nerves that are often found attached to the tumors. In addition, if the tumor can be truly identified as benign, superfluous adjuvant radiation and chemotherapy should not be given to the patient.

▶ The striking hypercellularity, increased mitotic activity, nuclear hyperchromasia and pleomorphism of "cellular schwannomas" are troublesome features that suggest malignant behavior to many. This study reemphasizes important behavioral (bony erosion and recurrence) and histologic features (increased cellularity, nuclear atypia, mitoses ≤4 per 10 high-power fields, rare circumscribed necrosis, and an absence of Verocay bodies) that characterize these lesion. It also underscores the broad cytologic repertoire of benign schwannomas. Initial follow-up of these cases reaffirms the temperate nature of this neoplasm.—M. Johnson, M.D.

Differentiation in Embryonal Neuroepithelial Tumors of the Central Nervous System

Cruz-Sanchez FF, Rossi ML, Hughes JT, Most TH (Univ of Barcelona, Spain; Midland Ctr for Neurology and Neurosurgery, Birmingham; Radcliffe Infirmary, Oxford; Frenchay Hosp, Bristol, England)

Cancer 67:965–976, 1991 15–3

Introduction.—Embryonal neuroepithelial tumors of the CNS have been variously classified. The current WHO classification proposes that all embryonal tumors be included in the category of primitive neuroectodermal tumors (PNET). Their constituent cells may derive from a single primitive multipotential neuroepithelial cell that can differentiate into one or more cell types.

Study.—Ninety-six tumors meeting the description of PNET were examined histologically and immunohistologically with a panel of antibodies that included glial, neuronal, epithelial, mesodermal, and myelin markers. Two pinealocytomas and 2 gangliocytomas were also reviewed. About two thirds of patients were less than 15 years old. About three fourths of the tumors were in the cerebellum.

Findings.—Seventy-one tumors exhibited glial and neuronal differentiation and expressed both an S (photoreceptor) antigen and vimentin. Twenty tumors had only neuronal differentiation, and 5 had only glial differentiation. None of the tumors exhibited reactivity for myelin or epithelial markers. Most tumors exhibited both glial and neuronal differentiation histologically. Fifty-eight lesions had the features of classic medulloblastoma.

Conclusions.—The WHO classification was supported, except that ependymoblastoma was thought to deserve a distinct designation. The embryonal neuroepithelial tumors of the CNS differentiate along glial and/or neuronal lines. Some medulloblastomas contain stem cells and retain bipolar differentiation, and others differentiate along one line only.

▶ This large series of embryonal neuroepithelial tumors confirms a smaller series of reports that demonstrated the capacity of these neoplasms to differentiate along glial and/or neuronal cell lines (1,2). These authors suggest that such differentiation may be normal or aberrant and agree with the WHO classification.—A.J. Garvin, M.D., Ph.D.

References

1. Coffin CM, et al: *Am J Surg Pathol* 7:555, 1983.
2. Burger PC, et al: *Acta Neuropathol* 73:115, 1987.

Primitive Neuroectodermal Tumors of the Central Nervous System: Patterns of Expression of Neuroendocrine Markers, and All Classes of Intermediate Filament Proteins

Gould VE, Jansson DS, Molenaar WM, Rorke LB, Trojanowski JQ, Lee VMY, Packer RJ, Franke WW (Rush Med College, Chicago; Swedish Univ of Agricultural Sciences, Uppsala; Children's Hosp, Philadelphia; Univ of Pennsylvania; German Cancer Research Ctr, Heidelberg)

Lab Invest 62:498–509, 1990 15–4

Background.—Comparatively little is known of the cytoskeletal features of those CNS tumors designated as primitve neuroectodermal tumors (PNETs). A panel of antibodies to intermediate filaments and desmoplakins were used to analyze snap-frozen samples from 22 PNETs primary in the CNS.

Methods.—Sections were immunostained using the avidin-biotin peroxidase complex method and indirect immunofluorescence microscopy. Some cases also were examined by double- and triple-label immunofluorescence microscopy, 2-dimensional gel electrophoresis, and immunoblot analysis.

Observations.—All PNETs extensively expressed synaptophysin and all expressed vimentin. All but 1 of the tumors expressed glial filament protein, and 16 of the 22 tumors expressed neurofilament proteins. Four tumors expressed desmin, and 3 expressed cytokeratins.

Discussion.—Significant phenotypic features are shared by PNETs of the CNS and neuroendocrine tumors. The present findings are very compelling evidence of neuroendocrine differentiation for these tumors as a group, and distinguish them from other types of CNS tumor.

▶ The precise meaning and classification of PNETs have been difficult to delineate. Whether tumors that are similar morphologically should be classified under 1 rubric (PNET) or should retain more classic definitions according to site of occurrence and type of differentiation has been debated by many respected authors in the field. This article by virtue of an evaluation of an extensive immunohistochemical profile and range of tumor types, presents a strong argument for the condensation of many currently differently designated tumor types into the PNET designation.—P. Garen, M.D.

Cerebellar Hemangioblastoma: Immunohistochemical Distinction From Metastatic Renal Cell Carcinoma

Mills SE, Ross GW, Perentes E, Nakagawa Y, Scheithauer BW (Univ of Virginia Health Sciences Ctr, Charlottesville; Mayo Clinic and Found, Rochester, Minn)

Surg Pathol 3:121–132, 1990 15–5

Background.—Hemangioblastomas are uncommon benign neoplasms that usually occur in the cerebellum, although they rarely have been found in the cerebral hemispheres, retina, spinal cord, and medulla oblongata. The clear stromal cells associated with hemangiomas can lead to confusion in diagnosis, and as a result, metastatic renal-cell carcinoma or the possibility of a second primary hemangioblastoma may be overlooked. Nine hemangioblastomas and 9 renal clear-cell carcinomas that had metastasized to the CNS were studied immunohistochemically to determine how these 2 conditions can be differentiated in clinical practice.

Methods.—Nine hemangioblastomas and 9 kidney cancer metastases (3 cerebellar, 4 cerebral, and 2 spinal) were studied by immunostaining of biopsy specimens obtained from files. All of the tissue samples had been fixed in 10% formalin and embedded in paraffin. Immunostaining was accomplished by the peroxidase-antiperoxidase (PAP) method in conjunction with monoclonal antibodies for antihuman glial fibrillary acidic protein (GFAP), antiepithelial membrane antigen (EMA), and antivimentin.

Findings.—Both the hemangioblastomas and the metastatic renal-cell carcinomas possessed histologic characteristics of clear cells. Immunohistochemical findings showed tht GFAP-reactive cells resided in near astrocytes but were found rarely in neoplastic stromal cells of thehemangioblastomas. No GFAP staining was observed in the cells of the metastatic renal carcinomas, but reactive astrocytes did stain for this protein. All 9 hemangioblastomas were EMA negative, and all 9 metastatic renal-cell carcinomas showed some degree of EMA staining. Six samples strongly stained with EMA (Fig 15–3); the cell membranes and the cytoplasm reacted positively in 7. All 8 hemangioblastomas and all 9 renal-cell carcinomas reacted positively to vimentin.

Conclusion.—The EMA antibody immunohistochemistry appears to offer an effective method of differentiating between hemangioblastomas

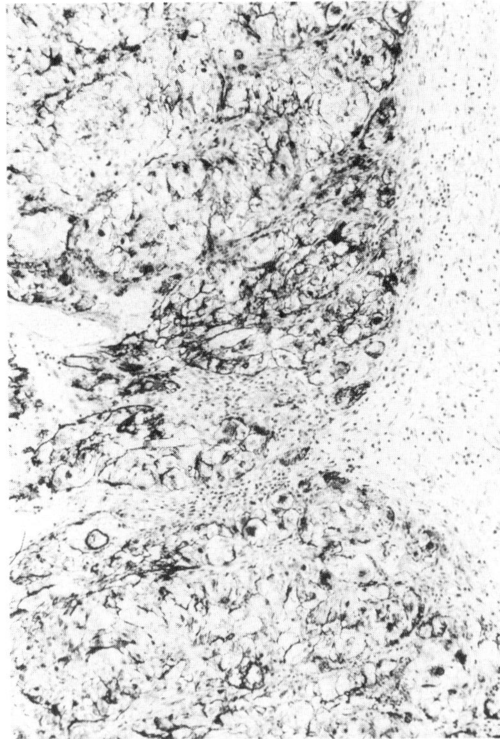

Fig 15–3.—Metastatic renal cell carcinoma shows strong staining, predominantly along cell membranes, for epithelial membrane antigen (anti-EMA and hematoxylin; original magnification, ×125). (Courtesy of Mills SE, Ross GW, Perentes E, et al: *Surg Pathol* 3:121–132, 1990.)

and metastases associated with renal-cell carcinoma. The patterns of immunohistochemistry for vimentin and, to a more limited extent, GFAP may also aid in distinguishing between these 2 types of cancer.

▶ This article addresses the sometimes difficult differential diagnosis of cerebellar hemangioblastoma vs. metastatic clear cell carcinoma. The discrimination of the "foamy" stromal cells of hemangioblastoma from the clear cell of renal carcinoma may cause problems, especially on small or stereotactic biopsies. Clinical and radiographic clues may also be confusing in these patients because they are both vascular, and hemangioblastomas may be multiple. The article stresses the importance of EMA as a discriminator, with all the renal carcinomas tested revealing a degree of positive EMA staining. It also points out the potential pitfall of staining with GFAP, which may stain reactive astrocytes within the tumor.—P. Garen, M.D.

Intraspinal Neurothekeoma (Nerve Sheath Myxoma): A Report of Two Cases

Paulus W, Jellinger K, Perneczky G (Ludwig Boltzmann Inst of Clinical Neurobiology, Vienna; Univ of Tuebingen, Germany; Rudolfstiftung Hosp, Vienna)

Am J Clin Pathol 95:511–516, 1991 15–6

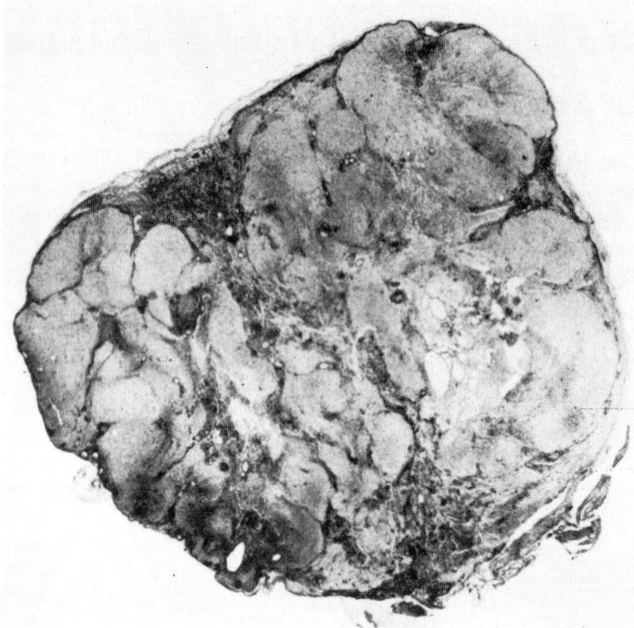

15–4.—A low-power view of the myxomatous tumor, revealing a prominent multinodular pattern. Hematoxylin-eosin; original magnification, ×9. (Courtesy of Paulus W, Jellinger K, Perneczky G: *Am J Clin Pathol* 95:511–516, 1991.)

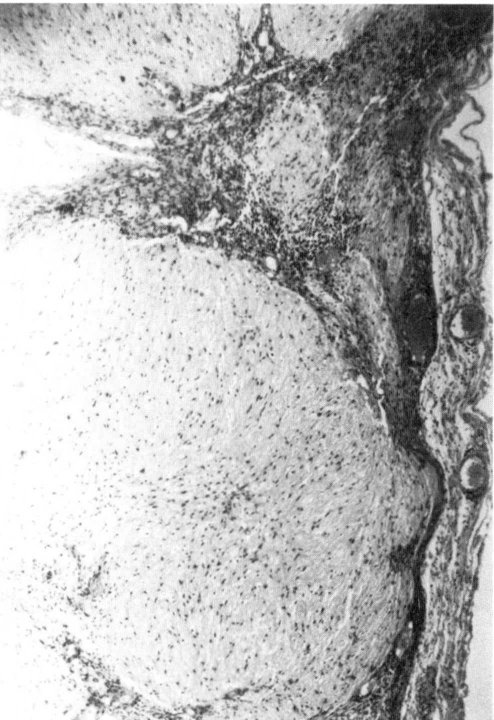

Fig 15–5.—Lobules composed of sparsely distributed tumor cells. Note inflammatory infiltrates within capsule *(right)* and intervening connective tissue septa. Hematoxylin-eosin; original magnification, ×45. (Courtesy of Paulus W, Jellinger K, Perneczky G: *Am J Clin Pathol* 95:511–516, 1991.)

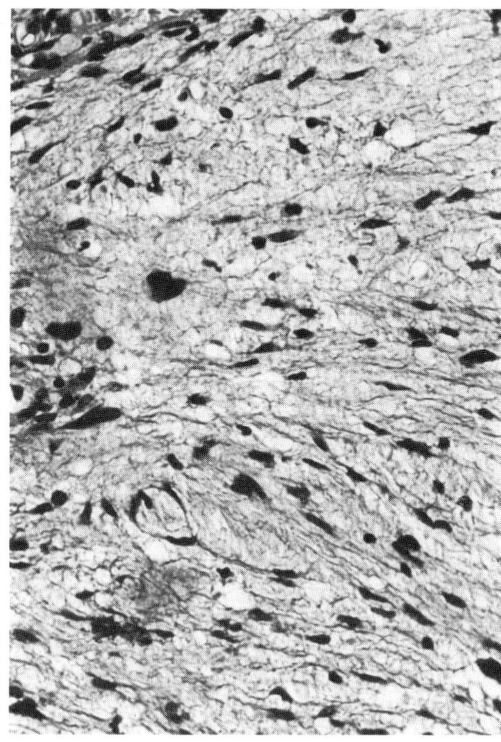

Fig 15–6.—High-power view showing some variation in nuclear size and shape. Hematoxylin-eosin; original magnification, ×320. (Courtesy of Paulus W, Jellinger K, Perneczky G: *Am J Clin Pathol* 95:511–516, 1991.)

Introduction.—Nerve sheath myxomas are rare benign cutaneous neoplasms most often found on the face or arms of young adults. Two spinal intradural tumors with histologic, ultrastructural, and immunohistochemical features identical to those of cutaneous neurothekeomas were found.

Case 1.—Woman, 32, with progressive back pain for 6 months had a nearly complete myelographic block at L4 representing an intradural mass. Magnetic resonance imaging demonstrated a well-delineated tumor at this level with marked peripheral contrast enhancement.

Case 2.—Man, 47, with progressive left thoracic back pain and mild weakness and numbness of both legs had an incomplete Brown-Séquard syndrome. Myelography showed a total block at T6, and a highly vascular intradural tumor was completely removed. The woman and the man were doing well 20 and 8 months, respectively, after tumor removal. Neither patient had signs of neurofibromatosis.

Pathology.—The tumors were multinodular and exhibited lobules of tumor cells with inflammatory cell infiltration (Figs 15–4 and 15–5). A few large pleomorphic nuclei were seen (Fig 15–6), but there were no mitoses. Vascular fibrosis was a prominent feature. Myxoid areas were

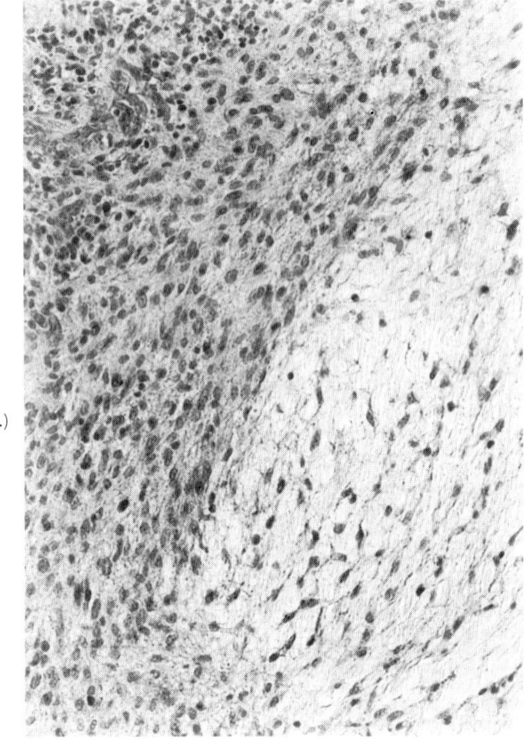

Fig 15–7.—Myxoid areas *(lower right)* clearly delimited from cellular epithelioid areas *(upper left)*. Hematoxylin-eosin; original magnification, ×170. (Courtesy of Paulus W, Jellinger K, Perneczky G: *Am J Clin Pathol* 95:511–516, 1991.)

delimited from cellular epithelioid areas (Fig 15–7). Tumor cells were positive for vimentin and S-100 protein but negative for neurofilament protein and desmin. The spindle-shaped tumor cells had long interdigitating cytoplasmic processes and exhibited infoldings of the cell membrane.

Interpretation.—The features of the neoplasms corresponded with descriptions of cutaneous neurothekeomas. As with cutaneous tumors, it is likely that intraspinal neurothekeomas can be cured by total removal.

▶ Neurothekeoma is a rare, benign tumor that has been described primarily in a cutaneous location. This neoplasm is often thought to arise in association with cutaneous nerves, leading to one of its other common designations, nerve sheath myxoma. Since the early descriptions of this lesion, it has been noted to occur in noncutaneous sites such as oral cavity and breast. This article discusses 2 intraspinal neoplasms connected to nerve roots. These neuroplasms have the characteristic lobulation and myxoid quality of neurothekeomas. Neither patient had evidence of von Recklinghausen's disease. This finding expands the reported sites of occurrence of neurothekeoma and the differential diagnosis of intraspinal benign tumors. Tumor immunostaining failed to resolve the question of Schwannian or perineurial origin.—P. Garen, M.D.

Melanotic Ependymoma and Subependymoma

Rosenblum MK, Erlandson RA, Aleksic SN, Budzilovich GN (Mem Sloan-Kettering Cancer Ctr, New York; New York Univ-Bellevue Hosp Med Ctr)

Am J Surg Pathol 14:729–736, 1990 15–7

Introduction.—Melanogenesis in the developed human CNS generally is limited to leptomeningeal melanocytes and selected neurons in brainstem nuclei and in the roof of the fourth ventricle. Production of melanin by primary intracranial tumors other than malignant melanomas and melanocytomas is rare.

Case 1.—Girl, 13 years, had right hemiparesis and muscle atrophy and had a grossly pigmented, well-differentiated ependymoma resected from the left frontoparietal region. She received radiotherapy and was well 12 years later. Little cytologic pleomorphism was present in the tumor (Fig 15–8). Fine brown pigment granules were seen in the tumor-cell cytoplasm (Fig 15–9). Premelanosomes were not identified.

Case 2.—Man, 52, died of complications of hyperparathyroidism caused by a functional parathyroid adenoma. At autopsy, a pigmented subependymoma was incidentally discovered. An intracytoplasmic pigment meeting histochemical criteria for melanin was present in the tumor cells.

Interpretation.—The mechanism of melanogenesis in these tumors is not clear, but the neoplasms do support the potential ability of glial derivatives to produce melanin. Melanogenesis in ependymal and

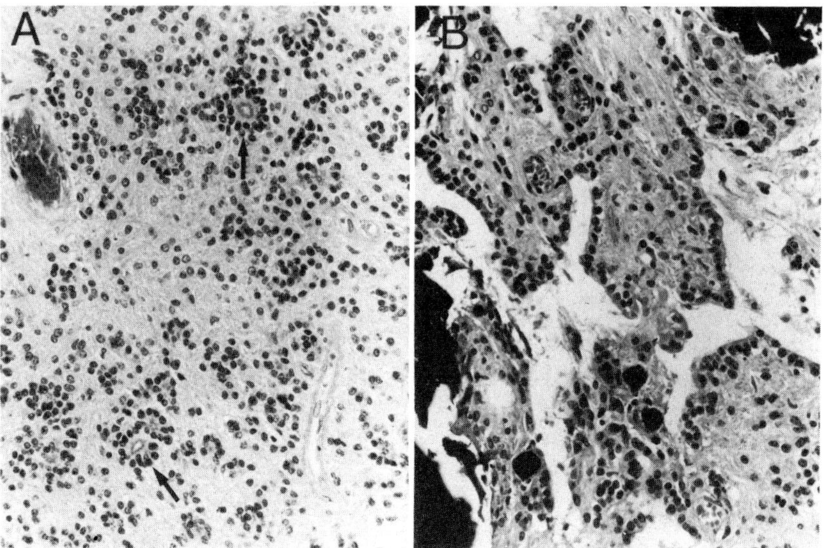

Fig 15–8.—Features indicative of ependymal differentiation are illustrated in these views of a tumor. **A,** formation of ependymal rosettes *(arrows);* **B,** lining of cleftlike spaces by cuboidal tumor cells resembling mature ependyma. Note also the calcifications. (Courtesy of Rosenblum MK, Erlandson RA, Aleksic SN, et al: *Am J Surg Pathol* 14:729–736, 1990.)

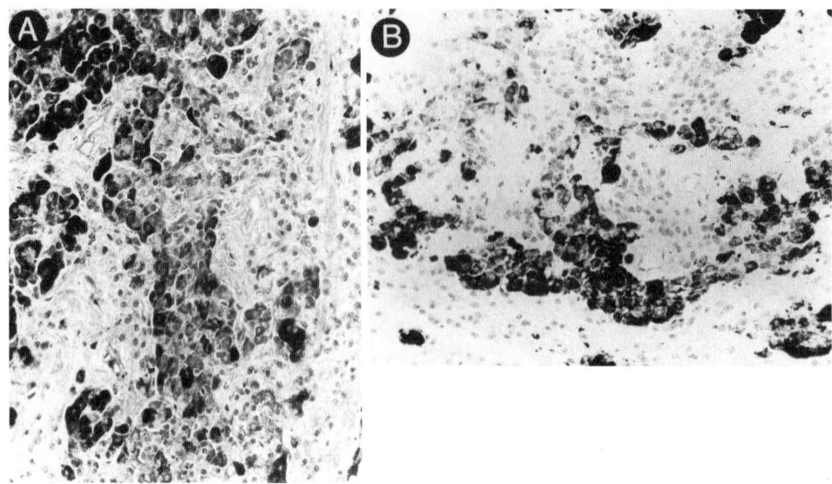

Fig 15–9.—Appearance of pigment-laden tumor cells in hematoxylin-eosin (**A**) and Fontana-Masson (**B**) preparations. (Courtesy of Rosenblum MK, Erlandson RA, Aleksic SN, et al: *Am J Surg Pathol* 14:729–736, 1990.)

subependymal neoplasms may lack adverse prognostic significance. These tumors contrast markedly with the anaplastic, rapidly fatal pigmented choroid plexus neoplasms.

▶ Melanotic tumors of the CNS are uncommon and are confined primarily to those arising in the leptomeninges. These consist of melanomas and melanocytomas. This article draws attention to some even rarer forms of tumors that produce melanin or a melanin-like substance, including choroid plexus and ependymal neoplasms, thus expanding the differential diagnosis. In addition, the cause of the melanotic pigment is investigated. Although these tumors share the histochemical profile of melanin, no ultrastructural evidence of premelanosomes was discovered. This suggests to the authors the possibility of an alternative pathway of production of the melanin-like pigment in these tumors. No evidence of lipofuscin pigment was present to indicate the possibility of pseudoperoxidation.—P. Garen, M.D.

Chordomas With Malignant Spindle Cell Components: A DNA Flow Cytometric and Immunohistochemical Study With Histogenetic Implications

Hruban RH, Traganos F, Reuter VE, Huvos AG (Mem Sloan-Kettering Cancer Ctr, New York)

Am J Pathol 137:435–447, 1990 15–8

Background.—Chordomas having a high-grade malignant spindle-cell population often are called "dedifferentiated" and tend to behave aggressively, frequently metastasizing. Possible explanations include a collision of unrelated tumors, postradiation sarcoma, and a tumor with differing rates of growth, causing 2 distinct morphological patterns.

Methods.—Paraffin-embedded tissue samples from 4 chordomas with a malignant spindle-cell component and 12 conventional chordomas underwent DNA flow cytometry. Immunohistochemical staining also was done to detect a range of epithelial and mesenchymal markers.

Findings.—All 4 tumors with a malignant spindle-cell component contained areas of conventional chordoma and all had an aneuploid-multiploid DNA content. The areas of conventional chordoma differed in DNA content from those containing the malignant spindle cells. Only 3 of the 11 conventional chordomas that could be analyzed had an aneuploid-multiploid DNA content. The malignant spindle cell areas stained strongly for vimentin and weakly for cytokeratin, S-100 protein, and epithelial membrane antigen. In contrast, the areas of conventional chordoma stained moderately for vimentin and S-100 protein and strongly for cytokeratin and epithelial membrane antigen, as did the conventional chordomas.

Conclusion.—Some chordomas that contain a malignant spindle-cell component are multipotential neoplasms in which the tumor cells can differentiate along both epithelial and mesenchymal paths.

▶ The cause of the spindle component of chordomas has been a matter of interest in the literature. These tumors frequently have been classified as "dedifferentiated" chordomas. The suggested causes have included a collision of unrelated tumors, an irradiation effect on chordomas, differing rates of tumor cell growth, and the origination of a sarcoma in a preexisting chordoma. Using a combination of DNA ploidy and calculation of proliferative indices in conjunction with the findings of both histologic features in metastatic lesions, the authors find that none of these explanations account fully for the behavior of the tumor. They suggest that, because the cell of putative origin for the tumor, the notochordal remnants, displays both epithelial and mesenchymal characteristics, so do the tumors arising from them. Thus, the tumors are not truly dedifferentiating but are expressing both aspects of their multipotential heritage.—P. Garen, M.D.

Cerebral Lymphomas: Review of 70 Cases

Adams JH, Howatson AG (Southern Gen Hosp, Glasgow; Royal Infirmary, Glasgow)

J Clin Pathol 43:544–547, 1990 15–9

Introduction.—Controversy continues over the nature of lymphomas in the CNS. The tumors tend to occur in older persons, except for those who are immune deficient. The incidence of these tumors appears to be increasing in the West of Scotland. Seventy cerebral lymphomas were examined and reclassified using the modified Kiel system. Only 2 patients were known to be immune deficient.

Findings.—The gross appearance varied substantially. Microscopically, the tumors consisted of sheets of lymphoid-type cells. Many monocyte-phagocyte cells also were present. Many of the tumors were of high-grade/large cell types. Twelve tumors contained very pleomorphic cells that did not fit any subtype of the Kiel classification. Sixteen of 47 autopsied patients had systemic tumor. Positive immunocytologic studies consistently showed the tumor cells to be of B cell origin. There were no T cell neoplasms, although reactive T cells frequently were present.

Discussion.—All of these tumors were classic diffuse non-Hodgkin's lymphomas. The findings fail to distinguish between 2 proposed hypotheses: that reactive lymphocytes are attracted to the CNS by latest Epstein-Barr virus or other herpesviruses, and that B lymphocytes are transformed elsewhere and develop specific binding markers for the CNS.

▶ Lymphomas of the CNS have received renewed attention, especially in relation to immunosuppression. Increased numbers of such lymphomas have been associated with organ transplantation and with AIDS. This article points out the apparent increase in CNS lymphomas being seen in Scotland, both in association with immunosuppression and as sporadic cases. The authors confirm the previously documented finding that primary CNS lymphomas are almost exclusively B cell in origin. Frequently, cells are present, but are reactive. These lymphomas are almost always diffuse and frequently are difficult to classify.—P. Garen, M.D.

Clues and Pitfalls in Stereotactic Biopsy of the Central Nervous System

Taratuto AL, Sevlever G, Piccardo P (Instituto de Investigaciones Neurologicas "Raul Carrea," Buenos Aires)

Arch Pathol Lab Med 115:596–602, 1991 15–10

Background.—Stereotactic biopsy specimens of the CNS were studied. Two different surgical teams performed the biopsies using the systems of Leksell and Talairach et al. independently and either Leksell or Sedan needles.

Methods.—In a 6-year period, 307 biopsies were performed. Patients with deep cerebral lesions, with lesions in highly functional areas, or with lesions that were poorly defined on imaging studies, and candidates for brachytherapy, were selected for stereotactic biopsy of the CNS. Smear examination during surgery was done routinely, followed by conventional histologic techniques.

Results.—Fifty-seven percent were astrocytic tumors; 9.7%, oligodendroglial; 2.3%, ependymal; 5.5%, pineoblastomas; 1.2%, medulloblastomas; 2.7%, lymphomas; 2.7%, meningiomas; 1.6%, schwannomas; 3.1%, craniopharyngiomas; 4.7%, germinomas; and 7.8%, metastases. Nontumors were arteriovenous malformations in 6 cases, pyogenic lesions in 6, infarcts in 7, hematomas in 2, multiple sclerosis plaque in 1, Fahr in 1, progressive multifocal leukoencephalopathy in 1, tuberculosis in 1, cysticercosis in 1, and Chagas' encephalitis in 1. An awareness of the cerebellar granular layer in infratentorial targets and glial reaction around craniopharyngiomas was essential for correct diagnosis. The differential diagnosis between well-differentiated astrocytomas vs. glial reaction and between poorly differentiated neoplasms vs. metastases was difficult. Smear cytologic assessment and myelin techniques in the former along with basic immunohistochemistry in the latter enabled correct diagnosis confirmed later at follow-up.

Conclusions.—When representative material is obtained, stereotactic biopsy is a reliable way to diagnose brain tumoral conditions histologically. It is the method of choice for deep-seated lesions.

▶ Stereotactic brain biopsy in the field of neurosurgery has proved to be reliable, precise, and reproducible. Placement of instrumentation is possible practically anywhere within the intracranial space. In this article, the authors presented 307 smear biopsies. Ninety-three percent of the cases correctly concurred with conventional histologic methods.

Pitfalls in stereotactic brain biopsies can be minimized by working closely with the neurosurgeon. Good representative materials, which are the first priority for accurate diagnosis, also help to minimize errors. This method should be used not only in well appointed medical centers but also in established community hospitals. With that in mind, residents in pathology should be exposed more often to this method because it will benefit their later practice of pathology.—S.W. Wong, M.D.

Diagnostic Value of Anti-Neuronal Antibodies for Paraneoplastic Disorders of the Nervous System

Moll JWB, Henzen-Logmans SC, Splinter TAW, van der Burg MEL, Vecht ChJ (Dr Daniel den Hoed Cancer Ctr, Rotterdam; Univ Hosp Dijkzigt, Rotterdam, The Netherlands)

J Neurol Neurosurg Psychiatry 53:940–943, 1990 15–11

Background.—It may be difficult to diagnose paraneoplastic disorders of the nervous system during life because symptoms and findings tend to be nonspecific. Several antineuronal autoantibodies have been identified in these patients, including antinuclear nucleoprotein antibody and anti-Purkinje cell antibody (APCA).

Objective.—The diagnostic value of antineuronal antibodies was examined in 21 patients suspected of having paraneoplastic disorders. Antibody was estimated using the indirect immunofluorescence technique. Control subjects included 25 patients with neurologic disease but not cancer, 27 with neurologic disorder and cancer but no signs of paraneoplastic disorder, and 94 patients with cancer alone.

Findings.—Eight of the 21 study patients (38%) had serum antineuronal nuclear antibody. In 5 of these patients, neurologic symptoms preceded the diagnosis of neoplasm. Among control subjects, only 2 patients with neurologic disease and cancer had increased titers of antineuronal nuclear antibody. Both of them had small-cell lung cancer.

Conclusion.—The presence of antineuronal nuclear antibody in serum is moderately sensitive and highly specific for paraneoplastic disorder of the nervous system. In particular, the presence of APCA has been shown to be highly specific for paraneoplastic cerebellar degeneration.

▶ The cause of paraneoplastic syndromes is one of many unanswered questions relating to relatively common clinical problems. In many cases these syndromes produce greater morbidity than their underlying neoplasm, and their treatment is purely symptomatic. The demonstration in this paper that immunologic mechanisms may be responsible for at least some of the paraneoplastic disorders opens up new possibilities for therapy and for a clearer understanding of these phenomena. Diagnostic use of tests such as the one described in this paper may also be of value in cases where the diagnosis is suspected but initial screening for neoplasm is negative.—B.D. Bennett, M.D., Ph.D.

Autopsy Study of Unruptured Incidental Intracranial Aneurysms

Inagawa T, Hirano A (Shimane Prefectural Central Hosp, Izumo, Japan; Montefiore Med Ctr, Bronx)
Surg Neurol 34:361–365, 1990 15–12

Introduction.—In a series of more than 10,000 autopsies done at Montefiore Medical Center between 1951 and 1987, 84 patients had 102 unruptured aneurysms, for a prevalence of .8%.

Findings.—Sixteen of the subjects had multiple aneurysms. The mean age was 67 years. Nearly two thirds were women. Middle cerebral artery and internal carotid aneurysms were most frequent. Unruptured aneurysms were most frequent in those aged 60 and above. Fifty-four percent of the aneurysms were 4 mm or less in diameter, and 35% measured 5 to 99 mm in diameter. Aneurysm size could not be related to age, aneurysm site, or wall thickness.

Conclusions.—Small aneurysms may be at a low risk of rupturing, but this low risk probably cannot be adequately explained by morphologic features alone. Hemodynamic studies might cast light on why these aneurysms rarely rupture.

▶ This paper examines the unruptured saccular aneurysms present in a series of 10,000 autopsies at Montefiore Medical Center. Eighty-four patients had aneurysms, some of which were multiple. The authors examined multiple factors in an effort to isolate any that would correlate with increased probability of rupture with its associated high mortality. The authors could find no correlation between rupture and age or sex of patients, location, size, or thickness of aneurysm wall. No morphologic finding could be found that corresponded to an increased likelihood of rupture. The authors suggest that other studies, such as hemodynamic indices, may be more helpful in indicating which aneurysms may rupture.—P. Garen, M.D.

Hyaline Globules Reacting Positively With Zidovudine Antibody in Brain and Spinal Cord of AIDS Patients

Artigas J, Arastéh K, Averdunk R, Bachler B, Hornscheidt M, Grosse G, L'age M, Niedobitek F (Auguste-Victoria-Krankenhaus, Berlin)
Lancet 337:1127–1128, 1991 15–13

Background.—A previously unreported extracellular material in the white matter of the brain and spinal cord was observed in 9 of 40 patients who died of AIDS. To identify the composition of these hyaline globules, an immunohistochemical study was performed. These spherical or lobulated collections were confined to the white matter especially in patients with vascular leucoencephalopathy. They were randomly distributed throughout the brain.

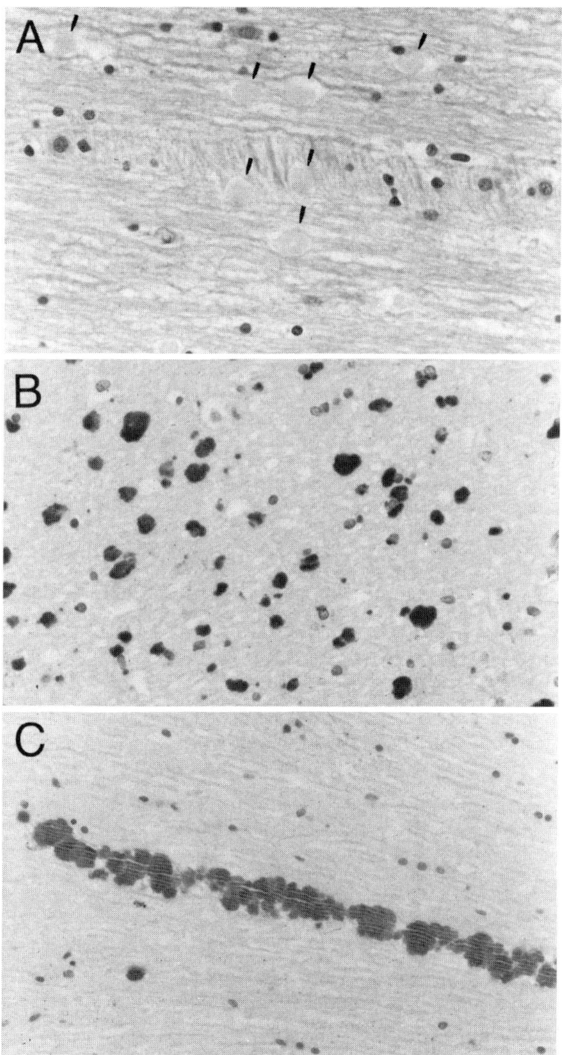

Fig 15–10.—Histopathology of globules. **A,** globules *(arrowheads)* in white matter of brain showing weak stain with PAS. Patient aged 27 years. Internal capsule reduced by 40% from ×800. **B,** droplets of different sizes with positive zidovudine staining in area with signs of vacuolar leukoencephalopathy. Patient aged 39 years. Parietal white matter, anti-zidovudine reduced by 40% from ×800. **C,** collections of droplets with positive zidovudine staining forming large chain in white matter of spinal cord. Patient aged 26 years. Longitudinal section through posterior columns of cervical spinal cord, anti-zidovudine reduced by 40% from ×600. (Courtesy of Artigas J, Arastéh K, Averdunk R, et al: *Lancet* 337:1127–1128, 1991.)

Methods.—Antibodies against a wide variety of viruses, proteins, and AIDS medications were tested. Biochemical studies were done by using tissue from patients who had received zidovudine and whose tissue stained positively with antizidovudine and from patients who had not received zidovudine. High-performance liquid chromatography (HPLC) was used to test for the presence of zidovudine.

Results.—Only antizidovudine showed strong positive staining with the globules (Fig 15–10). Tissue from patients without HIV infection did not stain with antizidovudine. Although HPLC showed a peak at 9,61 in AIDS patients who had received zidovudine, no peak was observed in those who did not receive the drug. The globules were easily distinguished from corpora amylacea and from degenerating or dystrophic axons.

Conclusions.—Zidovudine can enter the brain from the CSF and in AIDS patients through a disrupted blood-brain barrier. All these patients had neurologic deficits, but the effects of the droplets could not be assessed because the patients had died of other neurologic conditions. Further studies of the clinical significance of these globules are needed.

▶ This study suggests that zidovudine crosses a disrupted blood-brain barrier in AIDS patients to produce these inclusions.—A.J. Garvin, M.D.

Squamous Cell Carcinoma of the Cornea

Cameron JA, Hidayat AA (King Khaled Eye Specialist Hosp, Riyadh, Saudi Arabia; Armed Forces Inst of Pathology, Washington, DC)

Am J Ophthalmol 111:571–574, 1991 15–14

Introduction.—Squamous cell carcinoma of the cornea has been described in conjunction with a lesion of the adjacent limbus. The 2 patients studied had no limbal involvement.

Case 1.—Man, 40, was seen with left eye pain and a blood-tinged discharge. Vision had declined gradually during the past 3 years, and the right eye had been totally blind since childhood. Only light perception was present on the left. A central corneal lesion 10 mm wide and 88 mm high was seen on the left cornea; the peripheral cornea and corneoscleral limbus were free of gross disease. Microinvasive carcinoma was managed by superficial keratectomy and cryotherapy with a good outcome.

Case. 2.—Man, 57, had a corneal white spot for 1 year and perceived hand motion only. Both eyes exhibited elastotic degeneration, corneal scarring, and advanced immature cataracts. An elevated white lesion was found centrally in the left cornea. Penetrating keratoplasty was done with extracapsular cataract extraction and posterior chamber intraocular lens implantation. Microscopic study showed normal corneal epithelium at the periphery of the surgical specimen. The patient was well 9 months after surgery.

Discussion.—Ultraviolet exposure is considered the major cause of squamous cell carcinoma of the conjunctiva, and it also probably has a major role in primary squamous cell carcinoma of the cornea. Evidence of actinic damage was seen in both of these patients.

▶ The stratified squamous epithelium of the cornea can give rise to corneal intraepithelial neoplasia and to squamous cell carcinoma. With some similarity to the process at the squamocolumnar junction of the uterine cervix, dysplastic lesions of the eye are thought to arise at the corneoscleral limbus. The 2 cases described are unusual because no limbal involvement is identified. The authors speculate that this could be the result of migration of dysplastic epithelium from the corneoscleral limbus to a more central position on the cornea.—J.A. Tucker, M.D.

Creutzfeldt-Jakob Disease in Pituitary Growth Hormone Recipients in the United States

Fradkin JE, Schonberger L, Mills JL, Gunn WJ, Piper JM, Wysowski DK, Thomson R, Durako S, Brown P (Natl Inst of Diabetes and Digestive and Kidney Diseases, Bethesda, Md; Ctrs for Disease Control, Atlanta; Natl Inst of Child Health and Human Development, Bethesda, Md; Food and Drug Admin, Rockville, Md; Westat Inc, Rockville, Md; Natl Inst of Neurological Disorders and Stroke, Bethesda, Md)

JAMA 265:880–884, 1991 15–15

Purpose.—With the 1985 report of 3 deaths from Creutzfeldt-Jakob disease (CJD) among hypopituitary patients treated in childhood with human growth hormone (hGH) provided through the National Hormone and Pituitary Program, distribution of hGH was immediately terminated. A systematic epidemiologic study was begun of 6,284 patients who received hGH from the beginning of the program in 1963 to assess their current health status.

Methods.—A total of 5,288 recipients (84%) were successfully contacted and interviewed. Available reports were reviewed for 254 deaths, excluding previously reported cases of CJD. By using statistics and experimental injection of primates with samples of hGH thought to be contaminated, attempts were made to identify the batches of pituitary glands and lots of hormone that may have been contaminated.

Results.—Among the total cohort hGH therapy had begun at an average age of 9.6 years and continued for an average of 2.9 years. A total of 7 cases of CJD have resulted thus far, only 2 of which were newly identified during the present study. The median duration of therapy was 100 months in this group of 7, compared with 41 months for those who did not have CJD. The mean intervals from the start and end of hormone therapy to the onset of symptoms of CJD were 20 and 10 years. Ominously, only 6% and 14% of the rest of the cohort have as yet fulfilled a posttreatment incubation period of this length. Although altered mentation is the initial symptom in most cases of sporadic CJD, the present patients first showed ataxia and imbalance and then had increasingly serious motor signs; dementia occurred very late in the process. No statistically significant relationship was found between CJD and a batch or lot of hGH; no injected animals have yet expressed the disease.

Discussion.—From the analysis it may be concluded that duration of hormone therapy was a major risk factor for infection with CJD, that contamination was probably random and diluted among many hormone preparations, and that because only a fraction of the patients who may have been exposed have fulfilled the incubation period for expression of CJD, there may be an increasing number of deaths caused by CJD among this cohort in the future.

▶ This paper is noteworthy because of the many pathologists who, especially during residency, unwittingly participated in this experiment (i.e., retrieving at autopsy 1.4 million pituitaries). Although the causative agent for CJD remains elusive, evidence continues to accumulate pointing to a strange life form—the so-called prion protein. The relationship of this protein to a genetic pathogenesis for some cases of CJD now seems to be established (1).—W.A. Gardner, Jr., M.D.

Reference

1. Hsiao K, et al: *N Engl J Med* 325:1091, 1991.

The Occult Aftermath of Boxing

Roberts GW, Allsop D, Bruton C (St Mary's Med School, London; Psychiatric Research Inst of Tokyo, Japan; Runwell Hosp, Wickford, England)

J Neurol Neurosurg Psychiatry 53:373–378, 1990 15–16

Background.—Repeated head trauma can cause dementia pugilistic (DP), or punch drunk syndrome, in boxers. Initial affective disorder and psychotic symptoms are superseded by social instability with memory loss, parkinsonian signs, and finally, decreased general cognitive functioning and pyramidal tract disease.

Study.—Temporal lobe specimens from 14 of the 15 cases of DP originally reported by Corsellis et al., who described neurofibrillary tangles in the absence of plaques, were reeexamined.

Observation.—Cases with substantial numbers of neurofibrillary tangles consistently had immunocytochemical evidence of extensive β-protein deposits. These diffuse "plaques" were not apparent on Congo red or standard silver staining. The degree of β-protein deposition was similar to that seen in Alzheimer's disease. No marked association was seen between the β-immunoreactivity of diffuse plaques and blood vessels.

Discussion.—There are many clinical and pathologic similarities between Alzheimer's disease and DP, and they likely share common pathogenic mechanisms that produce tangles and plaque. Head injury with secondary neuronal shearing or damage to vessels may precipitate the pathologic processes that give rise to Alzheimer's disease.

▶ Traditionally, Alzheimer's disease and dementia pugilistica have been regarded as 2 different processes linked by a common finding of neurofibrillary tangles. This study demonstrates "occult" plaques, which are seen in some Alzheimer's disease patients, in temporal lobes of patients with dementia pugilistica. This finding, coupled with the presence of β-amyloid raises some interesting questions about the cause of Alzheimer's disease. Trauma is implicated as a possible precipitating factor that results in neuronal and perhaps vascular damage with subsequent plaque and tangle formation and deposition of β amyloid.—P. Garen, M.D.

What's in a Burger?

Carr NJ, Machin LG (RAF Inst of Pathology and Tropical Medicine, Buckinghamshire, England; Royal Marsden Hosp, Surrey, England)

J Clin Pathol 44:164, 1991 15–17

Introduction.—Because of the potential for introducing the transmissible agent of bovine spongiform encephalopathy into the human food chain, government regulations in the United Kingdom prohibit the use of CNS tissue in foodstuffs. A recent report described the use of an immunoperoxidase stain for glial fibrillary acidic protein to demonstrate the absence of CNS tissue in beef sausages. The same staining technique was used to confirm the absence of CNS tissue in beef burgers.

Methods.—The study material consisted of 4 beef burgers. Two were well-known supermarket house brands, 1 was prepared by a butcher, and 1 was obtained from a hospital staff canteen. The burgers were processed by routine formalin fixation and paraffin wax embedding. At least 2 stained sections from each tissue block were examined.

Results.—None of the burgers contained CNS tissue. Skeletal muscle was the predominant component. The proportions of fat, fibrous tissue, and vegetable matter varied among burgers. This technique could be useful for monitoring adherence to government regulations in the meat industry in the United Kingdom.

▶ This very preliminary study is not as frivolous as might be suggested by the title. The level of anxiety about the possible hazards of eating beef has resulted in high British government officials publicly eating hamburgers to demonstrate their confidence in the safety of the product. Once again, basic pathology techniques to the rescue. Governmental and media attention together with the theoretical risk of transmission of bovine encephalopathy to human beings resulted in an international conference (1). This conference addressed the implications of bovine spongiform encephalopathy and related diseases on the use of human and animal-derived materials in the health and biological industries. Unfortunately, the answers to the questions remain almost as hypothetical as the risk.—W.A. Gardner, Jr., M.D.

Reference

1. Baron H: *Toxicologic Pathology* 19:293, 1991.

PART TWO
CLINICAL PATHOLOGY

16 Chemical Pathology

The Effect of Haematocrit on Reagent Strip Tests for Glucose
Wiener K (North Manchester Gen Hosp, England)
Diabetic Med 8:172–175, 1991 16–1

Introduction.—Reagent strip tests that measure glucose in whole blood are quick and convenient for checking blood glucose levels in diabetic patients. One factor that can affect results is the hematocrit of the specimen. To quantify the influence of this factor, 4 different tests systems were compared.

Method.—The reagent strips tested were the BM-Test 1-44, Glucostix, Hypoguard GA, and Exactech. All 4 use strips impregnated with glucose oxidase. Erythrocytes and plasma of fresh venous blood samples were separated and then remixed in different proportions to achieve a range of hematocrit values. The resulting specimens were subjected to glucose assay.

Findings.—All strip tests were affected to some degree by hematocrit, lower hematocrits producing higher glucose results. The BM-Test 1-44 was least affected. The Hypoguard GA and Glucostix behaved similarly to each other at hematocrits below .45. At higher hematocrits, Hypoguard GA was affected more. Glucose results differed by as much as 49% from one end of the normal adult hematocrit range to the other.

Conclusion.—Hematocrit may affect results by influencing the rate or amount of plasma absorption into the reagent pad. The manufacturers' quoted ranges of acceptable hematocrit were often inconsistent with recommended limits of total error. Even more pronounced effects may occur in patients with abnormal hematocrits. Prescribers of strip testing systems should be aware of possible errors, and manufacturers should attempt to reduce the influence of hematocrit. The strips are not recommended for glucose tolerance testing.

▶ This is a particularly timely paper when one considers the rapidly increasing interest in and use of bedside testing for monitoring a variety of parameters. Glucose, certainly the most common of these, is also frequently monitored by reagent strip testing on an outpatient basis. Given the outcome of inappropriate insulin therapy, whether too much or too little, the influence of hematocrit in reagent strip testing for glucose is of critical importance.

Of even greater importance, however, is the more general topic that this article should bring to mind, i.e., there are many pathologic and nonpathologic states that can affect laboratory tests. No one can be expected to keep up with all of the various potential influences on test results. It is critical, however, that physicians who are responsible for establishing laboratory values and those who make decisions about patient care based on these values be aware that such influences occur. Both groups should require confirmation and explanation of values that deviate from the expected rather than accepting these as indicators of disease. Similar situations have been addressed in recent studies regarding the effect of reticulocyte concentration on lactate dehydrogenase isoenzyme distribution (1) and the influence of EDTA-dependent antibodies on automated white blood cell counts (2). Such articles usually appear as isolated case reports and as such may not attract appropriate attention from practicing physicians.—B.D. Bennett, M.D., Ph.D.

References

1. Kazmierczak SC, et al: *Clin Chem* 39:1638, 1990.
2. Hillyer CD, et al: *Am J Clin Pathol* 94:458, 1990.

Preanalytical Handling of Stored Urine Samples, and Measurement of β_2-Microglobulin, Orosomucoid, Albumin, Transferrin, and Immunoglobulin G in Urine by Enzyme-Linked Immunosorbent Assays (ELISA)

Vittinghus E (Univ Hosp of Aarhus, Denmark)

Scand J Clin Lab Invest 50:843–849, 1990 16–2

Background.—In measurement of urine proteins by sensitive immunologic techniques, the results may depend on how the samples are stored. Five urine proteins, β_2-microglobulin, orosomucoid, albumin, transferrin, and IgG, were measured to optimize sample storage conditions for later recovery of proteins.

Methods.—The subjects were 6 healthy volunteers and 13 patients with juvenile diabetes. After the addition of various substances, part of each sample from the normal subjects was stored at −20°C, part at +4°C, and part at room temperature for a week or more. Samples from diabetic patients were stored at −20°C for several years before the enzyme-linked immunosorbent assay (ELISA) was carried out. Samples were thawed by different methods, and various surfactants or albumin were added to some before analysis.

Results.—Transferrin decreased by 81%, IgG by 39%, and albumin by 26% in samples stored at −20°C for 1 week with no surfactant. The values were not decreased in the samples with Tween-20. Adding Tween-20 after thawing also increased values in samples previously stored without surfactant. Transferrin decreased by 80%, IgG by 57%, albumin by 30%, and β_2-microglobulin by 26% in urine samples thawed at room temperature just before analysis compared to samples that were thawed at 37°C, had added Tween-20, and were stored a few days at room temperature. No significant changes were seen in previously frozen samples that were handled in this manner whether analysis occurred the day after thawing or 35 days later. Freezing and thawing appeared to have less effect on orosomucoid values.

Conclusions.—In measurement of urine proteins by ELISA, preanalytic handling of specimens causes problems related to the choice of additives and storage temperature. These variables may be chosen according to the storage period and the protein in question. To assess the effects of storage, a prestorage value of the protein should be measured.

▶ Effects of storage on the stability of chemistry analytes can be difficult to determine from a search of the literature. This paper demonstrates a careful approach to documentation of the effects of storage on several urinary proteins and notes that freezing without the addition of a surfactant produces more significant changes in these analyses than does storage at room or refrigerator temperature. Because there is a common belief that most substances can be stored frozen with little, if any, effect on their measurement, this paper provides important information and reemphasizes the importance of knowledge of preanalytical variables.—B.D. Bennett, M.D., Ph.D.

Serum CA 125 Levels During the Menstrual Cycle

Lehtovirta P, Apter D, Stenman U-H (Helsinki Univ Central Hosp)

Br J Obstet Gynaecol 97:930–933, 1990 16–3

Background.—More than 80% of women with ovarian cancer have increased serum CA-125 levels. Measurement of CA-125 may be an important component of a strategy for early detection of ovarian cancer. Serum CA-125 levels were measured in different phases of the menstrual cycle, and a possible association with ovarian sex steroids was investigated in a group of 16 females with ovulatory and a group of 12 females with anovulatory cycles.

Findings.—In both groups, CA-125 levels were significantly higher during menstruation. The highest CA-125 levels in ovulatory and anovulatory participants during this phase were 51 units per mL and 125 units per mL, respectively. The CA-125 levels were already significantly increased before the beginning of menstruation in the anovulatory group. The overall CA-125 levels were slightly higher in the anovulatory than in the ovulatory group, but the difference was significant only during phase 3. The serum progesterone concentration was negatively correlated with CA-125 expressed as a percentage of individual mean value. As the progesterone concentration decreased in ovulatory cycles, CA-125 concentrations increased. In anovulatory cycles, most CA-125 values were increased above the mean level throughout the last week of the cycle.

Conclusion.—Premenstrual serum CA-125 increases in women with anovulatory cycles may be related to premature endometrial vascular changes resulting from a low serum progesterone concentration leading to insufficient endometrial control. The effect of progesterone on CA-125 synthesis therefore appears to be indirect. When the CA-125 assay is used as part of the diagnostic workup for cancer, samples should not be taken just before or during menstruation, because the physiologic increase of CA-125 levels may give false positive results.

▶ This paper demonstrates the influence of physiologic and pathophysiologic events on laboratory findings. Although these influences are true for a large number of tests, the most serious potential harm may occur when dealing with tests used as "screens" for cancer. Failure to recognize events that produce high levels of these "tumor markers" may result in significant emotional and financial expense to the patient before the cause of these "false positive" findings are discovered. This paper points out that the CA-125 level, although useful as part of the diagnostic workup for patients with suspected ovarian cancer, should not be measured immediately before or during the menstrual cycle. A second recent paper demonstrates that abdominal surgery, performed for any reason, also results in significant elevations of this marker and interferes with its specificity in the postoperative period (1). (See also Abstract 10–7.)—B.D. Bennett, M.D., Ph.D.

Reference

1. Van Der Zee AGT: *Br J Obstet Gynaecol* 97:934, 1990.

Early Diagnosis of Acute Myocardial Infarction Based on Assay for Subforms of Creatine Kinase-MB

Puleo PR, Guadagno PA, Roberts R, Scheel MV, Marian AJ, Churchill D, Perryman MB (Baylor College of Medicine, Houston; Helena Labs, Beaumont, Tex)
Circulation 82:759–764, 1990 16–4

Background.—Early implementation of thrombolytic therapy is necessary for maximum reduction of mortality rates in acute myocardial infarction (AMI). However, the early accurate diagnosis of AMI remains problematic.

Methods.—A 25-minute assay for the creatine kinase (CK)-MB subforms was developed and validated. Using this assay, plasma MB2 (tissue subform) activity, MB1 (plasma-modified subform) activity, and MB2/MB1 ratio were measured in 56 healthy individuals, 50 hospitalized patients without cardiac disease, and 49 patients with AMI. The sensitivity and specificity of this assay for the early diagnosis of AMI were determined.

Findings.—In the 56 healthy volunteers, the mean MB2 activity was .61 units per liter, the mean MB1 activity was .63 units per liter, and the MB2/MB1 ratio was .94; only 1 individual had both MB2 activity of more than 1 unit per liter and an MB2/MB1 ratio of more than 1.5. The values were similar in the 50 hospitalized patients without cardiac disease. Only 2 patients had both MB2 activity and a MB2/MB1 ratio greater than the cutoff values in normal volunteers. Thus the specificity of an abnormal result with both MB2 activity and an MB2/MB1 ratio greater than the cutoff values was 98% for normal individuals and 96% in the hospitalized patients.

In the 49 patients with AMI, MB2 activity and the subform ratio began to increase 2 hours after AMI. The subform ratio reached a plateau of 3.1 within 4–6 hours. The first available blood sample was abnormal by the subform assay in 67% of patients compared to only 27% by the conventional CK-MB assay. The sensitivity of the subform assay was

59% in blood samples collected 2–4 hours after AMI, 92% at 4–6 hours, and 100% at 6–8 hours. In contrast, the conventional MB assay had a sensitivity of less than 50% during the first 6 hours of AMI and 93% at 10–12 hours after onset of symptoms. False negative results were obtained by the subform assay in 15 samples at a mean of 2.3 hours after onset of AMI, whereas false negative conventional assay results were obtained in 54 samples at a mean of 5.8 hours after AMI.

Discussion.—The plasma CK-MB subform assay provides a rapid and reliable diagnosis of AMI within 4–6 hours after the onset of symptoms, a time when the conventional CK-MB assay remains in the normal range. The clinical application of these findings remains to be established.

▶ Vast progress has been made in the diagnostic laboratory evaluation of MI since the initial description of an elevated serum CK level in these patients. Extensive efforts continue to devise better and faster ways of diagnosing MI, thus allowing for earlier intervention and support. In addition, the ability of laboratory tests to rule out the diagnosis of MI is an important tool in attempts to minimize health care resources tied up in the observation of patients with non-MI chest pain. This paper documents the utility of a rapid, accurate procedure for diagnosis of MI within a time frame that allows for thrombolytic therapy in patients who need it and less intensive observation and intervention in those who do not. Relatively limited laboratory availability of isoform determinations and lack of information regarding the isoform pattern in patients with ischemic, noninfarction heart disease currently restrict the utility of this test. Although investigation of cardiac isoforms progresses, the utility of more readily available cardiac enzymes procedures continues to be evaluated, especially in clinically complicated situations. Areas of study include the use of discriminant analysis in the prediction of perioperative MI (1) and review of the significance of macromolecule CK (2).—B.D. Bennett, M.D., Ph.D.

References

1. Griesmacher A: et al: Clin Chem 36:883, 1990.
2. Laureys M, et al: Clin Chem 37:430, 1991.

Effect of Long-Term Monitoring of Glycosylated Hemoglobin Levels in Insulin-Dependent Diabetes Mellitus

Larsen ML, Hørder M, Mogensen EF (Odense Univ Hosp, Denmark)

N Engl J Med 323:1021–1025, 1990 16–5

Introduction.—Although determinations of glycosylated hemoglobin (hemoglobin A_{1c}) are commonly used to assess glycemic control in patients with diabetes mellitus, it has never been shown that monitoring hemoglobin A_{1c} results in improved metabolic control, as reflected by decreases in hemoglobin A_{1c} levels.

Patients.—In all, 240 patients with type I diabetes were divided randomly into 2 groups matched for age, sex, duration of diabetes, and initial levels of hemoglobin A_{1c}. The patients in 1 group were regularly monitored for hemoglobin A_{1c} for 1 year, with hemoglobin A_{1c} values used to modify therapy. Patients in the other group were monitored only for blood or urine glucose levels to adjust treatment.

Findings.—When hemoglobin A_{1c} levels were monitored, they decreased significantly from 10.1% to 9.5% during the year. This decrease was caused mainly by a lowering of hemoglobin A_{1c} values in patients with poor glycemic control initially. In the control group the mean levels of hemoglobin A_{1c} increased during the year from 10% to 10.1%. Patients whose hemoglobin A_{1c} levels were monitored had more frequent outpatient visits and changes in insulin regimens, but they required fewer hospitalizations than patients in the control group.

Conclusions.—Routine measurements of hemoglobin A_{1c} in patients with type I diabetes can result in improvement of glycemic control. It is not known whether lowering levels of hemoglobin A_{1c} will delay complications of diabetes.

▶ The importance of hemoglobin A_{1c} determinations in evaluation and monitoring of the diabetic patient is reconfirmed in this study. Use of this laboratory test as a primary monitor of the diabetic patient can result in improved control with fewer episodes of hospitalization. As the relationship between control of serum glucose and development of diabetic complications becomes more apparent, use of glycated hemoglobin and other long-term assessments of glucose status will become even more critical in management of these patients.—B.D. Bennett, M.D., Ph.D.

Chromogranin A in Children With Neuroblastoma: Serum Concentration Parallels Disease Stage and Predicts Survival

Hsiao RJ, Seeger RC, Yu AL, O'Connor DT (Univ of California, San Diego; VA Med Ctr, San Diego; Children's Hosp of Los Angeles; Univ of Southern California; Children's Cancer Study Group, Pasadena)

J Clin Invest 85:1555–1559, 1990 16–6

Introduction.—Chromogranin A is an acidic monomeric protein costored in and co-released from storage vesicles with catecholamines. Increased serum levels of chromogranin A have been reported in patients with peptide-producing endocrine neoplasia. The role of chromogranin A as a diagnostic and prognostic tool for neuroblastoma was assessed.

Methods.—With a rapid modification of the double-antibody radioimmunoassay, serum chromogranin A was measured at the time of diagnosis in 34 children with all stages of neuroblastoma, as well as in 38 age-matched controls (23 normal; 15 with non–peptide-producing neoplasms). Serum chromogranin levels were correlated with disease stage and prognosis.

Findings.—All children with neuroblastoma had elevated chromogranin A levels. An elevated serum chromogranin A level had a sensitivity of 91% and a specificity of 100% for neuroblastoma. Mean serum chromogranin A levels strongly correlated with disease stages. Furthermore, the level of serum chromogranin A was a significant prognostic factor.

During a median follow-up period of 18 months (range, 1–48 months), the survival rate for patients with lower serum chromogranin A levels (<190 ng/mL at the time of diagnosis) was significantly higher than that for patients with higher levels (69% vs. 30%). This relationship was particularly strong in children older than 1 year at the time of diagnosis and in those with more advanced disease (stages III and IV).

Conclusions.—Serum chromogranin A as a diagnostic tool for evaluation of children with neuroblastoma is better than or comparable to other neuroblastoma markers, including ferritin, neuron-specific enolase, and dopamine-β-hydroxylase. Furthermore, serum chromogranin A levels correlate with tumor burden and are effective prognostic tools, especially in patients older than 1 year or with more advanced disease.

▶ The search for the perfect serum tumor marker continues. Numerous candidates such as carcinoembryonic antigen (CEA) and α-fetoprotein have been proposed. Over time, the initial enthusiasm for these substances as tumor markers has decreased, although each retains significant utility under certain circumstances. In a subset of the population, i.e., children, it appears that chromogranin A answers many of the requirements for the ideal tumor marker. Although present in normal serum and in the serum of patients with neoplasms other than neuroblastoma, there is a 2½ to threefold difference between chromogranin A levels in patients with even stage I neuroblastoma and the other groups.

Chromogranin levels increase with tumor burden and are strongly associated with prognosis. Chromogranin concentrations are elevated in a variety of peptide-producing endocrine tumors and are therefore less valuable as definitive screening techniques in adults. In children, however (in whom neuroblastoma is by far the most common endocrine tumor), it appears that chromogranin may come close to being the ideal marker. Recent projects designed at screening the newborn population for neuroblastoma have been reported (1), and it can be assumed that similar projects based on chromogranin levels will soon follow.

Chromogranin has also been suggested as a valuable diagnostic tool in the detection of pheochromocytomas, both familial and sporadic, and could prove useful as a marker for patients with multiple endocrine neoplasia (2). Although not routinely performed in hospital laboratories, it is anticipated that this test will shortly become more widely available. It will be interesting to see whether it maintains a higher visibility as a tumor marker than its predecessors.—B.D. Bennett, M.D., Ph.D.

References

1. Tuchman M, et al: *Pediatrics* 86:765, 1990.
2. Hsiao RJ: *Am J Med* 88:607, 1990.

Plasma and Serum G4 Isoenzyme of Acetylcholinesterase in Patients With Alzheimer-Type Dementia and Vascular Dementia

Yamamoto Y, Nakano S, Kawashima S, Nakamura S, Urakami K, Kato T, Kameyama M (Kyoto Univ; Tottori Univ, Yonago, Japan)

Ann Clin Biochem 27:321–326, 1990 16–7

Background.—Human plasma and serum show high activity of pseudocholinesterase derived from the liver and low activity of true acetylcholinesterase (AChE), probably from neural tissue. Because measuring plasma or serum AChE activity is difficult, a new method was developed for measuring activity of the G4 AChE isoenzyme in plasma or serum and applied to patients with Alzheimer-type dementia and vascular dementia.

Methods.—Twenty patients with Alzheimer's dementia aged 46–91 years and 19 with vascular dementia aged 49–81 years were studied. The control group consisted of 26 healthy persons and 17 patients without significant psychiatric or neurologic disorders. The method for measuring plasma and serum G4 AChE activity used polyacrylamide gel electrophoresis.

Results.—The G4 AChE activity in serum and plasma did not differ. In the control group, plasma AChE activity was independent of age. Compared with age-matched controls, serum G4 AChE activity was significantly elevated in patients with vascular dementia and significantly reduced in patients with probable Alzheimer's disease. The difference in activity between the 2 groups was significant.

Conclusions.—Measurement of plasma G4 AChE activity may aid in the differential diagnosis of dementia and in decisions about acetylcholinesterase-inhibitor treatment. It should also be possible to correlate the clinical course of dementia with changes in plasma or serum G4 AChE levels. The finding of reduced G4 AChE activity, however, is not diagnostic for Alzheimer's dementia. Clinical and radiologic methods will still be important elements in diagnosis and follow-up of demented patients.

▶ Alzheimer's disease is the subject of intense investigation, not only in etiology and treatment but also in early diagnosis and screening. The documentation of a serum test that produces significantly different results in patients with Alzheimer's disease and those with vascular dementia is another step on the road to clarification of this mysterious and debilitating illness. Although this test is not now, and may never become, routinely available in hospital laboratories, its discovery will undoubtedly lead to the development of more easily disseminated laboratory testing as well as possible clarification of underlying biochemical abnormalities in Alzheimer's disease.—B.D. Bennett, M.D., Ph.D.

Consensus Document: Hawk's Cay Meeting on Therapeutic Drug Monitoring of Cyclosporine

Kahan BD, Shaw LM, Holt D, Grevel J, Johnston A (Univ of Texas, Houston; Univ of Pennsylvania; St. George's Hosp Med School, London; St. Bartholomew's Hosp, London)

Clin Chem 36:1510–1516, 1990 16–8

Background.—Many questions remain regarding the best measurement method and clinical application for the therapeutic monitoring of cyclosporine. A workshop was held to discuss extant as well as new methods of measurement, their validation studies, applications of trough concentration monitoring, and alternative pharmacokinetic approaches.

Findings.—Validation of selective monoclonal antibodies that detect parent compound cyclosporine in ^{3}H, ^{125}I, fluorosceinated, and enzyme-linked immunoassays has advanced a great deal. Development of simple automated assays is promising, but strict quality assessment procedures are needed for use both within and between laboratories. Use of selective monoclonal antibodies to measure whole-blood trough concentrations of cyclosporine is diagnostically efficacious. A wide range of prognostically insignificant blood concentrations is seen in patients in a clinically quiescent phase after transplantation; however, trough measurements can help in determining whether deterioration of renal allograft function is the result of insufficient immunosuppression or of drug-induced toxicity. Cyclosporine measurement may only measure compliance or identify patients with poor drug absorption or unusual metabolism and elimination when the dose is low or the therapeutic effect can be readily assessed. The reference procedure for parent drug determinations is high-performance liquid chromatography, although it is technically demanding. Experimental models and clinical correlations have not established a convincing role for cyclosporine metabolites in the therapeutic or toxic activities of the drug. To standardize communications on these metabolites, it was agreed that a new shorthand code is needed to identify them. Pharmacokinetic measurements to estimate total drug exposure appear promising for prediction of appropriate initial doses and adjustment of subsequent doses. To explain differences in immunologic sensitivity between individuals, assay systems must be developed that can measure the biological activity of cyclosporine.

Discussion.—Numerous questions require further study, including whether measurement of cyclosporine concentrations is sufficiently sensitive, specific, and predictive to use in monitoring for adverse events in posttransplant patients.

▶ Although numerous methods have been developed for measuring cyclosporine and its metabolites, problems in interpretation of these measurements continue. The development of automated immunoassays represents a major advance in the general availability of cyclosporine measurement. Questions concerning the utility of random vs. trough levels, the role of metabolites in therapeutic effect and toxicity, measurement of metabolites, and determination of "total exposure" represent only a few of the controversies surrounding cyclosporine measurement that will be difficult to resolve.—D.J. Wells, Ph.D.

Differentiation of Hematuria by Quantitative Determination of Urinary Marker Proteins

Hofmann W, Schmidt D, Guder WG, Edel HH (Städtisches Krankenhaus München-Bogenhausen, Germany; Städtisches Krankenhaus München-Harlaching, Germany)

Klin Wochenschr 69:68–75, 1991 16–9

Introduction.—Numerous noninvasive and invasive diagnostic procedures for differentiating between prerenal, renal, and postrenal causes of hematuria are available, but results of existing noninvasive studies are not always specific. Proteins are specifically handled by the kidney according to their molecular size and charge. Whether quantitative chemical tests based on patterns of problem excretion can be used to differentiate various forms of hematuria was investigated.

Methods.—The automated turbidimetric assay method was used to quantitate α_2-macroglobulin, which has a molecular weight (MW) of 720,000; IgG (MW 150,000), albumin (MW 67,000), and α_1-microglobulin (MW 33,000). Ratios of serum and urinary α_2-macroglobulin: albumin and IgG: albumin were determined in 21 healthy controls aged 18–60 years to define the reference ranges. Serum and urinary proteins were then quantitated for 93 adults with hematuria.

Findings.—Excretion of urinary α_2-macroglobulin, IgG, and albumin showed broad overlapping between patients with renal and postrenal hematuria and was not diagnostic. Moreover, concentrations of protein were not dependent on the degree of hematuria. The use of protein ratios, however, differentiated between renal and postrenal hematuria, with only a 20% overlap. When urines with albumin concentrations of less than 100 mg/L were excluded, this overlap disappeared. Measurement of the α_1-microglobulin concentration allowed further differentiation between postglomerular hematuria caused by interstitial nephropathy from glomerular and postrenal disease.

Conclusion.—Independent clinical examination confirmed that criteria derived from quantitative turbidimetric assay of urine protein can correctly localize the source of hematuria, provided urinary excretion of albumin exceeds 100 mg/L.

▶ The authors of this study propose a simple but previously unexplored hypothesis for evaluation of hematuria that could prove extremely useful in an era of medical cost containment. Quantitation of urinary albumin, α_2-macroglobulin, and IgG allows development of ratios that can accurately distinguish postrenal from renal causes of hematuria. These ratios may narrow the choice of other testing procedures, invasive or otherwise, required to allow a definitive diagnosis to be made. At present, urinary IgG and α_2-macroglobulin are not routinely analyzed in most hospital laboratories. If subsequent studies confirm these initial observations, clinical demand will probably make testing for these proteins considerably more common. It is also of note that quantitation of another protein, α_1-macroglobulin, shows promise in differentiating interstitial nephritis from glomerular and postrenal diseases without the necessity for renal biopsy.—B.D. Bennett, M.D., Ph.D.

Diagnostic Value of Synovial Fluid Microscopy: A Reassessment and Rationalisation

Freemont AJ, Denton J, Chuck A, Holt PJL, Davies M (Univ of Manchester, England)

Ann Rheum Dis 50:101–107, 1991 16–10

Objective.—Synovial fluid microanalysis is a potentially useful diagnostic procedure. Synovial fluids from patients with different arthropathies were examined microscopically to form criteria for analysis of synovial specimens. The scheme was then tested in a blind prospective study.

Methods.—Using techniques routinely available in pathology laboratories, the synovial fluid from 1,892 patients with 14 different arthropathies was examined microscopically. Wet preparations were analyzed for crystals, cartilage, fibrocartilage fragments, and ragocytes. The total nucleated cell count and differential cell count also were evaluated. Microscopic diagnostic criteria for each arthropathy were identified to form an algorithm that could be applied to the examination of synovial fluids from 200 patients without knowledge of the clinical diagnosis. Cytologic and clinical diagnoses were compared at the end of the study.

Findings.—Crystals of different types were identified among the various categories of arthritis. Certain cytologic features were unique to individual arthropathies, and other clinically distinct arthropathies shared similar patterns of synovial fluid cell content. In 71 patients (35.5%) the cytologic diagnosis correctly matched the clinical diagnosis. In another 43 patients (21.5%), a short list of differential diagnoses, which included the correct clinical diagnosis, was made. In 63 patients (31.5%) the arthropathies were correctly identified as inflammatory or noninflammatory. No diagnosis was made in 5 patients, and an inaccurate cytologic diagnosis was made in only 7 (3.5%). Overall, an appropriate working diagnosis was made on the basis of microscopic analysis of the synovial fluid alone in 62.5% of patients.

Conclusions.—Synovial fluid microanalysis is a potentially more important diagnostic screening test than previously acknowledged.

▶ This paper emphasizes the fact that despite the development of technologically sophisticated laboratory tests, much of the information important for timely clinical management of patients with joint disease can be obtained by use of the "old-fashioned" light microscope. More glamour and complexity do not necessarily indicate a better test.—B.D. Bennett, M.D., Ph.D.

Value of Retesting Subjects With a Positive Hemoccult in Screening for Colorectal Cancer

Kewenter J, Engarås B, Haglind E, Jensen J (Sahlgrenska Hosp, Göteborg, Sweden)

Br J Surg 77:1349–1351, 1990 16–11

Introduction.—The Hemoccult II is the most widely used method to screen for colorectal cancer. Rehydrating the test before development, which increases sensitivity but decreases specificity, has been done in some studies to avoid false negative results. Whether retesting of patients with a positive Hemoccult II might increase the test's specificity without lowering its sensitivity was investigated.

Methods.—In all, 5,692 patients were offered testing with Hemoccult II. Two tests were to be performed on each of 3 consecutive stools during a period of dietary restriction. The test was returned by 3,561 individuals and rehydrated before development. Patients with 1 or more positive slides were asked to repeat a similar test series. All with a positive test in the initial series underwent rectosigmoidoscopy and had a double-contrast barium enema. All of those in the test group and an additional screened group of 6,204 patients were invited to undergo rescreening 17–19 months later.

Results.—Those with a positive retest had significantly more neoplasms, including carcinomas and adenomas with a diameter of at least 1 cm, than those with a negative repeat test. One in 7 in the positive retest group, but only 1 in 108 of the negative retest group, had carcinoma. The repeat test increased the specificity of Hemoccult II from 95% to 98% without altering sensitivity. Patients with a negative retest after an initial positive result tended to be those who had not kept to the recommended diet during the first test.

Conclusion.—Rehydration results in an acceptable level of sensivity for the Hemoccult test. The loss of specificity can be offset by a combination of dietary restriction immediately before and during the test, and retesting those with an initial positive result.

▶ This paper serves to reinforce the concepts that laboratory tests, whether positive or negative, should not be accepted uncritically, and that factors outside of the laboratory may have a significant impact on test results. The screening test for occult blood in the stool is an example of an extremely important test that can be influenced by a number of dietary factors. Additional papers addressing this issue have been published recently (1,2).—B.D. Bennett, M.D., Ph.D.

References

1. Feinberg EJ, et al: *Ann Intern Med* 113:403, 1990.
2. Anderson GD, et al: *Am J Gastroenterol* 85:558, 1990.

Thyroid Hormone Resistance Syndrome: Inhibition of Normal Receptor Function by Mutant Thyroid Hormone Receptors

Chatterjee VKK, Nagaya T, Madison LD, Datta S, Rentoumis A, Jameson JL (Massachusetts Gen Hosp, Boston; Harvard Med School)

J Clin Invest 87:1977–1984, 1991 16–12

Background.—The syndrome of generalized thyroid hormone resistance (GTHR) is characterized by increased circulating free thyroxine and triiodothyronine levels and inappropriately normal or even increased levels of thyroid-stimulating hormone (TSH). Patients are variably resistant to the metabolic effects of increased thyroid hormone. Quantitative and qualitative defects in thyroid-hormone binding to fibroblast nuclear receptors have been described in patients with GTHR. Resistance usually is inherited in an autosomal dominant manner.

Objective.—Because single amino acid substitutions have been described in the ligand-binding domain of the β form of thyroid hormone receptor in 2 kindreds with GTHR, transient expression assays were used to characterize these receptor mutants: 1 with a Gly to Arg change at amino acid 340 (G340R), and 1 with a Pro to His change at amino acid 448 (P448H).

Observations.—Receptor mutants were unable to mediate thyroid hormone–dependent activation or repression of reporter genes, compared with wild-type receptors. The mutants inhibited normal α and β receptor isoforms in coexpression assays. The G340R mutant failed to bind triiodothyronine, and the P448H mutant bound hormone with reduced affinity. Inhibition by this mutant was reversed by high concentrations of triiodothyronine.

Discussion.—Mutant β receptors in patients with GTHR have a lowered affinity for triiodothyronine and are functionally deficient. More significantly, they inhibit the activity of normal receptors, explaining the dominant mode of inheritance of this disorder.

▶ This publication is an excellent example of the application of molecular biological techniques to the understanding of clinical dysfunctions with a genetic component.—D.J. Wells, Ph.D.

17 Clinical Microbiology

The Clinical Microbiology Laboratory as an Aid in Infection Control: The Application of Molecular Techniques in Epidemiologic Studies of Methicillin-Resistant *Staphylococcus aureus*

Pfaller MA, Wakefield DS, Hollis R, Fredrickson M, Evans E, Massanari RM (Univ of Iowa)

Diagn Microbiol Infect Dis 14:209–217, 1991 17–1

Background.—Once methicillin-resistant *Staphylococcus aureus* (MRSA) strains have been introduced into the hospital environment, it can be very difficult to control and eradicate them. The emergence of this problem at a Veterans Affairs medical center prompted a microbiologic surveillance program to estimate the point prevalence, source, and nosocomial acquisition of MRSA.

Methods.—All medical and surgical patients were tested for nasal carriage of MRSA in the 327-bed hospital in a 30-day prospective microbiologic survey. All patients were tested again before discharge. After this study was completed, the surgical service detected a cluster of nosocomial MRSA by routine infection control surveillance. Restriction endonuclease analysis of plasmid DNA (REAP) was then done on all MRSA isolates detected in the microbiologic surveillance study and on the subsequent cluster of nosocomial infections.

Results.—During the surveillance study, 1.5% of 473 patients were colonized at admission and an additional 1.1% acquired MRSA during hospitalization. The isolates showed similar antibiotypes. Of 24 infected or colonized patients, 10 distinct subtypes were identified on REAP subtyping. Subtype A2 was documented in 9 surgical patients, of whom 8 were hospitalized in the surgical intensive care unit. These findings suggested a breakdown of infection control practices in that unit. This was controlled by strict enforcement of handwashing and redirecting infected or colonized patients to a specific unit of the hospital. Colonization with MRSA was not found in any of the workers in the unit.

Conclusions.—Investigation and control of MRSA in the hospital environment can be effectively achieved by molecular typing methods in conjunction with careful epidemiologic investigation. Different subtypes can be well defined by use of REAP, allowing direction of infection control efforts to specific problem areas. Although REAP subtyping is not inexpensive, the cost is less than that attributable to nosocomial infection.

▶ Restriction endonuclease analysis of plasmid DNA (REAP) provides an additional method of epidemiologic surveillance for hospital-acquired cases of methicillin-resistant *Staphylococcus aureus.* The significant cost of this procedure is mentioned as a factor, and indeed this must be considered. Additional infection control precautions may be instituted in the hospital when isolates of methicillin-resistant *Staphylococcus aureus* are encountered without instituting any additional laboratory testing. Where multiple cases arise and patterns of the spread of nosocomial infections are being sought, antimicrobial susceptibility profiling may be useful in some cases at no additional cost. Furthermore, no comparison is made regarding the cost of REAP compared with previously available phage typing methods.—R.M. Austin, M.D., Ph.D.

A Three-Year Study of Positive Blood Cultures, With Emphasis on Prognosis

Roberts FJ, Geere IW, Coldman A (Vancouver Gen Hosp, BC; Univ of British Columbia; British Columbia Cancer Agency, Vancouver, BC, Canada)
Rev Infect Dis 13:34–46, 1991 17–2

Objective.—Bacteremia remains a significant medical problem. Factors that may affect prognosis in bacteremia include the causative organism, the source, treatment, complications, and underlying diseases or conditions. A 3-year study of positive blood cultures was conducted with emphasis on prognosis. Mortality curves were calculated for clinically significant bacteremia according to causative organism and source.

Data Analysis.—Between 1984 and 1987, 37,156 blood cultures were performed, yielding 1,972 positive cultures. Of these, 63% were classified as clinically significant, 7% were caused by transient bacteremia, 26% were from contamination, and 3% were of indeterminate significance. The incidence of clinically significant bacteremia was 14.6 cases per 1,000 acute admissions.

Mortality.—Mortality associated with clinically significant bacteremia was significantly higher than that for the other groups. In patients with clinically significant bacteremia, examination of mortality according to source and organism yielded a variety of curves. Mortality was 0 in bacteremia of bone and joint origin. Mortality from endocarditis, bacteremic pneumococcal pneumonia, β-hemolytic streptococcal bacteremia, and bacteremia associated with *Escherichia coli* urinary tract infection showed an early plateau effect and a drop before day 20. In bacteremia arising from intravascular sources other than endocarditis, there were no deaths until day 5, when mortality rose progressively. Bacteremia caused by most organisms and sources was associated with mortality that continued until at least day 20.

Conclusions.—Both the source and the type of organism appear to be major factors in mortality associated with bacteremia, and the influence of bacteremia on survival appears to extend beyond 7 days.

▶ Positive blood cultures may represent clinically significant disease, transient bacteremias, or contaminants. This paper points out that all clinically significant bacteremias do not have the same implications. Risk of mortality can be stratified based on the organism involved and the site of the originating infection. The authors also have demonstrated that the effect of clinically significant bacteremia on mortality persists for a much longer period of time than is generally appreciated. This effect undoubtedly bears some relationship to underlying disease, and the paper indicates that physicians should be aware of possible complications of bacteremic episodes occurring up to 30 days after initial documentation of bacteremia.—B.D. Bennett, M.D., Ph.D.

The Validity of Acid-Fast Smears in the Diagnosis of Pulmonary Tuberculosis

Gordin F, Slutkin G (San Francisco Gen Hosp; Univ of California)
Arch Pathol Lab Med 114:1025–1027, 1990 17–3

Background.—The validity of the acid-fast smear has been questioned as a diagnostic tool for tuberculosis when prevalence is low. The relationship between prevalence and predictive value of sputum smears was assessed in periods of both high and low *Mycobacterium tuberculosis* prevalence.

Methods.—Smears were evaluated by fluorescence, and Kinyoun stain was used to confirm the results. Of 2,956 samples studied from 1975 to 1978, 128 (4.3%) were positive for mycobacteria. Of 2,347 samples examined from 1979 to 1982, 197 (9.4%) were positive.

Results.—Only 1 of the 47 positive smears in the first period was a false positive. None of the positive smears studied in the second period was a false positive.

Thus, the positive predictive value of acid-fast microscopy was 97.9% in the earlier period and 100% for the later period.

Conclusions.—A shift in prevalence has a small effect on the positive predictive value of an acid-fast smear when specificity is maintained. The ability of an acid-fast smear to predict culture growth accurately depends on a laboratory method that maintains a specificity of 99.9% or greater.

Mycobacteremia in Acquired Immune Deficiency Syndrome: Rapid Diagnosis Based on Inclusions in the Peripheral Blood Smear

Godwin JH, Stopeck A, Chang VT, Godwin TA (The New York Hosp Cornell Med Ctr)
Am J Clin Pathol 95:369–375, 1991 17–4

Introduction.—*Mycobacterium avium-intracellulare* complex (MAC) can cause widely disseminated infection in patients with AIDS. The clinical diagnosis of MAC infection is difficult to confirm because patients do not show specific signs or symptoms. The laboratory diagnosis of MAC is time-consuming and expensive. A simple laboratory technique that may facilitate the diagnosis of MAC is reported.

Methods.—Bone marrow aspirates and peripheral blood smears obtained from 16 patients with HIV-associated MAC infection were examined for the presence of inclusion bodies. The diagnosis was made in 9

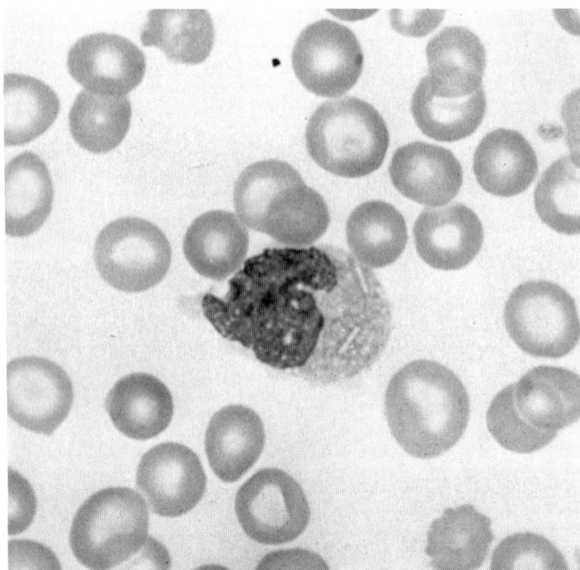

Fig 17–1.—Monocyte containing 2 linear, rod-shaped, negatively staining intracytoplasmic inclusions. PBS, Wright's stain; original magnification, ×1,000. (Courtesy of Godwin JH, Stopeck A, Chang VT, et al: *Am J Clin Pathol* 95:369–375, 1991.)

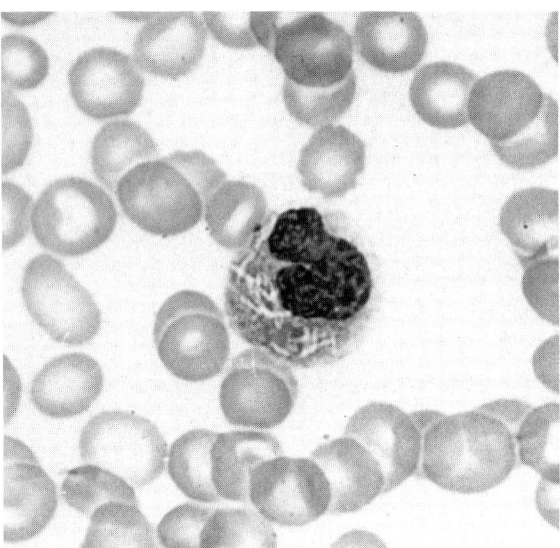

Fig 17–2.—Neutrophilic band containing multiple forked, crisscrossing, and parallel inclusions. PBS, Wright's stain; original magnification, ×1,000. (Courtesy of Godwin JH, Stopeck A, Chang VT, et al: *Am J Clin Pathol* 95:369–375, 1991.)

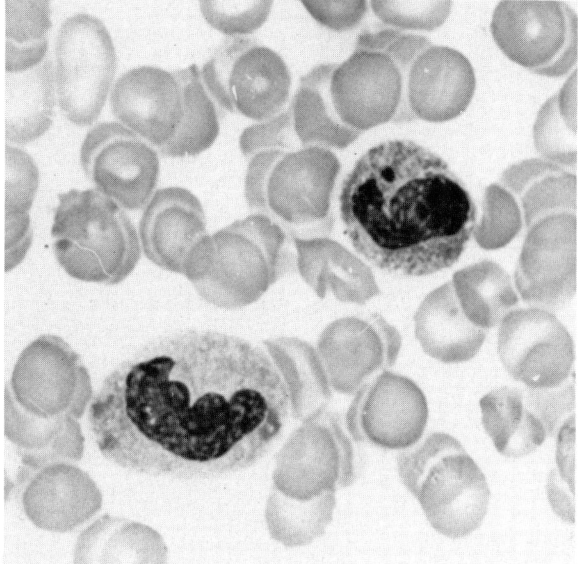

Fig 17–3.—Neutrophilic bands with 3 large Dohle bodies *(left)* and nuclear fragment *(right)*. PBS, Wright's stain; original magnification, ×1,000. (Courtesy of Godwin JH, Stopeck A, Chang VT, et al: *Am J Clin Pathol* 95:369–375, 1991.)

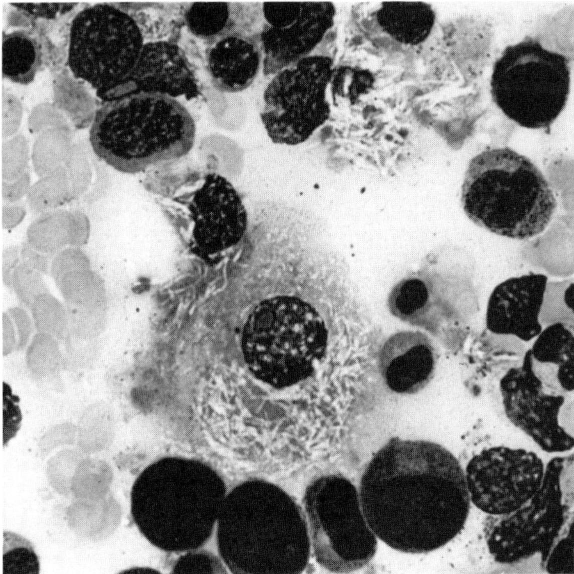

Fig 17–4.—A histocyte with its nucleus resting as an egg within a cytoplasmic nest of bacillary twigs. BM aspirate, Wright-Giemsa stain; original magnification, ×1,000. (Courtesy of Godwin JH, Stopeck A, Chang VT, et al: *Am J Clin Pathol* 95:369–375, 1991.)

patients after finding characteristic intracytoplasmic, negatively staining linear inclusions in histiocytes on bone marrow smears stained with Romanovsky-type stains. The inclusion-congested histiocytes often resembled a bird's nest (Fig 17–1). Wright's stain on peripheral blood smears showed negatively staining inclusions within monocytes (Fig 17–2) and neutrophils (Fig 17–3) in 4 patients. The number of inclusions per cell usually ranged from 1–15. All patients had abnormal white cell morphology, including large Dohle bodies, marked granulation, and vacuolation. Dohle bodies often were larger, more numerous, and more basophilic than usual (Fig 17–4). These signs of toxicity were most prominent in patients who showed MAC inclusions in their peripheral blood smear. Infection with MAC was diagnosed in the remaining 7 patients by positive bone-marrow culture. None of these patients had inclusions on peripheral blood smears or on bone marrow smears.

Conclusion.—The inclusions found in the monocytes and neutrophils of patients with HIV-associated MAC are characteristic of mycobacteria and can be confirmed by acid-fast stains and mycobacteriologic culture. Identification of these inclusions on peripheral blood smear offers a rapid, minimally invasive, and cost-effective method for diagnosing MAC infection in HIV-infected patients.

Relation of *Helicobacter pylori* to the Human Gastric Mucosa in Chronic Gastritis of the Antrum

Thomsen LL, Gavin JB, Tasman-Jones C (Univ of Auckland, New Zealand)
Gut 31:1230–1236, 1990 17–5

Background.—Spatial relationships between bacteria and affected tissue may indicate pathogenic mechanisms. The spatial relationship of *Helicobacter pylori* to the human gastric mucosa was investigated.

Methods.—Antral biopsy specimens were obtained from 8 patients with *H. pylori* infection. Antibodies against gastric mucus and ruthenium red were used to stabilize the glycoprotein structure of the mucus and glycocalyces in the specimens. Systematic scanning and transmission electron microscopy were used to determine the location of organisms and ultrastructural features.

Results.—Ninety-two percent of *H. pylori* were in the pit mucus, and 7% were in the surface mucus. Sixty percent of *H. pylori* were close to epithelial cells. Only 5% were located near the epithelial intercellular junctions. Fine filamentous strands extended between the organisms and nearby epithelial cells. Few organisms were in membrane-to-membrane contact. No *H. pylori* were seen between, beneath, or inside cells of the gastric mucosa.

Conclusions.—Virtual membrane-to-membrane contact, accumulation at intercellular junctions, and incorporation into epithelial cells or lamina propria are not important features of the pathogenic action of *H. pylori*. Physicochemical changes in the protective gastric mucus layer probably are more important.

▶ This rather elegant study provides exhaustive, finely detailed ultrastructural confirmation of impressions gained from light microscopic evaluation of gastric biopsies (i.e., that these organisms are essentially confined to the mucus).—W.A. Gardner, Jr., M.D.

A Cluster of *Pneumocystis carinii* Pneumonia in Adults Without Predisposing Illnesses

Jacobs JL, Libby DM, Winters RA, Gelmont DM, Fried ED, Hartman BJ, Laurence J (New York Hosp-Cornell Med Ctr)

N Engl J Med 324:246–250, 1991 17–6

Introduction.—Pneumocystis carinii pneumonia is the most common infection complicating AIDS. Before 1981 it occurred in small clusters of hospitalized patients with a predisposing or immunocompromising illness or in children. During a 3-month period a cluster of cases of *P. carinii* pneumonia was observed in 5 elderly patients without AIDS or other identifiable risk factors.

Patients.—In all patients *P. carinii* was discovered on bronchoscopy with bronchoalveolar lavage. Patient 1, a woman aged 78 years with a history of chronic obstructive lung disease and congestive heart failure, was admitted to the hospital after a minor trauma at home. Patient 2, a previously healthy man aged 66 years, had a 3-day history of fever, malaise, and frontal headache. Patient 3, a woman aged 73 years with a history of adult-onset diabetes mellitus, asthma, gastritis, and congestive heart failure, was admitted with a 3-week history of anorexia, nausea, and vomiting. Patient 4, a man aged 70 years, had a history of adult-onset diabetes mellitus and alcohol abuse. Surgery was performed for squamous cell carcinoma of the cervical esophagus. Patient 5, a woman aged 78 years with a history of aortic valve replacement and long-term anticoagulant therapy, was admitted after a traumatic head injury at home. Patients 1, 3, and 4 died in the hospital.

Findings.—There was no evidence of undetected predisposing illness in the 5 patients, and the method of transmission of the organism is unclear. Hypotheses include increased likelihood of exposure in the community or hospital or increased susceptibility in the elderly.

Discussion.—Although rare, clusters of *P. carinii* have occurred in adults without predisposing disease. Bronchoalveolar lavage with staining for *P. carinii* should be performed on patients with undiagnosed pneumonia that is not responsive to empirical antibiotic therapy. This group of 5 elderly patients with *P. carinii* may be unique or may indicate a shift in the epidemiologic nature of *P. carinii* infection.

▶ This intriguing study raises the possibility that, in some instances, *P. carinii* pneumonia may be acquired from another person rather than arising from organisms already present in salivary glands or elsewhere in the body. In New York City, with a high rate of AIDS and massive numbers of organisms available, *P. carinii* pneumonia and other AIDS-related infections may occasionally be spread to persons not overtly immunosuppressed. Follow-up conversation with the senior author indicates that the cluster of pneumocystosis described in this report has not enlarged over the past year, with no further cases being noted.—R.A. Harley, M.D.

Comparison of Four Methods for Rapid Detection of *Pneumocystis carinii* in Respiratory Specimens

Cregan P, Yamamoto A, Lum A, VanDerHeide T, MacDonald M, Pulliam L (Univ of California, San Francisco; VA Med Ctr, San Francisco)

J Clin Microbiol 28:2432–2436, 1990 17–7

Background.—*Pneumocystis carinii* pneumonia is the most common index diagnosis for AIDS. Four different staining methods for *P. carinii* in respiratory specimens were compared: the modified silver stain, the Diff-Quick (DQ) method, and the direct and indirect immunofluorescence staining methods. Fifty sputum specimens and 50 bronchoalveolar lavage specimens were analyzed.

Findings.—Two or more of the 4 methods were positive in 58% of cases. Rates of positivity were 74% for sputum specimens and 42% for lavage specimens. The silver stain and direct fluorescence method were somewhat more sensitive in analyzing bronchoalveolar lavage specimens. Three of 10 patients with initially negative findings on DQ (Giemsa) staining were later found to be positive by using method on lavage specimens. All 3 initially negative smears were positive by 1 or both fluorescence assays. Cost was lowest for DQ and highest for the silver stain and direct fluorescence assay.

Conclusions.—Any of these tests can reliably be used to identify *P. carinii* in respiratory specimens. It may be reasonable to use the rapid, inexpensive DQ test for screening purposes and to confirm negative smears by using a more sensitive assay.

Blinded Comparison of a Direct Immunofluorescent Monoclonal Antibody Staining Method and a Giemsa Staining Method for Identification of *Pneumocystis carinii* in Induced Sputum and Bronchoalveolar Lavage Specimens of Patients Infected With Human Immunodeficiency Virus

Wolfson JS, Waldron MA, Sierra LS (Massachusetts Gen Hosp, Boston; Harvard Med School)

J Clin Microbiol 28:2136–2138, 1990 17–8

Objective.—The spread of HIV infecting requires methods of identifying *Pneumocystis carinii* that are rapid, minimally invasive, and inexpensive. A new direct immunofluorescence monoclonal antibody (DFA) technique was compared with an established Giemsa staining method.

Methods.—A total of 148 sputum and bronchoalveolar lavage specimens were examined by the 2 methods. Sixty-seven patients (64% of

Comparison of 2 Methods for Identification of *P. carinii* in IS and BAL Specimens From HIV-Infected Patients

DFA result/ Giemsa result	No. with result			
	Specimens		Patients*	
	IS	BAL	IS	BAL
Positive/positive	12	10	10	2
Positive/negative	9†	3†	6	0
Negative/positive	0	0	0	0
Negative/negative	60	11	47	2

*For patients evaluated by both IS and BAL, the first test performed was tallied.
†Discrepancies between the DFA and Giemsa methods that occured on evaluation of different clinical specimens from the same patient or that occurred on evaluation of a clinical specimen obtained after evaluation of a specimen with no discrepancy are included.
(Courtesy of Wolfson JS, Waldron MA, Sierra LS: *J Clin Microbiol* 28:2136–2138, 1990.)

those evaluated) had HIV infection. There were 109 induced sputum specimens and 39 bronchoalveolar lavage specimens.

Findings.—Specimens from 49 of the 67 HIV-infected patients were initially negative by both methods (table), and 12 were positive by both methods. All 6 patients whose initial specimens were positive by DFA only had positive results for subsequent specimens by both methods.

The DFA method was simple to use and required less time in scoring stained slides than did the Giemsa technique. Care was needed to avoid false positive readings based on extraneous fluorescence.

Conclusions.—The DFA method is a simple, expeditious means of diagnosing *P. carinii* infection. It may be more sensitive than the Giemsa method in HIV-infected patients. Whether all positive results represent clinically significant disease remains uncertain.

Comparison of Papanicolaou's Stain With the Gomori Methenamine Silver (GMS) Stain for the Cytodiagnosis of *Pneumocystis carinii* in Bronchoalveolar Lavage (BAL) Fluid

Schumann GB, Swensen JJ (Univ of Utah Health Sciences Ctr)
Am J Clin Pathol 95:583–586, 1991 17–9

Background.—The Papanicolaou (Pap) stain is the most common cytologic staining technique, but it does not stain the walls of *Pneumocystis carinii* (PC) cysts. The GMS technique is expensive, time-consuming, and difficult to perform. If the foamy alveolar casts that accompany PC cysts are identifiable on Pap-stained slides of lavage specimens with positive GMS reactions, cyst staining might be unnecessary.

Observations.—Of 318 bronchoalveolar lavage specimens, PC was found in 20%. Both Pap and GMS staining studies were positive in 86% of those with PL. The Pap stain was positive for 11% of specimens that were GMS negative. Restaining by the GMS technique showed that these were not false positive results. Only 2 GMS-positive specimens had negative Pap stain findings.

Conclusions.—The Pap stain appears to be a very sensitive means of detecting PC in bronchoalveolar lavage specimens. It is important that experienced workers examine an adequate amount (about 6 cytocentrifuge slides) of properly prepared material. Staining with GMS should be necessary only occasionally to confirm the diagnosis.

▶ Contrasting views are expressed in these 2 articles (Abstracts 7–8 and 7–9) regarding proper evaluation of respiratory cytologic specimens for *Pneumocystis carinii.* The article by Wolfson et al. (Abstract 7–8) advocates a relatively "high tech" procedure, using an immunofluorescent monoclonal antibody stain, and the article by Schumann and Swensen (Abstract 7–9) advocates a "less is more" position, using only Pap-stained slides. As the control, Wolfson et al. used the Giemsa stain, which does not stain the cell wall of the organism and, in our opinion, is less sensitive than the GMS stain. Schumann and Swensen claim that the GMS technique is expensive, time-consuming, and technically difficult. They show excellent results reviewing Pap-stained slides of lavage specimens, but these results may not be reproducible in sputum specimens if the casts are disrupted by the Saccomano technique.

Our opinion is that the GMS technique is still the "gold standard." It has not been technically difficult to perform in our laboratory, and at 30 minutes for the microwave method (1), is hardly time-consuming.

Another important factor influencing cost that is not clearly addressed in the study by Schumann and Swensen is the amount of screening time required for each method. We would suspect that screening times may be reduced in both GMS and immunofluorescent methods.

The choice of staining methods for this increasingly common opportunistic infection will likely remain based on personal experience and volume of material.—G.F. Worsham, M.D.

Reference

1. Brinn NT: *J Histotechnology* 6:125, 1983.

Use of the Gen-Probe PACE System for the Detection of *Neisseria gonorrhoeae* in Urogenital Samples

Granato PA, Franz MR (Crouse Irving Med Hosp; Community-General Hosp, Syracuse, NY)

Diag Microbiol Infect Dis 13:217–221, 1990 17–10

Background.—Noncultural methods of diagnosing gonorrhea have been made in which *Neisseria gonorrhoeae* is directly detected in urogenital samples. One commercially available test, the Gen-Probe Assay-Chemiluminescent Enhanced (PACE) System, uses an acridinium ester-labeled DNA probe that binds with gonococcal target rRNA. The effectiveness of this kit was compared with Martin-Lewis medium in JEMBEC plates for direct detection of *N. gonorrhoeae.*

Methods.—In all, 412 urethral and endocervical specimens were collected from consecutive high-risk walk-in patients at a sexually transmitted disease clinic. Each specimen was cultured for 72 hours and examined daily for the appearance of microbial growth. The PACE assay consisted of sample preparation, hybridization, separation of hybridized and unhybridized probe, and chemiluminescent measurement. Batch runs were performed on up to 80 samples and took about 2 hours to perform.

Results.—Overall correlation was 97.3% between the 2 tests. There were 11 discrepant probe results, 9 false negative results, and 2 false positive results. Excluding test of cure samples, the prevalence of disease in the study population was 24%. Compared with culture, the PACE system had a sensitivity of 90%, specificity of 99%, positive predictive value of 98%, and negative predictive value of 97%.

Conclusions.—The Gen-Probe PACE System appears to be a reasonable alternative to culture for detecting *N. gonorrhoeae* directly in urogenital specimens. The technique is conducive to both small- and large-batch analyses. False negative results are a concern, but they likely result from bias associated with the order of specimen collection and or sampling error.

▶ The Gen-Probe system for the detection of *Neisseria gonorrhoeae* has several advantages over the older chocolate agar culture techniques. A single thin probe may be used to test for both chlamydia and *N. gonorrhoeae,* a particular advantage in male urethral swab material. The false positive results reported may be the result of the fastidious nature of the organism and culture techniques requiring rapid production of a carbon dioxide laden gas environment. Other studies have found sensitivity to be higher than the 90% reported here (1). The probe system can replace culture and sensitivity testing, because most isolates are now recommended to be treated presumptively as if they are β-lactamase resistant (2).—R.M. Austin, M.D., Ph.D.

References

1. Gruninger R, et al: Comparison of two DNA probes using a single swab with culture in detection of *N. gonorrhoeae* and *Chlamydia trachomatis* in women. American Society of Microbiology National Meeting, 1990, Abstract C-367.
2. Schwarcz SK, et al: *JAMA* 264:1413, 1990.

Detection of Circulating Candida Enolase by Immunoassay in Patients With Cancer and Invasive Candidiasis

Walsh TJ, Hathorn JW, Sobel JD, Merz WG, Sanchez V, Maret SM, Buckley HR, Pfaller MA, Schaufele R, Sliva C, Navarro E, Lecciones J, Chandrasekar P, Lee J, Pizzo PA (Natl Cancer Inst, Bethesda, Md; Duke Univ; Wayne State Univ; Johns Hopkins Med Insts; Becton Dickinson Advanced Diagnostic, Baltimore, et al)

N Engl J Med 324:1026–1031, 1991 17–11

Objective.—Invasive candidiasis can be difficult to diagnose, yet it is an important cause of morbidity and death in patients with cancer. The value of blood enolase was examined as a marker for invasive candidiasis in 170 patients at high risk because of cancer and neutropenia.

Patients.—Twenty-four of the patients had invasive candidiasis manifested as tissue infection in 13 cases and as fungemia in 11. Controls included 50 patients with candidal colonization and 96 patients with no evidence of candidiasis.

Method.—Antigen testing was done in a blinded manner using a double-sandwich liposomal immunoassay for candida enolase in serial serum specimens.

Findings.—More than half of sera from patients with proved invasive candidiasis were positive; the assay was 54% sensitive. Multiple sampling was positive in 85% of proved cases of deep tissue infection and in 64% of patients with fungemia. The assay was 96% specific. Enolase antigenemia occurred in all but 1 of 5 patients in whom invasive disease was established by tissue diagnosis alone.

Conclusions.—The presence of candida enolase in the blood may be a useful indicator of deep infection in patients with cancer who are neutropenic. Limiting testing to those at high risk of invasive disease will maximize its specificity and help control costs.

▶ A major diagnostic difficulty lies in identifying disseminated candidiasis: In more than 50% of cases, routine blood cultures either are negative or take a long time to turn positive, even when the most sensitive method, lysis centrifugation, is used (1). Several studies have shown that an antemortem diagnosis of dissemenated candidiasis is made in only 15% to 40% of patients (2). Consequently, much effort has been devoted to developing immunologic techniques for earlier diagnosis. Studies proving that survival is increased after early diagnosis and treatment with tests such as candida enolase immunoassay are still awaited.—R.M. Austin, M.D., Ph.D.

References

1. Rubin RH: *Sci Am Med* 7:X:12, 1991.
2. Edwards JE Jr, et al: *Ann Intern Med* 89:91, 1978.

The Agent of Bacillary Angiomatosis: An Approach to the Identification of Uncultured Pathogens

Relman DA, Loutit JS, Schmidt TM, Falkow S, Tompkins LS (Stanford Univ; Indiana Univ)

N Engl J Med 323:1573–1580, 1990 17–12

Introduction.—Bacillary angiomatosis (BA) is a vascular proliferative disorder initially described in the skin and nodes of HIV-seropositive patients. Lesions contain clusters of bacilli that stain positively by the Warthin-Starry technique and resemble the lesions of cat scratch disease. The histologic findings, however, differ from those of classic cat scratch disease.

Methods.—The polymerase chain reaction (PCR) technique was used to analyze tissues from 4 patients with a diagnosis of BA. Oligonucleotide primers complementary to the 16S ribosomal RNA genes of eubacteria amplified 16S ribosomal gene fragments directly from tissue samples. The target DNA was from a recent case of disseminated BA. The DNA sequence of the ribosomal gene fragments was analyzed for phylogenetic relatedness to known organisms.

Findings.—Tissues from 3 unrelated patients yielded a unique 16S gene sequence, and the sequence from the fourth patient differed at only 4 of 241 base positions. No related 16S gene fragment was found in normal tissues. The sequences found in tissues from BA appeared most closely related to *Rochalimaea quintana,* an organism that is transmitted by the body louse and causes trench fever.

Conclusion.—This approach may prove helpful in investigating other infectious diseases whose cause is uncertain.

▶ This article and the accompanying editorial in the same issue (1) raise some of the most exciting prospects regarding the application of new molecular biological technology to the study of infectious disease and to pathology in general. The authors used PCR technique to determine that the small bacillus identified in the tissue of bacillary angiomatosis, a peculiar vascular proliferation affecting AIDS patients and initially confused with Kaposi's sarcoma, is a rickettsia-like organism closely related to *Rochalimaea quintana.* Two additional articles in the same journal issue (2) described similar small bacilli identified in the tissue of AIDS patients with peliosis hepatis and associated with a septicemic illness in AIDS and immunocompromised patients, respectively.

There has been much speculation about whether the organism of bacillary angiomatosis is the same organism that causes cat scratch disease or Carrion's disease (Bartonellosis). Carrion's disease results in septicemic illness (Arroyo fever) and a more indolent skin disease (verruga peruana) that closely resembles the histologic lesion of bacillary angiomatosis. However, these studies suggest that they are not the same organism. Whether all of the authors in this issue of the *New England Journal of Medicine* are describing the same organism is not clear, but there are overlapping similarities in each of the investigator's findings.

In the future, the PCR technique to identify "signature rRNA sequences" will prove to be a powerful taxonomic tool, and as shown here, will enable us to more easily and more clearly recognize new illnesses associated with previously identified organisms as well as to relate newly identified organisms to their relatives already associated with existing diseases.—G.F. Worsham, M.D.

References

1. Eisenstein BI: *N Engl J Med* 323:1625, 1990.
2. Perkocha LA, et al: *N Engl J Med* 323:1581, 1990.
3. Slater LN, et al: *N Engl J Med* 323:1587, 1990.

Rapid Dysplastic Transformation of Human Genital Cells by Human Papillomavirus Type 18

Barnes W, Woodworth C, Waggoner S, Stoler M, Jenson AB, Delgado G, DiPaolo J (Georgetown Univ Med Ctr; Natl Cancer Inst, Bethesda, Md; Cleveland Clinic Found)

Gynecol Oncol 38:343–346, 1990 17–13

Background.—The role of human papillomavirus (HPV) in the development of genital tract lesions has been the focus of much recent attention. An in vitro model has been developed to study the interaction between HPV types 16 and 18 recombinant DNA and normal cervical epithelial cells. This model was used to assess differences between HPV-16 and HPV-18 xenografts in the development of epithelial neoplasia.

Methods.—The experiment began by isolation, culture, and grafting of human cervical and foreskin epithelial cells. The cultured cells were then transfected with recombinant HPV-16 and HPV-18 DNA, which resulted in immortalized cell lines. Female athymic mice then received transplanted normal epithelial cells and HPV-16- and HPV-18-immortalized cells. Cell lines of both early passage—less than 40 population doublings—and late passage—more than 180 population doublings—were used.

Results.—Stratified squamous tissue formed at the sites of normal epithelial cell grafts. In HPV-immortalized cell grafts, either normal-appearing epithelium or dysplastic changes were seen. None of the 13 early-passage HPV-16 grafts resulted in dysplastic changes, whereas 9 of 14 early-passage HPV-18 grafts resulted in dysplasia. In both HPV types, most of the late-passage grafts resulted in dysplasia.

Conclusions.—Experimental study supports clinical observations that HPV-18 is associated with a more aggressive and rapidly progressive cervical neoplasia. Both HPV-16 and HPV-18 cell lines will cause dysplastic epithelium in mice, but HPV-16 grafts have about the same ability to cause dysplasia with early- and late-passage grafts.

▶ Dysplastic transformation of early passage HPV-18 infected cultured cervical epithelial cell grafts provides an interesting in vitro model for further studies on the underlying mechanisms of dysplastic and malignant transformation associated with HPV infection. It will be interesting to see whether this in vitro model can yield additional information regarding the effects of possible cocarcinogenic factors (1).—R.M. Austin, M.D., Ph.D.

Reference

1. Iwasaka T, et al: *Am J Obstet Gynecol* 159:1251, 1988.

Comparison of Southern Transfer Hybridization and Dot Filter Hybridization for Detection of Cervical Human Papillomavirus Infection With Types 6, 11, 16, 18, 31, 33, and 35

Kiviat NB, Koutsky LA, Critchlow CW, Galloway DA, Vernon DA, Peterson ML, McElhose PE, Pendras SJ, Stevens CE, Holmes KK (Univ of Washington; Fred Hutchinson Cancer Research Center, Seattle)
Am J Clin Pathol 94:561–565, 1990 17–14

Background.—Detection of human papillomavirus (HPV) for research and possible clinical uses is of great interest. Polymerase chain reaction amplification is sensitive, but the technique is not routinely available or standardized. A commercially available dot hybridization test kit was compared with Southern transfer hybridization for detection of 7 types of HPV.

Methods.—Cervical specimens from 450 consecutive females at a sexually transmitted disease clinic were tested with both dot filter hybridization using the Virapap Kit and Southern transfer hybridization. Both tests were evaluated for interobserver and intraobserver reproducibility. The patients' mean age was 24 years, 69% were white, and 92% were single.

Results.—Either method was positive in 91 cases (20%). Of the 91, 68% were found to be positive by both methods, 24% by dot filter only, and 8% by Southern blot only. Compared with Southern transfer hybridization, the dot filter kit had a sensitivity of 90%, specificity of 94%, positive predictive value of 74%, and negative predictive value of 98%. Forty-seven women had cytologic changes suggesting dysplasia; HPV DNA was detected in 45% of these by dot filter hybridization and 36% by Southern transfer hybridization. Cervical dysplasia was found in 25% of 20 patients with HPV DNA detected by dot filter hybridization alone compared with 8% of those in whom neither method gave definite evidence of HPV, and 16% in whom HPV DNA was detected by both methods. The 2 methods had similar reproducibility.

Conclusions.—The Virapap dot filter hybridization kit appears to be an acceptable alternative to Southern transfer hybridization for detecting HPV DNA in cervical specimens. Under the conditions of the present study, dot filter hybridization appears to be the more sensitive method. Combining hybridization tests with polymerase chain reaction will be useful in studying the natural history and transmission of genital HPV infection.

▶ Some previous reports of HPV analysis from public clinics using sensitive techniques have reported the presence of HPV DNA in up to 80% to 90% of cases tested (1). The most important unanswered question regarding these findings is whether HPV DNA studies will significantly predict disease progression separate from classical cytologic screening in large prospective studies.—R.M. Austin, M.D., Ph.D.

Reference

1. Tidy JA, et al: *Lancet* 1:434, 1989.

18 Diagnostic Immunology

Cardiac Abnormalities in Systemic Lupus Erythematosus: Association With Raised Anticardiolipin Antibodies

Nihoyannopoulos P, Gomez PM, Joshi J, Loizou S, Walport MJ, Oakley CM (Hammersmith Hosp, London)

Circulation 82:369–375, 1990 18–1

Background.—Patients with systemic lupus erythematosus (SLE) have a high incidence of cardiac abnormalities and an increased frequency of anticardiolipin antibodies. The possible relationship between these abnormalities has not been explored. A group of 93 consecutive patients with SLE were examined to determine the relationship between cardiac involvement and the presence or absence of anticardiolipin antibodies.

Methods.—The patient group included 84 females and 9 males (median age, 32 years). Twelve additional patients with increased anticardiolipin antibodies but who did not meet the American College of Rheumatology criteria for SLE also were examined. All participants underwent 2-dimensional and Doppler echocardiographic studies.

Results.—Of the patients with SLE, 43 had normal cardiac anatomy. Valvular lesions were observed in 26 patients, pericardial involvement in 20, and myocardial dysfunction in 5. Patients with normal intracardiac anatomy were unlikely to have increased anticardiolipin antibodies, but abnormal cardiac findings were strongly associated with increased anticardiolipin antibodies. Of the 12 patients with increased anticardiolipin antibodies whose disease did not fulfill the American College of Rheumatology classification criteria for SLE, 8 had cardiac abnormalities similar to those observed in patients with SLE.

Conclusions.—This study demonstrates a strong correlation between the presence of increased anticardiolipin antibodies and cardiac pathology in patients with SLE and lupus-like syndromes. The possibility of a causal link between the increased anticardiolipin antibodies and cardiac damage should be further explored because it may have therapeutic implications.

Prenatal Screening for Anticardiolipin Antibody

Bendon RW, Hayden LE, Hurtubise PE, Getahun B, Siddiqi TA, Glueck HI, Luggen ME, Gartside PS (Univ of Cincinnati)

Am J Perinatol 7:245–250, 1990 18–2

Objective.—Anticardiolipin antibodies have predicted fetal loss in patients with systemic lupus erythematosus and also have been associated with maternal deaths. Whether antibody titers are a useful prenatal screening measure for identifying pregnancies at high risk was investigated.

Methods.—Anticardiolipin titers were estimated at the initial clinic visit in 686 women at a mean of 20 weeks' gestation. Titers of IgG and IgM anticardiolipin antibody were estimated using an enzyme-linked immunoassay.

Findings.—Titers of IgG anticardiolipin antibody correlated inversely with birth weight but not with gestation. The IgM titers correlated closely and inversely with age, positively with essential hypertension, and negatively with the 1-minute Apgar score. Most of the patients tested with increased IgG or IgM anticardiolipin titers had low-level increases in antibody to double-stranded DNA. No placental infarcts were observed.

Conclusion.—This study failed to relate convincingly anticardiolipin antibody titers in pregnant women to uteroplacental ischemia or to a population of high-risk patients.

▶ The presence of antiphospholipid antibodies (anticardiolipin and lupus anticoagulant) is well documented in patients with SLE and related disorders. Anticardiolipin antibody, when present in these patients, is a predictor of fetal loss and also demonstrates a strong association with recurrent vascular thromboses. Extensive investigation into the association of these antibodies with various thrombotic syndromes and other immunologic and nonimmunologic diseases has been undertaken (1–4), along with standardization of anticardiolipin assays (5). When taken as a group, these articles seem to indicate that in the subset of patients with SLE and associated or similar disorders, the presence of anticardiolipin antibodies can indeed be a predictor of significant vascular complications, including fetal demise.

Outside of this particular subset of patients, however, anticardiolipin antibodies, when present, are usually in low titer and do not show a predictive relationship for vascular events (e.g., myocardial infarction) or for increased obstetric complications. These data would indicate that use of anticardiolipin as a screening device for these problems is not indicated and should be discouraged. Ongoing investigation into the techniques of measurement and mechanism of action of anticardiolipin antibodies and lupus anticoagulant (6–8) may provide insight into therapeutic mechanisms that may be of value in these patients.—B.D. Bennett, M.D., Ph.D.

References

1. Eber B, et al: *Klin Wochenschr* 68:594, 1990.
2. Gronhagen-Riska C, et al: *Br Med J* 300:1696, 1990.
3. Griesman SG, et al: *Arch Intern Med* 151:389, 1991.
4. Espinoza LR, et al: *Am J Med* 90:474, 1991.
5. Harris EN: *Am J Clin Pathol* 94:476, 1990.
6. Tsakiris DA, et al: *J Rheumatol* 17:785, 1990.

7. Watson KV, et al: *Am J Med* 90:47, 1991.
8. Kaczor DA, et al: *Am J Clin Pathol* 95:408, 1991.

Sensitivity of Treponemal Tests for Detecting Prior Treated Syphilis During Human Immunodeficiency Virus Infection

Haas JS, Bolan G, Larsen SA, Clement MJ, Bacchetti P, Moss AR (San Francisco Gen Hosp; Univ of California, San Francisco; Centers for Disease Control, Atlanta)

J Infect Dis 162:862–866, 1990 18–3

Background.—There is some evidence that HIV-infected persons may not have a typical clinical or serologic response to syphilitic infection. The use of serologic tests for syphilis in these persons has not been assessed.

Objective.—The sensitivity of treponemal tests as markers for past syphilis was examined in 109 homosexual men with a documented history of treated syphilis.

Observations.—No HIV-seronegative subject lost reactivity to a treponemal test, but 7% of seropositive subjects without symptoms and 38% of those with symptomatic HIV infection exhibited loss of reactivity. Reactivity was lost regardless of the stage at which the last documented episode of syphilis was diagnosed and treated. The chance of losing test reactivity increased as the T4 lymphocyte count and the T4 to T8 ratio declined. A VDRL of 1:32 or lower in the most recent episode of syphilis also was an independent predictor of loss of treponemal test reactivity.

Conclusion.—Treponemal tests may not be a sensitive marker of past syphilitic infection in persons infected by HIV. The sensitivity of these tests for the diagnosis of active syphilis in this population should be evaluated.

▶ This paper points out that one cannot necessarily rely on laboratory tests based on immunologic response in patients with disordered immune systems. The study demonstrates loss of reactivity to treponemal antigens in HIV-positive patients. Similar changes in antibody responses to various components of the immunodeficiency virus itself have also been noted (1).

Inability to rely on skin tests in patients with depressed cell-mediated immunity has been recognized for many years. A similar situation, described in this article, points out the potential fallibility of laboratory tests done under inappropriate or unclear circumstances and reemphasizes the importance of an accurate history. The effect of immunodeficiency on the immunologic diagnosis of active infections in patients with AIDS and other immune disorders must be evaluated further. Until clarified, such diagnostic methods should be used in conjunction with other technologies.—B.D. Bennett, M.D., Ph.D.

Reference

1. Allain JP: *Blood* 77:1118, 1991.

Infection of Monocytes by Human Immunodeficiency Virus Type 1 Blocked by Inhibitors of CD4-gp120 Binding, Even in the Presence of Enhancing Antibodies

Perno C-F, Baseler MW, Broder S, Yarchoan R (Natl Cancer Inst, Bethesda and Frederick, Md)

J Exp Med 171:1043–1056, 1990 18–4

Introduction.—Although it has been demonstrated that CD4 is the predominant T cell receptor for HIV binding, other receptors may be important in other cell types. Human peripheral blood monocyte-macrophages (M/M) can be infected by certain strains of HIV, and this infection has been reported to be enhanced by low titers of anti-HIV antibodies. This suggests that Fc or complement receptors may be involved in HIV binding in these cells. Enhancement of HIV infection of M/M by anti-HIV antibodies and the binding mechanism involved were studied in fresh and percultured peripheral human M/M.

Results.—When M/M were exposed to HIV-1 in the absence of anti-HIV antibodies, soluble CD4 or anti-CD4 monoclonal antibody (OKT4A) interfered with infection of M/M by HIV-1. As had been reported, the addition of low titers of anti-HIV antibodies enhanced infection of M/M by HIV-1. However, under these conditions, CD4 and OKT4A still inhibited infection of M/M by HIV-1.

Conclusion.—It appears that CD4 binding by HIV-1 is an essential step in the infection of M/M. Enhancement of HIV-1 binding of M/M by low titers of anti-HIV antibodies does not seem to indicate the presence of an alternative binding and infection mechanism.

▶ This paper points out what may be a fundamental difficulty in effective immunotherapy for HIV. Not yet understood are the full implications of this paradoxical enhancement of HIV infection by antibodies to HIV.—W.A. Gardner, Jr., M.D.

Review of Laboratory Findings for Patients With Chronic Fatigue Syndrome

Buchwald D, Komaroff AL (Harborview Med Ctr, Seattle; Brigham and Women's Hosp, Boston)

Rev Infect Dis 13:S12–S18, 1991 18–5

Background.—Because chronic fatigue syndrome (CFS) is so ill defined, it is difficult to compare the results of various reports. This may explain in part why no previous review article on CFS has appeared. The various laboratory abnormalities in cases of CFS reported in the literature were examined.

Discussion.—Hematologic tests showed leukocytosis and leukopenia in about 20% of patients, relative lymphocytosis in 22%, and lymphopenia in 28%. Atypical lymphocytosis has been found in none to 30% of patients. Eighteen percent of patients have elevated erythrocyte sedimentation rates, and 20% have modestly increased levels of transaminases.

About 7% have signs of hypothyroidism. The most impressive abnormalities were thought to be those involving the immune system. Various authors have reported evidence of diffuse immunologic dysfunction. Some parameters indicate deficient function, and others show hyperreactivity. These immunologic findings were not correlated with CFS symptomatology or with changes in symptoms over time. It is also not known whether these findings distinguish CFS patients from those with illnesses that mimic CFS clinically, e.g., systemic lupus erythematosus, multiple sclerosis, and major depressive disorder. Allergies are a common feature of patients with CFS, and several authors have found increased cutaneous reactivity to allergens, increased levels of circulating IgE and IgE-bearing T and B cells, greater lymphocyte responsiveness to allergens, and greater numbers of EBNA-bearing B cells in response to stimulation with specific antigens. Muscle studies in patients with postviral fatigue syndrome have shown no increase in levels of muscle enzymes and the absence of antibodies to the acetylcholine receptor. In most patients, muscle biopsy samples demonstrated type II fiber atrophy or necrosis and abnormalities in tubular and mitochondrial structures. Three-fourths had abnormal single-fiber electromyographic results.

Conclusions.—Several laboratory tests for assessing patients with possible CFS are recommended. These include tests to determine the complete blood cell count, with manually done differential white blood cell count, erythrocyte sedimentation rate, blood chemistry, thyroid-stimulating hormone level, antinuclear antibodies activity, presence of circulating immune complexes, and immunoglobulin levels. Such tests may be useful in supporting the diagnosis of CFS or in excluding other disorders that can produce chronic fatigue.

▶ Chronic fatigue syndrome is frequently described but poorly characterized. This paper reinforces the fact that, despite numerous laboratory abnormalities found in patients with this syndrome, there is no definitive set of changes that can be considered diagnostic. With the exception of more intensive evaluation of the immune system, the laboratory tests recommended are those that would generally be done on any patient complaining of fatigue. Immunologic disorders appear to be the most significant and most characteristic findings in this and other studies of patients with CFS (1). As yet, however, the laboratory is of limited importance in confirming or discarding this diagnosis.—B.D. Bennett, M.D., Ph.D.

Reference

1. Morrison LJA: *Clin Exp Immunol* 83:441, 1991.

Development of Vascular Neoplasia in Castleman's Disease: Report of Seven Cases

Gerald W, Kostianovsky M, Rosai J (Yale Univ; Thomas Jefferson Univ)
Am J Surg Pathol 14:603–614, 1990 18–6

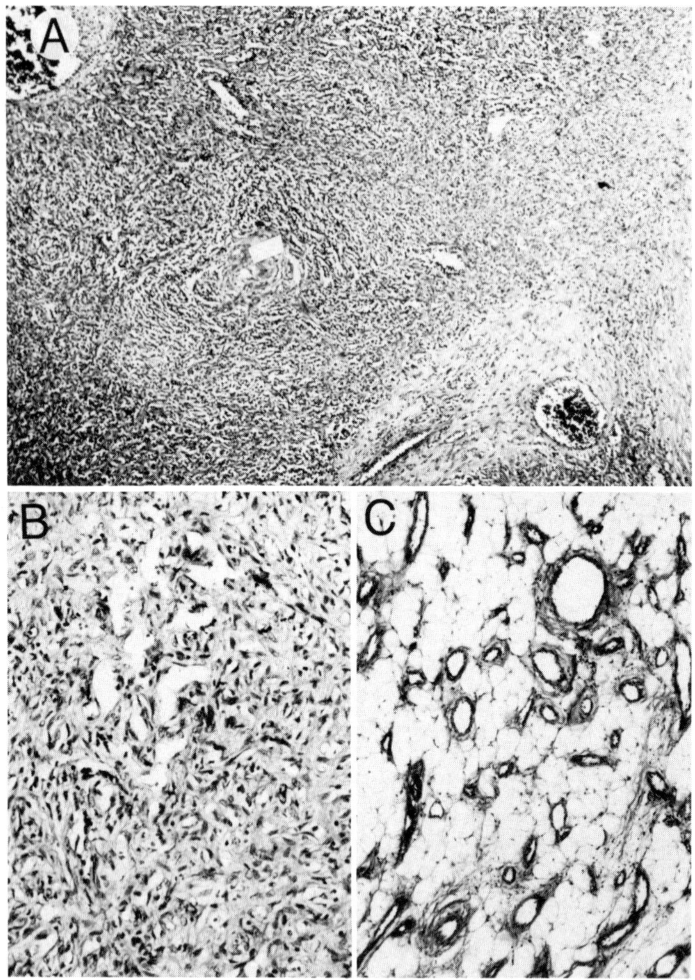

Fig 18–1.—**A,** panoramic view showing lesion with morphological features of Castleman's disease merging with spindle cell proliferation associated with large vessels *(right lower corner)*. **B,** high-power view of spindle proliferation showing numerous neoformed vascular structures. C, medium-sized mature vessels haphazardly arranged in adipose tissue located around main mass. (Courtesy of Gerald W, Kostianovsky M, Rosai J: *Am J Surg Pathol* 14:603–614, 1990.)

Background.—Hypervascular follicular hyperplasia (HFH), a distinct pattern of lymph node hyperplasia characterized by combined proliferation of lymphoid elements and blood cells, is designated as Castleman's disease in its fully developed form. It is sometimes attributable to rheumatoid arthritis, and now to AIDS, but the cause is usually unknown. In 7 patients, Castleman's disease was complicated by the development of a neoplastic vascular proliferation.

Patients.—The 5 male and 2 female patients ranged in age from 8 to 48 years. All fulfilled the microscopic criteria for vascular hyaline Castleman's disease. Five masses occurred in the retroperitoneum, 1 in the mediastinum, and 1 in the axilla. No patient had any evidence of AIDS or other immunologic disorder. Patients were usually treated with surgery alone; 1 died with local recurrence, and another died with spinal metastases at 1 year. All of the other patients were well 1–3 years after operation.

Pathology.—On gross examination the tumors appeared variegated and were up to 20 cm in size. Each was a mesenchymal spindle-cell neoplasm with evidence of vascular differentiation and Castleman's disease of hyaline vascular type (Fig 18–1). These processes had a blended appearance, with the neoplasm appearing to be continuous with the interfollicular proliferation of small vessels typical of Castleman's disease. Immunohistochemically, the cells showed diffuse cytoplasmic reactivity for vimentin. Two cases examined ultrastructurally contained a preponderance of poorly differentiated mesenchymal cells.

Conclusions.—The findings in these 7 patients with combined features of HFH and vascular neoplasia reflect a remarkable pathologic manifestation of the close relationship between the immune and vascular systems. Castleman's disease may also be associated with Kaposi's sarcoma, vascular hamartoma, and other vascular conditions. Production of angiogenic factors by activated lymphoid cells may mediate these pathologic associations.

▶ Castleman's disease is usually regarded as a peculiar abnormal immune reaction. Malignant lymphomas and plasmacytomas are noted to occur rarely in the setting of Castleman's disease, usually the plasma cell variant. Also, patients with AIDS have been described with nodal lesions similar to Castleman's disease. Kaposi's sarcoma has been reported to occur in the background of hyaline vascular follilcular hyperplasia. The current study demonstrates another category of vasoformative neoplasms occurring in Castleman's disease.—J.B. Cousar, M.D.

19 Blood Banking

Reports of 355 Transfusion-Associated Deaths: 1976 Through 1985

Sazama K (Ober, Kaler, Grimes and Shriver, Baltimore, Md)

Transfusion 30:583–590, 1990 19–1

Introduction.—Since 1975 the Center for Biologics Evaluation and Research has required reporting of all mortalities associated with blood transfusions. Previous studies have generally agreed that clerical errors were involved in most of the deaths reported under this regulation. The initial decade of mandatory reporting was reviewed to identify prophylactic measures that could reduce the number of transfusion-related deaths.

Methods.—Food and Drug Administration regulations do not currently specify the information to be included in these reports; age, gender, correct ABO blood group, and details of the incident were sometimes not available. Of the 355 deaths reported between 1976 and 1985, the following were not included in the present analysis; 16 deaths unrelated to transfusion, 12 of which occurred during or as a result of blood or plasma donation; 68 caused by hepatitis; and 3 resulting from AIDS. The latter 2 groups have been thoroughly addressed in other reports.

Results.—Of the remaining 256 patients, 51% died of acute hemolysis after ABO-incompatible transfusions—85% of ABO-related deaths were type O patients who received non-O transfusions; delayed hemolysis caused by a variety of antigens accounted for another 10%. Acute pulmonary damage was responsible for 15% of the deaths, bacterial contamination of the transfused component for 10%, nonserologic in vitro hemolysis for 2%, and graft-vs.-host disease for .4%.

Discussion.—In every aspect of the management of blood products where there was a possibility for error, errors were made. This study shows a shift in the nature of the errors leading to deaths from acute hemolysis. The shift is away from "clerical error" (improper observation and recording of information) to "management system error." Such errors include inadequate training of persons responsible for actual administration of the transfusion, inadequate standardization of procedures, and failure to clearly assign responsibility for various aspects of transfusion. The change in type of errors is most clearly reflected in the category "blood given to the wrong person," which accounted for 38% of errors in an earlier review and for 49% of errors in the current review. The site of occurrence of these errors has moved from the Operating Room to Intensive Care areas, the Emergency Room, and regular patient rooms. No system will ever totally eliminate errors resulting in transfusion-associated deaths. It is suggested, however, that an increased emphasis on hospital-wide systems of transfusion practice, rather than on programs that target only the Blood Bank, are necessary to reduce the majority of errors resulting in acute hemolytic transfusion deaths. More extensive involvement of the nursing service, in particular, in the establishment and monitoring of these policies, is suggested.

▶ Deaths directly related to transfusion of blood products remain rare events occurring in about 1/100,000 patients transfused. Human error in the collection, processing, and especially administration of these products is responsible for more than half of these cases. Such error cannot be eliminated totally, but ongoing quality assurance activities designed to reduce mistakes associated with blood transfusion are vital, primarily from the standpoint of patient survival but also from that of hospital liability. Although from a regulatory standpoint the hospital laboratory is held responsible for transfusion procedures, many of these aspects are beyond the control of pathology and laboratory personnel, i.e., the great majority of such errors are made outside the blood bank. This article reminds us that information regarding transfusion-associated deaths and their causes must be disseminated to nursing personnel and physicians, and their involvement in quality assurance activities in these areas must be expanded.—B.D. Bennett, M.D., Ph.D.

Safety and Cost-Containment Data That Advocate Abbreviated Pretransfusion Testing

Cordle DG, Strauss RG, Snyder EL, Floss AM (Univ of Iowa Hosps and Clinics)
Am J Clin Pathol 94:428–431, 1990 19–2

Introduction.—Although the American Association of Blood Banks Standards permit abbreviated pretransfusion testing for nonimmunized patients, this is not widely practiced. The procedure is cost effective, but many blood centers remain reluctant to adopt this approach.

Methods.—A total of 3,380 serum samples were tested prospectively. Antibody screens for 2,000 samples, performed with a 2-cell screen, were compared with those for 1,380 samples studied using a 3-cell screen. In addition, major cross-matches were done on all 3,380 samples through the antiglobulin phase.

Findings.—About 5% of samples had positive findings on antibody screening regardless of which reagent screening set was used. The rate of reactive antiglobulin cross-matching was .69% for samples with negative antibody screens and .65% overall. Among the antibodies detected by antiglobulin testing, the only 1 of definite significance was anti-Kp^a. The immediate spin (IS) cross match took only half as long to complete as the antihuman globulin cross-match.

Conclusion.—Use of the 2-cell or 3-cell reagent antibody screening procedure plus the IS abbreviated cross-match provides safe pretransfusion testing at substantial cost savings when nonimmunized patients are screened.

▶ Abbreviated pretransfusion testing of nonimmunized patients is an appealing alternative to the complete antiglobulin cross-match in terms of cost effectiveness, efficient use of labor, and inventory management. Despite this appeal, only about 30% of hospital laboratories in the United States currently use this approach (1). Part of this reluctance probably stems from the fact that reliance on a negative antibody screen, plus a compatible immediate major cross-match, does not guarantee the absence of red blood cell (RBC) antibodies in the recipient's serum. The issue of clinically significant RBC antibodies missed by abbreviated pretransfusion testing is addressed in this paper. The results show that clinically significant RBC antibodies are rarely missed by this procedure. Also, a carefully selected 2-cell screening panel was as effective as a 3-cell panel for antibody detection. Abbreviated pretransfusion testing, if performed properly (2), is a safe and cost-effective approach.—J.R. Stubbs, M.D.

References

1. Schmidt PJ: *Comprehensive Blood Bank 1990 Survey, Set J–A*. Chicago, College of American Pathologists, 1990.
2. Shulman IA, Calderon C: *Transfusion* 31:197, 1991.

Antibody to Hepatitis C Virus and Liver Disease in Volunteer Blood Donors

Alberti A, Chemello L, Cavalletto D, Tagger A, Dal Canton A, Bizzaro N, Tagariello G, Ruol A (Clinica Medica II, Padua; Istituto di Virologia, Milan; Ospedale di Castelfranco Veneto; Ospedale di S Dona di Piave, Italy)

Ann Intern Med 114:1010–1012, 1991 19–3

Introduction.—The etiology of parenterally acquired non-A, non-B hepatitis was identified as a single-strand RNA virus, the hepatitis C virus (HCV). Soon afterward, an antibody assay for HCV was developed to a nonstructural protein of the virus, which had a reputation of generating false positive results. The outcome of a study of 50 blood donors seropositive for anti-HCV by enzyme-linked immunosorbent assay (ELISA) was evaluated.

Methods.—All sera were tested by recombinant immunoblotting assay (RIBA) to assess the specificity of anti-HCV.

Findings.—Both the ELISA and RIBA test results for anti-HCV reactivity correlated with the ALT concentrations. One of 14 patients with an ELISA optical density (OD) value below 1.5 had a positive RIBA test, whereas 12 of 36 individuals with an OD of more than 1.5 had a positive RIBA result. The ALT level was increased in 18 of 36 patients (50%) with an OD value greater than 1.5, a significant difference. The 13 patients with a confirmed seropositive RIBA test for anti-HCV and the 6 with an indeterminate RIBA pattern and raised ALT level all underwent liver biopsy to determine the type and degree of liver disease. None of the 6 with an indeterminate RIBA pattern had histologic evidence of liver problems, but 8 of the 13 seropositive for anti-HCV had chronic active hepatitis.

Conclusions.—These findings indicate that, at least in blood donors, the anti-HCV RIBA technique is more specific than anti-HCV ELISA methodology in monitoring for liver disease. The RIBA method is also useful in identifying patients who have an underlying chronic liver disorder.

▶ Blood donor screening for antibodies to HCV with enzyme immunoassay (EIA) has been a major advance in transfusion medicine. Hepatitis C virus is the major cause of posttransfusion non-A, non-B hepatitis. The addition of this assay to blood donor testing may result in a 50% to 70% reduction in transfusion-associated hepatitis. False positive results, attributable to the questionable specificity of the anti-HCV EIA, have been a concern, especially in low-risk populations, e.g., blood donors. The use of more specific assays for HCV may provide valuable information that will aid in distinguishing true positives from false positives. These investigators found that the HCV RIBA provided improved specificity over the identification of patients with chronic liver disease. The RIBA assay promises to be a helpful aid in the identification, notification, and medical follow-up of blood donors who are true positives for HCV.—J.R. Stubbs, M.D.

Reference

1. Alter HJ, et al: *Transfusion* 31:771, 1991.

20 Hematology

Prognostic Importance of Immunophenotyping in Adults With Acute Myelocytic Leukaemia: The Significance of the Stem-Cell Glycoprotein CD34 (My10)

Geller RB, Zahurak M, Hurwitz CA, Burke PJ, Karp JE, Piantadosi S, Civin CI (Johns Hopkins Oncology Ctr)

Br J Haematol 76:340–347, 1990 20–1

Objective.—A panel of 23 monoclonal antibodies reactive with differentiation antigens on normal myeloid and lymphoid cells was used to characterize acute myelocytic leukemia (AML) in 96 adults. The central question was whether antigen expression can predict the response to intensive chemotherapy. Two courses of intensive therapy, including daunorubicin, ara-C, and amsacrine, were given.

Findings.—Of patients whose leukemic cells expressed CD34, 59% experienced complete remission, compared with 87% of those whose blasts did not express this antigen. After adjusting for disease category and the white blood cell count, patients with CD34-positive AML were only a third as likely to enter complete remission as those lacking the antigen. The CD34-positive patients more often had abnormalities involving chromosomes 5 and/or 7, and they had a higher incidence of secondary AML and preceding hematologic disorder. In all of these cases, immunophenotyping at the time of relapse again showed CD34-positive leukemia. Some patients seen with CD34-negative AML had CD34-positive disease at the time of relapse. The absence of HLA-DR was associated with complete remission and also with CD34 positivity.

Conclusions.—Intensive cytoreductive treatment is relatively ineffective in patients having CD34-positive AML. Such patients may require a different therapeutic approach to totally eradicate disease. Possibilities include early cytoablative therapy followed by marrow transplantation, and the use of biomodulating or differentiating agents.

▶ Immunophenotypic analysis of acute leukemias by flow cytometry is critical for precise classification. Also, expression of certain differentiation antigens by leukemic blasts appears to be of prognostic significance. Several studies have now shown that expression of CD34 by AML blasts is an important predictor of response to chemotherapy.—J.B. Cousar, M.D.

Prognostic Value of Lymphocyte Surface Markers in Acute Myeloid Leukemia

Ball ED, Davis RB, Griffin JD, Mayer RJ, Davey FR, Arthur DC, Wurster-Hill D, Noll W, Elghetany MT, Allen SL, Rai K, Lee EJ, Schiffer CA, Bloomfield CD (Dartmouth-Hitchcock Med Ctr, Hanover, NH; Cancer and Leukemia Group B, Lebanon, NH)

Blood 77:2242–2250, 1991 20–2

Objective.—In 1982 the Cancer and Leukemia Group B (CALGB) began a prospective study of the expression of surface antigens defined by monoclonal antibodies (MoAbs) on acute myeloid leukemia (AML) cells. The prognostic significance of the lymphocyte-associated surface antigens on AML cells was examined.

Methods.—Bone-marrow-derived blast cells from 339 patients with newly diagnosed de novo AML were examined by immunofluorescence

Clinical/Pathologic Characteristics of Patients

		Lymphoid Antigen		
	All Patients	Positive (68)	Negative (114)	*P* Value
Age (median)	51	52	46	.70
Sex (M:F)	1.08	0.89	1.28	.28
Extramedullary disease	132 (39%)	22 (32%)*	42 (37%)	.63
CNS	13 (4%)	2 (3%)	3 (3%)	1.00
Splenomegaly	38 (11%)	6 (9%)	9 (8%)	1.00
Hepatomegaly	34 (10%)	5 (7%)	8 (7%)	1.00
Lymphadenopathy	45 (13%)	8 (12%)	17 (15%)	.66
Skin/gingival	59 (17%)	8 (12%)	20 (18%)	.40
Other	14 (4%)	2 (3%)	4 (4%)	1.00
WBC/μL				
Median	24,800	20,500	28,100	.31
Range	500-500,000	700-500,000	500-409,000	
Platelets/μL				
Median	59,000	51,000	59,000	.83
Hemoglobin (g/dL)				
Median	9.6	10.0	9.1	.03
FAB				.08
M1*	68 (20%)	17 (25%)	27 (24%)	
M2	71 (21%)	10 (15%)	33 (29%)	
M3	29 (9%)	8 (12%)	6 (5%)	
M4†	107 (32%)	20 (29%)	28 (25%)	
M5	45 (13%)	6 (9%)	16 (14%)	
M6	12 (4%)	3 (4%)	3 (3%)	
M7	1 (0%)	0 (0%)	0 (0%)	
Undifferentiated	2 (1%)	2 (3%)	0 (0%)	
Unclassified	4 (1%)	2 (3%)	1 (1%)	

*Number of patients in category and the percentage of the total in either the lymphocyte antigen-positive or antigen-negative groups.

†Of the 12 patients classified as M4E whose lymphoid antigen status was evaluable, 10 were lymphoid antigen-positive.

(Courtesy of Ball ED, Davis RB, Griffin JB, et al: *Blood* 77:2242–2250, 1991.)

with a panel of MoAbs that were reactive to known myeloid cell-associated antigens and selected pan-lymphocyte antigens associated with B cells and T cells. The expression of cell surface antigens was correlated with response to therapy, time to failure, length of remission, and survival. All patients were treated according to CALGB protocols for AML.

Findings.— A T cell marker, CD2, was the most common lymphocyte-associated antigen, being present in 45 of 211 patients (21%). A B-lymphocyte marker CD19, was found in 41 of 298 patients (14%). Overall, 56 (33%) of 170 patients studied for both CD2 and CD19 were positive. A review of the French-American-British (FAB) Cooperative Study Group morphology of the CD2- or CD19-positive patients showed that FAB M4Eos was 8 times and M3 twice as common in CD2- or CD19-positive patients as in CD2- or CD19-negative patients (table). Cytogenetic analysis showed that lymphocyte antigen-positive patients had karyotypes commonly seen in AML, including t(8;21)(q22;q22), inversion 16(p13q22), t(15;17)(q22;q12), or t(9;11)(p22,q23). These karyotypic abnormalities were significantly more common in patients with lymphocyte markers than those with lymphocyte negative-antigen AML. Studies of Ig and T cell antigen receptor (TCR) gene rearrangements in 22 patients with lymphocyte markers showed germline configuration in 20, rearranged Ig heavy chain gene in 1, and rearranged TCRb and Ig heavy chain genes in 1. Northern blot analysis showed the presence of messenger RNA for CD2 in 3 of 4 CD2-positive patients.

Outcome.— Compared with patients without lymphocyte antigens, patients with CD2- or CD-19 positive leukemia had higher complete remission rates (75% vs. 59%), a significantly longer time to failure (32.4% vs. 18% at 2 years), and superior survival (43.8% vs. 29.8% at 2 years). There were no significant differences between groups in age, leukocyte count at diagnosis, incidence of extramedullary disease, or FAB classification.

Conclusion.— A significant proportion of adults with AML express lymphoid cell-associated antigens (CD2 and CD19) in the absence of other features of lymphocytic leukemia. These patients have a more favorable prognosis.

▶ The more we study acute leukemia immunologically, the more diversity we find. These mixed phenotypic leukemias are important to recognize because of apparent prognostic differences.— J.B. Cousar, M.D.

Monoclonal Nature of Transient Abnormal Myelopoiesis in Down's Syndrome

Kurahashi H, Hara J, Yumura-Yagi K, Murayama N, Inoue M, Ishihara S, Tawa A, Okada S, Kawa-Ha K (Osaka Univ, Japan)

Blood 77:1161–1163, 1991 20–3

Background.— Neonates with Down's syndrome sometime have an excess of blasts in peripheral blood. This disorder, transient abnormal myelopoiesis (TAM), resolves spontaneously in several months. It is not known, however, whether the blast excess in TAM results from clonal proliferation or a polyclonal reactive condition.

Methods.—From 1987 through 1989, peripheral blood samples obtained from 8 neonates with Down's syndrome associated with TAM were referred for phenotypic analysis. Four infants were females. Of these, 3 had polymorphic restriction sites on the hypoxanthine phosphoribosyltransferase (HPRT) and/or phosphoglycerate kinase (PGK) genes. These genes were used to analyze the methylation patterns through restriction fragment length polymorphism (RFLP).

Results.—Analysis of the methylation patterns of these genes showed a clonal nature for the blasts. Lymphocytes with a normal appearance in samples from these 3 female infants also demonstrated a monoclonal pattern.

Conclusions.—These findings indicate that TAM is a clonal proliferative disorder. The monoclonal pattern found in lymphocytes with a normal appearance suggests that it may be a disorder of multipotent stem cells.

▶ The incidence of leukemia in children with Down's syndrome is higher than that in the normal population. In addition, an excess of blasts is occasionally observed in the blood in neonates with Down's syndrome. These authors, utilizing molecular techniques, have demonstrated that these transient blasts arise from the same clone of cells. Because the blasts exhibit different lineage markers, it suggests that they originate from a stem cell population. Thus transient abnormal myelopoiesis appears to represent transient clonal expansion of stem cells, which would predispose to another "hit" or mutation to give rise to a malignant clone of cells.—A.J. Garvin, M.D., Ph.D.

Leukopenia, Neutropenia, and Reduced Hemoglobin Levels in Healthy American Blacks

Reed WW, Diehl LF (Walter Reed Army Med Ctr, Washington, DC; Uniformed Services Univ of the Health Sciences)

Arch Intern Med 151:501–505, 1991 20–4

Background.—American blacks have lower mean white blood cell and mean neutrophil counts than American whites, but separate hematologic reference values for blacks and whites have not been widely adopted. Blacks also have lower mean hemoglobin concentrations than whites. An attempt was made to establish normal hematologic values in a sample of healthy American blacks, mostly active-duty service members, and to determine whether morbidity from infection in this group was related to the neutrophil count.

Methods.—The study population consisted of 462 blacks and whites who volunteered to participate. All were asked to a complete a questionnaire while undergoing routine physical examinations. Questions included medication use, infectious illness within the previous 10 days, history of leukemia, cancer, or blood disease, and whether they had had fever, pneumonia, skin abscess, hospitalization for infection, or work lost because of infection within the previous year. All participants also had complete blood counts performed. Complete profiles were available for 166 blacks, including 102 men and 64 women, and for 296 whites, including 200 men and 96 women.

Findings.—Whites had significantly greater mean concentrations of leukocytes and neutrophils than blacks. The differences could be largely explained by relatively symmetric shifts in the frequency distributions for these cell concentrations. Whites also had greater mean hemoglobin levels than blacks. There was no significant correlation between neutrophil count and morbidity from infection, or between hemoglobin concentration and neutrophil count when controlling for age, gender, and race.

Conclusion.—Separate hematologic reference values for blacks and whites should be considered.

▶ This paper points out that our interpretation of laboratory values is only as good as the reference ranges against which such values are measured. The report confirms the previously documented lower white blood cell count, neutrophil count, and hemoglobin levels in blacks compared with whites and points out differences in mean corpuscular volume as well. It extends previous studies by demonstrating that lower neutrophil counts are not associated with a significant increase in infection in this population. The authors correctly point out that, by using identical reference ranges for blacks and whites, not only are numerous blacks subjected to unnecessary evaluations for low cell counts, but they may not be appropriately evaluated for increased white blood cell counts and hemoglobin.

Reasonable arguments may be made on both sides of the question as to whether or not separate reference ranges should be used for evaluation of these parameters in blacks and whites. It is obvious, however, that these differences and their implications should be incorporated into the working knowledge of all physicians. It should also be noted that the overall population can be divided into numerous groups whose reference values for certain biochemical and hematologic parameters may be significantly different. A recent evaluation of 55 parameters in elderly patients indicated that a lower reference interval for thyrotropin, B_{12}, and calcium might be appropriate in this group (1).—B.D. Bennett, M.D., Ph.D.

Reference

1. Lantz B, et al: *Scand J Clin Lab Invest* 1990.

Radioimmunoassay of Erythropoietin: Analytical Performance and Clinical Use in Hematology

Schlageter M-H, Toubert M-E, Podgorniak M-P, Najean Y (Hôpital Saint-Louis, Paris)

Clin Chem 36:1731–1735, 1990 20–5

Objective.—Immunoassays for erythropoietin (EPO) are easier and less expensive to perform than bioassays. The performance and clinical significance of a newly available radioimmunoassay kit for EPO determination in serum or plasma were evaluated.

Methods.—Pure recombinant EPO was used as standard and tracer. The radioimmunoassay kit developed by Incstar Corp was used. The sensitivity, precision profile, and linearity of the method were assessed, and its clinical usefulness evaluated in 51 normal individuals without anemia, 77 patients with polycythemia vera, 57 patients with pure erythrocytosis, 79 patients with chronic anemia (excluding those with malignant and renal diseases), 14 patients with chronic renal failure receiving hemodialysis, and 27 patients with myeloma, macroglobulinemia, or lymphoma.

Results.—The sensitivity of the method was good, with a lower detection limit of 3 units per liter. The method was accurate, recovery and dilution tests showing a good correlation between the calculated and the observed EPO concentrations. Furthermore, the coefficient of variation was less than 10%. In normal individuals with a hematocrit between 39% and 49%, the mean EPO value was 13.5 units per liter (range, 10–20 units per liter; 95% confidence interval, 8.7–18.3 units per liter). Among patients with chronic anemia whose hematocrit was between 18% and 39%, a logarithmic relationship was observed between EPO values and hematocrit, with a relatively large dispersion around the regression line. Patients with chronic renal failure had low EPO values regardless of the severity of anemia. Similarly, half of the patients with malignant disease had significantly low EPO values. In patients with polycythemia vera (hematocrit between 51% and 70%), the mean EPO level was below normal for 95% of patients regardless of clinical stage, and none had EPO values above 17 units per liter. In contrast, 91% of the patients with pure erythrocytosis had a normal or increased EPO value, even when the etiology was unknown.

Conclusion.—Measurement of the EPO concentration in serum is useful in distinguishing between polycythemia vera and pure erythrocytosis. A limit of 14 units per liter would include 98% of patients with polycythemia vera and exclude 86% of those with pure erythrocytosis.

▶ The development of a commercially available radioimmunoassay for EPO allows this hormone to join the long list of substances present in nanogram or smaller quantities in plasma that can be assayed in routine hospital laboratories. The availability of recombinant EPO for treatment of EPO-deficient anemias makes it important to be able to diagnose this category of chronic anemia with certainty. In addition, determination of EPO levels appears to be of significant value in discrimination between patients with polycythemia vera and primary erythrocytosis, even when those with polycythemia vera are in remission.

Although bioassays are being developed that are stated to be suitable alternatives for immunoassay of EPO (1), it is not likely that the complexity required by these bioassays will ever become a routine part of the hospital laboratory. In contrast, as we have seen with other hormones, immunoassay of EPO is likely to move from the highly technique-dependent, personnel-intensive radioimmunoassay to an automated method of measurement, provided the volume of requests supports development of such technology.—B.D. Bennett, M.D., Ph.D.

Reference

1. Wognum AW: *Blood* 76:1323, 1990.

An Investigation of the Cause of the Eosinophilia-Myalgia Syndrome Associated With Tryptophan Use

Belongia EA, Hedberg CW, Gleich GJ, White KE, Mayeno AN, Loegering DA, Dunnette SL, Pirie PL, MacDonald KL, Osterholm MT (Minnesota Dept of Health Minneapolis; Mayo Clinic and Found, Rochester, Minn; Univ of Minnesota)

N Engl J Med 323:357–365, 1990 20–6

Introduction.—The eosinophilia-myalgia syndrome is a disorder of scleroderma-like changes and marked peripheral eosinophilia associated with consumption of tryptophan-containing products. A surveillance study was conducted in Minnesota, and a community survey of tryptophan use was made in Minneapolis–St Paul. In addition, a case-control study was carried out on 52 patients with eosinophilia-myalgia syndrome to delineate potential risk factors.

Observations.—The use of tryptophan increased from 1980 to 1989 and was higher in women than in men. All but 1 of 30 evaluable case patients and 21 of 35 controls had taken tryptophan made by a company that used a fermentation process involving *Bacillus amyloliquefaciens*. Lots used by case patients contained a new strain of the organism and also less powdered carbon in a purification step. An absorbance peak was present more often in retail lots used by patients than in control lots.

Conclusions.—This outbreak of eosinophilia-myalgia syndrome apparently resulted from ingestion of a chemical constituent, which may itself be a pathogenic factor or may represent a surrogate for another chemical that actually causes the syndrome.

▶ This study sheds considerable light on the pathogenesis of eosinophilia-myalgia syndrome. Another recent study (1) that emphasizes the clinicopathologic spectrum of the syndrome, including the connective tissue inflammatory infiltrate and microangiopathy, should be of interest to the practicing pathologist.—J.B. Cousar, M.D.

Reference

1. Martin RW, et al: *Ann Intern Med* 113:124, 1990.

Histopathologic Features of the L-Tryptophan-Related Eosinophilia-Myalgia (Fasciitis) Syndrome

Winkelmann RK, Connolly SM, Quimby SR, Griffing WL, Lie JT (Mayo Clinic, Scottsdale, Ariz)

Mayo Clin Proc 66:457–463, 1991 20–7

Background.—The syndrome of eosinophilia-myalgia and fasciitis-scleroderma was first linked to L-tryptophan ingestion in 1989. The histopathologic features of this syndrome were studied in a relatively large group of patients to elucidate the pathogenesis of the syndrome.

Methods and Findings.—Eighteen biopsy specimens were obtained from 11 patients with the syndrome. All specimens showed hyaline sclerodermoid changes. Dermal scleroderma was present in 8 of 9 punch biopsy specimens and in 8 of 9 excisional biopsy specimens. Fascial scleroderma was noted in 8 specimens in the latter group. Eleven biopsy specimens showed dermal edema. Thirteen demonstrated dilated lymphatic structures. Five excisional biopsy specimens showed mucinous fasciitis in conjunction with a large number of macrophages in 4. Eleven biopsy specimens had dermal mucinosis. Lymphocytic and macrophage inflammation was minimal in 14 specimens and marked in 4. Eight showed plasma cells. Substantial numbers of eosinophils were present in 3 specimens; occasional eosinophils were seen in 4. One patient had eosinophilic spongiosis. Lymphocytic inflammation occurred around a single muscle spindle and large nerve trunks in 3. The pathologic features were not associated with the duration or dosage of tryptophan, prednisone therapy, or symptom duration.

Conclusions.—The L-tryptophan syndrome is characterized pathologically by hyaline sclerodermoid collagen in the dermis, the septa, and the fascia. Additional features that may identify this event are edema, focal mucinosis, and macrophage inflammation.

▶ This report expands earlier observations on the histologic effects of massive doses of L-tryptophan on patients. These effects, combined with study of a single peak of the syndrome in patients using tryptophan from a single manufacturer (1), suggest a toxic factor as the etiologic agent.—A.J. Garvin, M.D., Ph.D.

Reference

1. (1) Mayens AN, et al: *JAMA* 264:1698, 1990.

21 Coagulation

Lack of Increased Bleeding After Paracentesis and Thoracentesis in Patients With Mild Coagulation Abnormalities
McVay PA, Toy PTCY (Univ of California, San Francisco)
Transfusion 31:164–171, 1991 21–1

Background.—Whether mild coagulopathy increases the risk of bleeding in patients requiring paracentesis or thoracentesis was examined in 608 consecutive procedures. Mild coagulopathy was defined as a prothrombin or partial thromboplastin time from the upper normal limit to 1.5 times the midnormal range or a platelet count of $50–99 \times 10^3$ μL. Moderate coagulopathy was a prothrombin or partial thromboplastin time 1.5 to 2 times the midnormal point.

Observations.—No increased bleeding was found in patients having mild to moderate coagulopathy. Those with a markedly increased serum creatinine levels, however, had a relatively large loss of hemoglobin. Only .2% of procedures were attended by bleeding necessitating red blood cell transfusion. The most frequent indication for paracentesis was alcoholic liver disease, and that for thoracentesis was infection.

Conclusions.—Prophylactic plasma or platelet transfusion is not necessary for patients with mild to moderate coagulopathy. Those with a high serum creatinine level should be observed closely after paracentesis or thoracentesis.

▶ This retrospective review analyzes the important issue of hemorrhagic risk associated with the performance of thoracentesis and paracentesis. These investigators found that mild to moderate abnormalities of prothrombin time, partial thromboplastin time, and platelet count are not associated with increased procedure-associated bleeding. Prophylactic transfusion of fresh-frozen plasma or platelets in this patient population appears to provide little or no benefit and should be avoided. Markedly elevated creatine levels, on the other hand, do appear to be associated with an increased bleeding tendency and thus may define an at-risk subpopulation of patients. This article is an excellent companion to the authors' previously published experience (1) in patients undergoing liver biopsy.—J.R. Stubbs, M.D.

Reference

1. McVay PA, Toy PTCY: *Am J Clin Pathol* 94:747, 1990.

The Changing Prognosis of Classic Hemophilia (Factor VIII "Deficiency")
Jones PK, Ratnoff OD (Case Western Reserve School of Medicine)
Ann Intern Med 114:641–648, 1991 21–2

Background.—The length of life of individuals with classic hemophilia has increased in developed countries since the turn of the century, an effect that parallels the increased longevity among all males in these nations. Applying survival and life-table analyses to hemophiliacs has been used only recently. The relative risk of mortality and median life expectancy were estimated in patients with classic hemophilia using life-table methods, which consider disease-related deaths during infancy or childhood before symptom onset.

Methods.—A retrospective analysis was made of patients with classic hemophilia attending the University Hospitals of Cleveland. A total of 701 patients, identified from 289 affected families, were classified as having mild, moderate, or severe hemophilia. Life-table analysis was performed using age-specific death rates for all males in the United States from 1900 to 1986; the age-specific death rates for males in 1986 were applied to the years 1987 to 1990. The person-year criteria and median life expectancy at selected ages were computed for both normal and hemophiliac males.

Results.—Some 60% of the patient population resided in Ohio or its 5 adjoining states and 36% had been born before 1941. Of the 701 patients identified, 239 had died by September 1990; 42% of these deaths were attributed to trauma or bleeding. No deaths occurred in the mildly affected group before 5 years of age, and no deaths were recorded in the moderately affected patients before 1 year of age. The crude relative mortality rate for hemophiliac males vs. that for all US males was 1.86; the adjusted estimate of relative mortality was 3.13 when corrected for unrecognized deaths caused by hemophilia in infants and children. In all patients there was a declining linear trend of adjusted relative mortality associated with age. Thus, as the overall male population experienced an increased life expectancy, so did hemophiliacs. Death rates among severely affected children aged 1–14 years decreased significantly from 1971 to 1980 compared to rates in the previous decade. A significant inverse relationship was found between the presence of circulating anticoagulants and death from either AIDS or liver disease.

Implications.—The findings of this retrospective analysis indicate improvement of survival for hemophiliacs from 1971 to 1980, during which time the use of antihemophilic factor became widespread. The relative mortality among hemophiliacs now appears to be increasing, however, largely because of AIDS.

▶ This analysis provides insight into factors determining the relative mortality risk and median life expectancy in a population of patients with hemophilia A studied for the years 1900 to 1990. Emphasis is placed on the accuracy of the adjusted, rather than the crude, estimate of relative mortality because it accounts for unrecognized hemophilia-A-related deaths in infancy and early childhood. The anaysis illustrates the trend of improved relative mortality and increased life expectancy for all patients with hemophilia A up to the year 1980. These findings probably represent a combination of improved treatment and an overall decrease in relative mortality of the US male population. In fact, relative mortality statistics and the average life expectancy of mild hemophilia A patients essentially mirrored the trends of the general US male population.

Another important finding was the marked improvement in relative mortality, especially in severely affected patients, during the decade of 1971–1980. This likely corresponded to the widespread use of factor VIII concentrates. This positive trend quickly reversed itself in the decade of 1981–1990, however, because of the high incidence of HIV infection in this patient population.

Relative mortality is on the rise in patients with hemophilia A, especially among those with severe disease, as a result of AIDS. The total impact of AIDS on mortality and life expectancy in patients with hemophilia A remains to be seen.—J.R. Stubbs, M.D.

Fibrin Fragment D-Dimer and Fibrinogen β Peptides in Plasma as Markers of Clot Lysis During Thrombolytic Therapy in Acute Myocardial Infarction

Lawler CM, Bovill EG, Stump DC, Collen DJ, Mann KG, Tracy RP (Univ of Vermont)

Blood 76:1341–1348, 1990 21–3

Background.—The balance between thrombin and plasmin activities is critical in the regulation of clot formation and dissolution. The validity of plasma markers of in vitro thrombolysis was assessed in patients with differing degrees of fibrinogen breakdown.

Study Design.—Twelve patients had fibrinogen breakdown of more than 80% after receiving 100 mg of recombinant tissue plasminogen activator (rt-PA) in 6 hours. Twelve others had fibrinogen breakdown of less than 20%. Levels of cross-linked fibrin degradation products (FDPs) were measured using 2 enzyme-linked immunosorbent assays, both of which include a fibrin fragment D-dimer-specific capture antibody. In 1 assay the tag antibody cross-reacted with fibrinogen, whereas in the other it was specific for fibrin fragment D.

Findings.—Most patients had normal levels of FDPs at baseline. Those with limited fibrinogen breakdown had a twofold to fourfold increase in cross-linked FDPs 8 hours after rt-PA. Those with extensive fibrinogen breakdown had significantly higher levels with the assay using a tag antibody cross-reactive with fibrinogen compared with that using the fibrin-specific tag. The rise in fibrinopeptide B 1-42 (a marker of fragment X formation) correlated with the extent of fibrinogen breakdown.

Implications.—Caution is necessary when analyzing the results of assays for cross-linked FDP in the setting of marked fibrinogenolysis. There appears to be persistent fibrinogen or fibrin I breakdown well after active rt-PA is cleared from the circulation.

▶ These investigators have conducted a careful assessment of plasma markers used to monitor the efficacy of thrombolytic therapy. They discovered that extensive fibrinogen degradation will lead to elevations of certain tests (e.g., the pan-specific D-dimer and fibrinopeptide B15-42 assays), which may not accurately reflect the degree of therapeutic fibrinolysis. The fibrin-specific D-dimer assay may provide a more accurate picture of fibrinolysis during thrombolytic therapy.—J.R. Stubbs, M.D.

Soluble Fibrin Degradation Products Potentiate Tissue Plasminogen Activator-Induced Fibrinogen Proteolysis

Weitz JI, Leslie B, Ginsberg J (McMaster Univ)

J Clin Invest 87:1082–1090, 1991 21–4

Background.—Tissue plasminogen activator (t-PA) produces systemic fibrinogenolysis despite its affinity for fibrin. Models for the interaction between t-PA and plasminogen predict that thrombolytic doses will have this effect. It also is possible that products of thrombolysis augment fibrinogen proteolysis. In vitro studies do, in fact, show that fibrin fragments accelerate plasminogen activation by t-PA in buffer systems.

Objective.—The mechanism of systemic fibrinogenolysis was examined by incubating t-PA with plasma, with or without a fibrin clot present, and estimating fibrinogenolysis by measuring the level of β1-42.

Findings.—Soluble fibrin degradation products appeared to potentiate fibrinogenolysis in the presence of fibrin. The extent of fibrinogenolysis correlated directly with clot lysis and, once lysis began, fibrinogenolysis continued despite removal of the clot. Lysates of cross-linked fibrin clots actively potentiated t-PA–mediated fibrinogenolysis. Degradation products stimulated fibrinogenolysis by binding t-PA and plasminogen, as evident from studies with plasminogen-Sepharose. The major potentiating species was (DD)E complex. D-dimer was the predominant species in fractions not binding to adsorbant; it lacked potentiating activity.

Conclusions.—Products of t-PA–induced degradation of cross-linked fibrin are able to potentiate t-PA–mediated fibrinogenolysis by providing a surface for t-PA and plasminogen binding, thereby inducing plasmin generation. This phenomenon may help to explain the limited fibrin selectivity of t-PA.

▶ The development of recombinant (r) t-PA as a thrombolytic therapy was eagerly awaited because of its fibrin selectivity. Expectations were that rt-PA would produce clot lysis without inducing systemic lysis. Unfortunately, this has not proven to be the case. Significant fibrinogen proteolysis often accompanied rt-PA thrombolytic therapy. These investigators, using t-PA, demonstrated one mechanism by which it stimulates fibrinogen proteolysis. They have shown that lysis of cross-linked fibrin produces soluble products that promote plasmin generation by providing a surface for t-PA and plasminogen binding. This study aids in the understanding of the limited fibrin selectivity of rt-PA.—J.R. Stubbs, M.D.

22 Laboratory Management

What Constitutes a Laboratory Quality Monitoring Program?
Bernstein LH (Bridgeport Hosp, Bridgeport, Conn)
Quality Assurance Utilization Rev 5:95–99, 1990 22–1

Introduction.—Quality assurance now is a major issue in managing laboratories. The Clinical Laboratory Improvement Amendments of 1988 impose stringent quality assurance requirements on clinical laboratories and assign professional responsibility to the pathologist for evaluating and upgrading laboratory services.

Observable Indicators.—The list of observable monitoring indicators includes improper labeling of specimens and incorrect reporting. Several quality indicators concern turnaround time, because preanalytic and postanalytic requirements for test performance significantly influence timely clinical decision-making. Other indicators may be needed for the blood bank and microbiology.

Evaluating Resource Application.—Staff competency requirements include the ability to carry out necessary tasks without difficulty, an understanding of the medical relevance of laboratory results, and a knowledge of quality control measures. A quality assurance program should help to reduce expenses.

Evaluating Utilization of Resources.—Physician utilization of the laboratory is an important aspect of quality assurance assessment. Heavy utilization is not an issue in the typical community hospital. Nevertheless, the effectiveness of laboratory information and its availability for use may be considered for audit purposes.

Summary.—Quality assurance offers an opportunity to structure a monitoring program that will ultimately benefit the laboratory and the hospital as well as the patient. In setting up such a program it should be remembered that all valid monitors must demonstrate some relationship (direct or indirect) to performance and/or outcome.

▶ The development of workable quality assurance programs in the hospital laboratory has become a permanent fact of life for laboratory directors. Although typically viewed as a thorn in the side, when properly established the system can provide considerable help to the laboratory in terms of test development, staffing, and laboratory utilization. This paper provides an excellent summary of a working approach to quality assurance and some practical suggestions for implementation of such a program.—B.D. Bennett, M.D., Ph.D.

Preoperative Screening: Value of Previous Tests

Macpherson DS, Snow R, Lofgren RP (Univ of Minnesota; Univ of Pittsburgh; Pittsburgh, VA Med Ctr)
Ann Intern Med 113:969–973, 1990 22–2

Background.—Although evidence indicates that selective testing of surgical patients on the basis of history and physical examination is an appropriate strategy, it is still common practice to screen all patients preoperatively for laboratory abnormalities. The frequency of tests done within the year before elective surgery that could serve as substitutes for preoperative screening was examined. The frequency of test results that change from a normal value to a value more likely to change perioperative management also was investigated.

Methods.—Data on 1,109 consecutive patients undergoing elective surgery in 1988 were analyzed retrospectively. Data included complete blood count; sodium, potassium, and creatinine levels; prothrombin time; and partial thromboplastin time.

Results.—Of 7,549 preoperative tests done, 47% duplicated tests performed in the previous year. Of 3,096 previous normal results, repeat values fell outside the range considered acceptable for surgery less than 1% of the tests (.4%). Most of the abnormalities could be predicted from the patients' history. In addition, most were not noted in the medical record. Of the 461 previous tests yielding abnormal findings, 17% had repeat values at admission that were outside the acceptable range.

Conclusions.—A high proportion of patients undergo tests in the year before elective surgery that could be substituted for preoperative screening tests. Changes in test values that would affect patient management during surgery are rare. If a patient's previous results are normal and his or her clinical status has not changed, repeat testing is not necessary.

▶ Obtaining a standard set of laboratory tests before surgery is common practice in many hospitals. These tests include electrolytes, complete blood count, coagulation studies, and, frequently, assessment of renal and liver function. Failure to obtain these tests on admission has often resulted in postponing scheduled surgery or the imposition on the laboratory of "STAT" testing. Previous studies have indicated that obtaining such tests adds virtually nothing to the surgical management of the patient. The current study serves to confirm these findings and indicates that data obtained within at least 2–4 months before surgery can be substituted for perioperative laboratory testing with no detriment to the patient. These results were confirmed in another recently published article (1).—B.D. Bennett, M.D., Ph.D.

Reference

1. Wagner JD, et al: *J Oral Maxillofac Surg* 49:177, 1991.

Inappropriate Use of Laboratory Services: Long Term Combined Approach to Modify Request Patterns

Bareford D, Hayling A (Dudley Road Hosp, Birmingham, England)
Br Med J 301:1305–1307, 1990 22–3

Background.—Hospital clinical laboratories receive many inappropriate requests for tests. Whether changes in request patterns for hematologic tests are affected in the long term by information released from a hematology department was investigated.

Methods.—Request patterns before and after the intervention, and the costs of intervention and savings, were analyzed in an inner-city district general hospital hematology laboratory. The intervention consisted of a monthly release of a comparison of clinicians' workload statistics, issue of on-call guidelines, and seminars and fact sheets on the appropriate use of tests.

Results.—In the year after the intervention, requests for tests dropped by at least a fifth. This reduction persisted over the next 2 years. The greatest reduction occurred in the division of medicine, in which requests fell from an average of 4 per patient in the 6 months before the intervention to 2.9 per patient in the 6 months afterward.

Conclusions.—An ongoing policy of intervention, including guidelines, fact sheets, and seminars, can reduce the number of inappropriate requests for laboratory tests. A positive attitude among senior consultant staff is essential.

▶ This study is an addition to the considerable body of literature concerning the efforts of laboratory personnel to alter request patterns of physicians on clinical services. A renewed emphasis on more appropriate use of laboratory data has been stimulated by recent governmental guidelines influencing the cost of numerous aspects of laboratory practice. This study appears to be more successful than many of its predecessors, probably because it targeted both attending physicians and housestaff and provided an ongoing, active form of intervention. A similar, although less active approach, has also been reported recently (1). The long-term effects of any education programs in a hospital with housestaff require active programs with continued efforts at resident and attending physician education. They tend to be more successful in Departments of Medicine, with less impact in Departments of Surgery and Obstetrics and Gynecology. These differences may be related to the less standardized types of emergency cases seen in the latter 2 specialties.—B.D. Bennett, M.D., Ph.D.

Reference

1. Gama R, et al: *Ann Clin Biochem* 28:143, 1991

The Advent of DNA Databanks: Implications for Information Privacy

de Gorgey A
Am J Law Med 16:381–398, 1990 22–4

Background.—Tests to identify DNA may provide critical evidence linking a suspect and the scene of a crime. Ways to enter DNA profiles into a centralized computer database are under study. The privacy implications of a mass cataloging of DNA codes was examined.

National Databank.—To realize the full law enforcement potential of DNA technology, a national coordination effort is essential. The DNA database would operate in a manner similar to the existing fingerprint identification system, requiring human judgment after the computer has narrowed the search. This method will be used mainly to solve sex crimes, but it may eventually be applied to other felonies in which bodily tissues are left behind. It is presumed that only the bare prints will be kept on file once the proper protocols for a databank are approved. Now, with the storage of whole blood required by law, extraneous information about the individual could be obtained. Eventually, certain chromosomal deficiencies indicating an inclination to violent crime may be identified. Also, a person's bloodprint may be easily accessible and liable to be called up in computer matching to detect sensitive information about the individual.

Privacy.—Privacy may be defined as the ability to control the circulation of information about oneself. The Supreme Court has been unwilling to apply the concept of privacy to personal information held by others in such areas as banking, so it seems likely that it would not apply this protection to biological materials. Advocates of privacy have turned to Congress, but the goals of the Privacy Act have consistently been undermined by the "routine use" exemption, permitting agencies to disclose information if disclosure is compatible with the purpose for which it was collected. The government's interest in bureaucratic efficiency could thus be used to justify disclosure of an individual's genetic defects to other interested agencies.

Conclusions.—Although the benefits of DNA databanks cannot be minimized, it appears that their advent will diminish the fundamental principle of presumption of innocence. Adequate safeguards are needed to protect this extremely sensitive information. Law enforcement officials have a responsibility to ensure that the information is not used for any purpose other than investigating the crime in question. Unless the confidentiality of the genetic information is insured, implementation of the DNA databank will not withstand constitutional scrutiny.

▶ This paper addresses another issue with broad societal implications. Pathologists will naturally be involved in (1) the collection of specimens, (2) analysis, and (3) storage and interpretation of data. This paper provides a sobering perspective of another area in which the social, moral, and legal implications have not been explored as vigorously as the analytical technology.—W.A. Gardner, Jr., M.D.

Selective Microscopic Examination of Gallbladders, Hernia Sacs, and Appendices

Wolkomir AF, Barone JE, Moser RL (Ferguson Clinic, Grand Rapids, Mich; St Francis Med Ctr, Trenton, NJ)

Am Surg 57:289–292, 1991 22–5

Objective.—Because of greater emphasis on cost containment, the usefulness of many routine medical procedures is being challenged. The utility of routine microscopic pathologic examination of 3 frequently submitted surgical specimens was evaluated.

Methods.—Pathology reports of 39,568 consecutive specimens, including 17,105 appendices, 14,654 hernia sacs, and 7,809 gallbladders, submitted during a 49-year period were reviewed to analyze the benefit of routine gross and microscopic pathologic examinations, particularly in terms of patient outcome.

Results.—There were few unexpected findings on microscopic examination of the specimens. Primary carcinoma of the bladder was detected in 45 specimens (.58%). Cancer was not diagnosed by the surgeon during celiotomy in 15 patients, although 8 had gross abnormalities noted by the pathologist. Microscopic examination was useful in establishing an unsuspected diagnosis of malignancy in 1 hernial sac and in 7 appendix specimens. In patients in whom unexpected findings were discovered, either the primary surgery was curative or additional surgery would not have altered the prognosis. In general, there was relatively little benefit to the patient from microscopic examination of these tissues.

Implications.—Greater selectivity in microscopic examinations of the hernial sac, appendix, and gallbladder should probably be implemented. A careful and thorough gross examination is usually sufficient. Microscopic examination of the gallbladder should be performed when extensive gross pathology (e.g., ulcer, abscess, gangrene, fistula, large stones, calcified walls, or polyps) is present. Similarly, microscopic examination of a hernial sac or appendix should be undertaken when unusual findings are present on gross examination, or when the diagnosis is uncertain.

▶ It may be noteworthy that this paper appeared in the surgical literature. Pathologists have been rather reluctant to open this particular can of worms, especially as it relates to historical standards of practice. In many practices there are now criteria for the selective microscopic examination of placentas. It is likely that the larger question of microscopic examination of tissues in general (e.g., tonsils, hemorrhoids) will not go away. As pathologists, we should come to grips with this question and provide some appropriate answers so that it will not be answered for us.—W.A. Gardner, Jr., M.D.

Selected Reviews

General

Bloch W: A biochemical perspective of the polymerase chain reaction. *Biochemistry* 30:2735–2747, 1991.

Epstein WL, et al: Mechanisms of granulomatous inflammation. *Immunol Ser* 46:687–721, 1989.

Heitz PU: Neuroendocrine markers in pathology. *Acta Histochem Suppl (Jena)* 38:35–43, 1990.

Heldin CH, et al: Platelet-derived growth factor: Mechanism of action and possible in vivo function. *Cell Regul* 1:555–566, 1990.

Hill RB, et al: Pathologists and the autopsy. *Am J Clin Pathol* S42–49, 1991.

The Association for Practitioners in Infection Control, The Society of Hospital Epidemiologists of America: Position paper: The HIV-infected health care worker. *Am J Infect Control* 18:371–382, 1990.

Smith RM, et al: Molecular basis of chronic granulomatous disease. *Blood* 77:673–686, 1991.

Thorstensen K, et al: The role of transferrin in the mechanism of cellular iron uptake. *Biochem J* 265:97–105, 1991.

van Kessel KP, et al: A view to a kill: Cytotoxic mechanisms of human polymorphonuclear leukocytes compared with monocytes and natural killer cells. *Pathology* 58:249–264, 1990.

Wardlaw A: Leucocyte adhesion to endothelium. *Clin Exp Allergy* 20:619–626, 1990.

Warford A, et al: In situ hybridisation in perspective. *J Clin Pathol* 44:177–181.

Yoon JW: The role of viruses and environmental factors in the induction of diabetes. *Curr Top Microbiol Immunol* 164:95–123, 1990.

Ferrara JL, et al: Graft-versus-host disease. *N Engl J Med* 324:667–674, 1991.

Gatti RA, et al: Ataxia-telangiectasia: An interdisciplinary approach to pathogenesis. *Medicine (Baltimore)* 70:99–117, 1991.

Hansen JA, et al: Autoimmune diseases and HLA. *Crit Rev Immunol* 10:307–328, 1990.

Mayr WR, et al: Paternity testing—Quo vadis? *Blood Rev* 5:51–54, 1991.

Mongey AB, et al: Antinuclear antibodies and disease specificity. *Adv Intern Med* 36:151–169, 1991.

Mozes E: The role of anti-DNA idiotype antibodies in systemic lupus erythematosus. *Crit Rev Immunol* 10:329–345, 1990.

Parkman R: Graft-versus-host disease. *Annu Rev Med* 42:189–197, 1991.

Provost TT, et al: Antinuclear antibodies in systemic lupus erythematosus. *Immunol Ser* 46:333–357, 1989.

Rose ML, et al: Mechanisms of cardiac allograft rejection and avenues for immunological monitoring. *Semin Thorac Cardiovasc Surg* 2:162–174, 1990.

Simmons RJ, et al: Altered immune status in the elderly. *Semin Respir Infect* 5:251–259, 1990.

Spickett GP, et al: Cellular abnormalities in common variable immunodeficiency. *Immunodefic Rev* 2:199–219, 1990.

Neoplasia

Beastall GH, et al: A review of the role of established tumour markers. *Ann Clin Biochem* 28:5–18, 1991.

Beuth J, et al: Lectins: Mediators of adhesion for bacteria in infectious diseases and for tumor cells in metastasis. *Int J Med Microbiol* 274:350–358, 1990.

Bishop JM: Molecular themes in oncogenesis. *Cell* 84:235–248, 1991.
Cerutti PA, et al: Inflammation and oxidative stress in carcinogenesis. *Cancer Cells* 3:1–7, 1991.
Cox PM, et al: Transcription and cancer. *Br J Cancer* 63:651–662, 1991.
Fojo AT Multidrug resistance. *Adv Intern Med* 36:195–218, 1991.
Kagan J, et al: Molecular biology of lymphoid malignancies. *Ann Oncol* 2:9–21, 1991.
Russo J, et al: Mammary tumorigenesis. *Prog Exp Tumor Res* 33:175–191, 1991.
Wiedemann LM, et al: Review article—Chromosome Pathology: Chromosome rearrangement, oncogene activation, and other clonal events in cancer: Their use in molecular diagnostics. *J Pathol* 163:7–12, 1991.

Genetics

Brown R: Review article—Chromosome pathology. Gene amplification and drug resistance. *J Pathol* 163:287–292, 1991.
Hooberman AL, et al: Molecular methods to detect the Philadelphia chromosome. *Clin Lab Med* 10:839–855, 1990.
Machnicki JL, et al: Chromosomal abnormalities in myelodysplastic syndromes and acute myeloid leukemia. *Clin Lab Med* 10:755–767, 1990.

Cytology

Alt ER, et al: The cytopathology of metal overload. *Int Rev Exp Pathol* 31:165–188, 1990.
Egidi MF: Fine-needle aspiration biopsy in renal transplantation: A review of cytologic features. *Diagn Cytopathol* 6:330–335, 1990.
Houn HY: Fine needle aspiration in the diagnosis of liver neoplasms: A review. *Ann Clin Lab Sci* 21:2–11, 1991.
Kline TS: Survey of aspiration biopsy cytology of the breast. *Diagn Cytopathol* 7:98–105, 1991.
Nguyen GK, et al: Fine needle aspiration biopsy cytology of the thyroid. Its value and limitations in the diagnosis and management of solitary thyroid nodules. *Pathol Annu* 26:63–91, 1991.
Suhrland MJ, et al: Fine needle aspiration biopsy in the diagnosis of lymphoma. *Cancer Invest* 9:61–68, 1991.

Pediatric Pathology

Broadway D, et al: Congenital malignant melanoma of the eye. *Cancer* 67:2642–2652, 1991.
Christian CL: Prenatal diagnosis of cystic fibrosis. *Clin Perinatol* 17:779–791, 1990.
DePalma L, et al: Blood component therapy in the perinatal period: Guidelines and recommendations. *Semin Perinatol* 14:403–415, 1990.
Ghodsian Fischel: Prenatal diagnosis of hemoglobinopathies. *N Clin Perinatol* 17:811–828, 1990.
Goren MP, et al: Pediatric soft tissue sarcomas. *Curr Opin Oncol* 2:481–485, 1990.
Iafolla AK, et al: Prenatal diagnosis of metabolic disease. *Clin Perinatol* 17:761–777, 1990.
Lacayo A, et al: Brain tumors in children: A review. *Ann Clin Lab Sci* 21:26–35, 1991.

Loft AG: Determination of amniotic fluid acetylcholinesterase activity in the antenatal diagnosis of foetal malformation: The first ten years. *J Chem Clin Biochem* 28:893–911, 1990.
Wu JT: Screening for inborn errors of amino acid metabolism. *Ann Clin Lab Sci* 21:123–142, 1991.

Transplantation

Lasky LC: The role of the laboratory in marrow manipulation. *Arch Pathol Lab Med* 115:293–298, 1991.
Moller E: Advances in and future of tissue typing. *Transplant Proc* 23:63–66, 1991.
Rose ML, et al: Mechanisms of cardiac allograft rejection and avenues for immunological monitoring. *Semin Thorac Cardiovasc Surg* 2:162–174, 1990.

Cardiovascular System

Anderson JW, et al: Lipoproteins and diet in the pathogenesis of atherosclerosis. *Adv Exp Med Biol* 273:245–258, 1990.
Billingham ME: The pathology of transplanted hearts. *Semin Thorac Cardiovasc Surg* 2:233–240, 1990.
Burke M: Viral myocarditis. *Histopathology* 17:193–200, 1990.
Davies MJ: The pathological basis of angina pectoris. *Cardiovasc Drugs Ther* 1:249–255, 1989.
Francis RB Jr, et al: Vascular occlusion in sickle cell disease: Current concepts and unanswered questions. *Blood* 77:1405–1414, 1991.
Hjelle B: Human T-cell leukemia/lymphoma viruses. Life cycle, pathogenicity, epidemiology, and diagnosis. *Arch Pathol Lab Med* 115:440–450, 1991.
Isner JM, et al: Cardiovascular complications of cocaine. *Curr Probl Cardiol* February 1991.
McCaffrey FM, et al: Sudden cardiac death in young athletes. A review. *Am J Dis Child* 145:177–183, 1991.
Snell RJ, et al: Cardiovascular dysfunction in septic shock. *Chest* 99:1000–1009, 1991.

Hematopoietic System

Dehner LP, Morphologic findings in the histiocytic syndromes. *Semin Oncol* 18:8–17, 1991.
Ferry JA, et al: Malignant lymphoma, pseudolymphoma, and hematopoietic disorders of the female genital tract. *Pathol Annu* 26:227–263, 1991.
Hjelle B: Human T-cell leukemia/lymphoma viruses. *Arch Pathol Lab Med* 115:440–450, 1991.
Kroese FG, et al: Germinal center reaction and B lymphocytes: Morphology and function. *Curr Top Pathol* 84:103–148, 1990.
Martinez C, et al: The thousand and one ways of being a T cell. *Thymus* 16:173–185, 1990.
Smith RE, et al: Myelofibrosis: A review of clinical and pathologic features and treatment. *Crit Rev Oncol Hematol* 10:305–314, 1990.
Suhrland MJ, et al: Fine needle aspiration biopsy in the diagnosis of lymphoma. *Cancer Invest* 9:61–68, 1991.
Thomas JA, et al: B-cell lymphoma in organ transplant recipients. *Semin Thorac Cardiovasc Surg* 2:221–232, 1990.
Walker AN, et al: Thymomas and thymic carcinomas. *Semin Diagn Pathol* 7:250–265, 1990.

Respiratory System

Burke AP, et al: The pathology of primary pulmonary hypertension. *Mod Pathol* 4:269–282, 1991.

Corrin B, et al: Histopathology of the pleura. *Respiration* 57:160–175, 1990.

Lillington GA, et al: Biopsies in patients with intrathoracic disease. *Clin Rev Allergy* 8:333–360, 1990.

Rosenthal SA, et al: The significance of histology in non-small cell lung cancer. *Cancer Treat Rev* 17:409–425, 1990.

Wick MR, et al: Neuroendocrine neoplasms of the mediastinum. *Semin Diagn Pathol* 8:35–51, 1991.

Alimentary System

Basser RL, et al: Recent advances in carcinoids and gastrointestinal neuroendocrine tumors. *Curr Opin Oncol* 3:109–120, 1991.

Beyer KL, et al: Primary small-cell carcinoma of the esophagus. Report of 11 cases and review of the literature. *J Clin Gastroenterol* 13:135–141, 1991.

Frable MAS, et al: Fine-needle aspiration biopsy of salivary glands. *Laryngoscope* 101:245–249, 1991.

Krutchkoff DJ, et al: Dysplasia of oral mucosa: A unified approach to proper evaluation. *Mod Pathol* 4:113–119, 1991.

Peterson WL: *Helicobacter pylori* and peptic ulcer disease. *N Engl J Med* 324:1043–1048, 1991.

Thomas CR Jr, et al: Gastrointestinal lymphoma. *Med Pediatr Oncol* 19:48–60, 1991.

Winawer SJ: Colorectal cancer screening. *J Natl Cancer Inst* 83:243–253, 1991.

Yang GC, et al: Mixed (composite) glandular-endocrine cell carcinoma of the stomach. Report of a case and review of the literature. *Am J Surg Pathol* 15:592–598, 1991.

Hepatobiliary System

Houn HY, et al: Fine needle aspiration in the diagnosis of liver neoplasms: A review. *Ann Clin Lab Sci* 21:2–11, 1991.

Ishak KG, et al: Alcoholic liver disease: Pathologic, pathogenetic and clinical aspects. *Alcohol Clin Exp Res* 15:45–66, 1991.

Ludwig J: Small-duct primary sclerosing cholangitis. *Semin Liver Dis* 11:11–17, 1991.

Schorr-Lesnick B, et al: Liver diseases unique to pregnancy. *Am J Gastroenterol* 86:659–670, 1991.

Pancreas

Kloppel G, et al: Histological typing of pancreatic and periampullary carcinoma. *Eur J Surg Oncol* 17:139–152, 1991.

Kidney

Neild GH: Cyclosporin nephrotoxicity. *Semin Thorac Cardiovasc Surg* 2:198–203, 1990.

Olumi AF, et al: Molecular analysis of human bladder cancer. *Semin Urol* 8:270–277, 1990.

Pappas PG: Laboratory in the diagnosis and management of urinary tract infections. *Med Clin North Am* 75:313–325, 1991.

Wilson DM: Clinical and laboratory evaluation of renal stone patients. *Endocrinol Metab Clin North Am* 19:773–803, 1990.

Zukerberg LR, et al: Transitional cell carcinoma of the urinary bladder with osteoclast-type giant cells: a report of two cases and review of the literature. *Histopathology* 17:407–411, 1990.

Male Genital System

Dilworth JP, et al: Non-germ cell tumors of testis. *Urology* 37:399–417, 1991.

Jorgensen N, et al: Clinical and biological significance of carcinoma in situ of the testis. *Cancer Surv* 9:138–142, 1990.

Osterling JE: Prostate specific antigen: A critical assessment of the most useful tumor marker for adenocarcinoma of the prostate. *J Urol* 145:907–923, 1991.

Female Genital System

Chang KL, et al: Primary uterine endometrial stromal neoplasms. *AJSP* 14:415–438, 1990.

Eichhorn JH, et al: Ovarian myxoma: Clinicopathologic and immunocytologic analysis of five cases and a review of the literature. *Int J Gynecol Pathol* 10:156–169, 1991.

Ferry JA, et al: Malignant lymphoma, pseudolymphoma, and hematopoietic disorders of the female genital tract. *Pathol Annu* 26:227–263, 1991.

Mandelblatt J, et al: Clinical implications of screening for cervical cancer under Medicare. The natural history of cervical cancer in the elderly: What do we know? What do we need to know? *Am J Obstet Gynecol* 164:644–651, 1991.

Pinedo F, et al: Primary malignant melanoma of the uterine cervix: Case report and review of the literature. *Gynecol Obstet Invest* 31:121–124, 1991.

Breast

Haslam SZ: Stromal-epithelial interactions in normal and mammary gland. *Cancer Treat Res* 53:401–420, 1991.

Kline TS: Survey of aspiration biopsy cytology of the breast. *Diagn Cytopathol* 7:98–105, 1991.

Leathem AJ: Biological, biochemical and morphological markers of breast disorders and of breast cancer. *Acta Histochem Suppl* 40:51–58, 1990.

Page DL: Prognosis and breast cancer. Recognition of favorable prognostic types. *Am J Surg Pathol* 15:334–349, 1991.

Russo J, et al: Mammary tumorigenesis. Prog Exp Tumor Res 33:175–191, 1991.

Stegner HE, et al: Breast carcinoma. *Curr Top Pathol* 83:459–474, 1991.

Endocrine Tumors

Cady B, Papillary carcinoma of the thyroid. *Semin Surg Oncol* 7:81–86, 1991.

Chao JC, et al: Null cell adenoma of the pituitary gland. *S Med J* 84:1239–1242, 1991.

Chow CC, et al: Thyroid disorders induced by lithium and amiodarone: An overview. *Adverse Drug React Acute Poisoning Rev* 9:207–222, 1990.

Jensen EV: Steroid hormone receptors. *Curr Top Pathol* 83:365–431, 1991.

Roubidoux M, et al: Adrenal cortical tumors. *Bull N Y Acad Med* 67:119–130, 1991.

Stein PP, et al: A simplified diagnostic approach to pheochromocytoma. A review of the literature and report of one institution's experience. *Medicine (Baltimore)* 70:46–66, 1991.
Watne AL, et al: Follicular carcinoma of the thyroid. *Semin Surg Oncol* 2:87–91, 1991.

Musculoskeletal System

Jozsa L, et al: Tumors and tumor-like lesions arising in tendons. A clinicopathologic study of 75 cases. *Arch Orthop Trauma Surg* 110:83–86, 1991.
Persselin JE, Diagnosis of rheumatoid arthritis. Medical and laboratory aspects. *Clin Orthop* 265:73–82, 1991.

Dermatopathology

Koh HK: Cutaneous melanoma. *N Engl J Med* 325:171–182, 1991.
Miller SJ: Biology of basal cell carcinoma (Part I). *J Am Acad Dermatol* 24:1–13, 1991.
Miller SJ: Biology of basal cell carcinoma (Part II). *J Am Acad Dermatol* 24:161–175, 1991.
Roth ME, et al: The histopathology of dysplastic nevi. Continued controversy. *Am J Dermatopathol* 13:38–51, 1991.
Shaw JH, et al: Merkel cell tumour: Clinical behaviour and treatment. *Br J Surg* 89:138–142, 1991.

Neuropathology

Black PM: Brain tumors. *N Engl J Med* 324:1471–1476, 1991.
Black PM: Brain tumors (2). *N Engl J Med* 324:1555–1564, 1991.
Dam AM: Neuropathology of epilepsy. *Acta Neurochir Suppl (Wein)* 50:20–25, 1990.
Horowitz MB, et al: Central nervous system germinomas. *Arch Neurol* 48:652–657, 1991.
Katzman R, et al: Advances in Alzheimer's disease. *FASEB J* 5:278–286, 1991.
Massaro AR, et al: Cerebrospinal fluid markers in neurological disorders. *Ital J Neurol Sci* 11:537–547, 1990.
Selkoe DJ: The molecular pathology of Alzheimer's disease. *Neuron* 6:487–498, 1991.
Shiraishi K, Glycogen-rich meningioma. Case report and short review. *Neurosurg Rev* 14:61–64, 1991.
Thompson EJ, et al: Laboratory investigation of cerebrospinal fluid proteins. *Ann Clin Biochem* 27:425–435, 1990.
Voelker JL, et al: Clinical, radiographic, and pathological features of symptomatic Rathke's cleft cysts. *J Neurosurg* 74:535–544, 1991.

Ophthalmology

Dutton JJ: Optic nerve gliomas and meningiomas. *Neurol Clin* 9:163–177, 1991.
Lee WH, et al: Molecular biology of the human retinoblastoma gene. *Immunol Ser* 51:169–200, 1990.

Chemical Pathology

Bennett MJ: The laboratory diagnosis of inborn errors of mitochondrial fatty acid oxidation. *Ann Clin Biochem* 27:519–531, 1990.

Greenlee JE: Approach to diagnosis of meningitis. Cerebrospinal fluid evaluation. *Infect Dis Clin North Am* 4:583–598, 1990.
Krantz SB: Erythropoietin. *Blood* 77:419–434, 1991.
Kohse KP, et al: Antibodies as a source of analytical errors. *J Clin Chem Clin Biochem* 28:881–892, 1990.
Lemann J Jr, et al: Hypercalciuria and stones. *Am J Kidney Dis* 17:386–391, 1991.
Pohl LR: Drug-induced allergic hepatitis. *Semin Liver Dis* 10:305–315, 1990.
Prusiner SB: Molecular biology of prion diseases. *Science* 252:1515–1522, 1991.
Righetti PG: Recent developments in electrophoretic methods. *J Chromatogr* 516:3–22, 1990.
Salem M, et al: Hypomagnesemia in critical illness. A common and clinically important problem. *Crit Care Clin* 7:225–252, 1991.
Sherman KE: Alanine aminotransferase in clinical practice. A review. *Arch Intern Med* 151:260–265, 1991.
Tunkel AR, et al: Pathogenesis and pathophysiology of meningitis. *Infect Dis Clin North Am* 4:555–581, 1990.
Thompson EJ, et al: Laboratory investigation of cerebrospinal fluid proteins. *Ann Clin Biochem* 27:425–435, 1990.
Wilson DM: Clinical and laboratory evaluation of renal stone patients. *Endocrinol Metab Clin North Am* 19:773–803, 1990.

Microbiology

Arends MJ, et al: Papillomaviruses and human cancer. *Hum Pathol* 21:686–698, 1990.
Beuth J, et al: Lectins: Mediators of adhesion for bacteria in infectious diseases and for tumor cells in metastasis. *Int J Med Microbiol* 274:350–358, 1990.
Bozzette SA, et al: Cryptococcal disease in AIDS. *AIDS Clin Rev* 193–213, 1990.
Curry A, et al: Opportunistic protozoan infections in human immunodeficiency virus disease: Review highlighting diagnostic and therapeutic aspects. *J Clin Pathol* 44:182–193, 1991.
Dance DA: Melioidosis: The tip of the iceberg? *Clin Microbiol Rev* 4:52–60, 1991.
Drumm B: *Helicobacter pylori. Arch Dis Child* 65:1278–1282, 1990.
Figueroa ME, et al: Molecular pathology and diagnosis of infectious diseases. *Am J Clin Pathol* S8–21, 1991.
Gentry LO, et al: Candida infections. *Complications Surg* 10:10–24, 1991.
Niu MT, et al: Meningitis due to protozoa and helminths. *Infect Dis Clin North Am* 4:809–841, 1992.
Pfaller MA: Diagnostic applications of DNA probes. *Infect Control Hosp Epidemiol* 12:103–110, 1991.
Snell RJ, et al: Cardiovascular dysfunction in septic shock. *Chest* 99:1000–1009, 1991.
Tunkel AR, et al: Pathogenesis and pathophysiology of meningitis. *Infect Dis Clin North Am* 4:555–581, 1990.
Wispelwey B, et al: Bacterial meningitis in adults. *Infect Dis Clin North Am* 4:645–659, 1990.

Blood Banking

DePalma L, et al: Blood component therapy in the perinatal period: Guidelines and recommendations. *Semin Perinatol* 14:403–415, 1990.

Mason PD, et al: Plasma exchange in nephrological diseases. *Curr Stud Hematol Blood Transfus* 57:152–166, 1990.
Triulzi DJ, et al: Association of transfusion with postoperative bacterial infection. *Crit Rev Clin Lab Sci* 28:95–107, 1990.
Uldry PA, et al: Plasma exchange in neurology. *Curr Stud Hematol Blood Transfus* 57:167–183, 1990.
Williams C, et al: Plasma exchange in idiopathic thrombocytopenic purpura. *Curr Stud Hematol Blood Transfus* 57:131–151, 1990.

Hematology

Beck WS: Diagnosis of megaloblastic anemia. *Annu Rev Med* 42:311–322, 1991.
Erselv AJ: Erythropoietin. *N Engl J Med* 324:1399–1344, 1991.
Ghodsian Fischel: Prenatal diagnosis of hemoglobinopathies. *N Clin Perinatol* 17:811–828, 1990.
Landaw SA: Polycythemia vera and other polycythemic states. *Clin Lab Med* 10:857–871, 1990.
Lee EJ, et al: Leukemias of indeterminant lineage. *Clin Lab Med* 10:737–754, 1990.
Liesveld JL, et al: State of the art: The hypereosinophilic syndromes. *Blood Rev* 5:29–37, 1991.
Smith BR: Regulation of hematopoiesis. *Yale J Biol Med* 63:371–380, 1990.
Thiele J, et al: Megakaryocytopoiesis in haematological disorders: Diagnostic features of bone marrow biopsies. An overview. *Virchows Arch (A)* 418:87–97, 1991.
Weller PF: The immunobiology of eosinophils. *N Engl J Med* 324:1110–1118, 1991.
Willman CL, et al: The molecular biology of acute myeloid leukemia. Proto-oncogene expression and function in normal and neoplastic myeloid cells. *Clin Lab Med* 10:769–796, 1990.

Laboratory Management

Bentley SA: Quality control and the differential leukocyte count. *Clin Lab Haematol* 1:101–109, 1990.
Connelly DP, et al: Expert systems and the clinical laboratory information system. *Clin Lab Med* 11:135–151, 1991.
Field MA: Testing for AIDS: Uses and abuses. *Am J Law Med* 16:33–106, 1990.
Hailey DM, et al: Developments in near-patient testing. *Med Lab Sci* 47:319–325, 1990.
Leggett RW, et al: Suggested reference values for regional blood volumes in humans. *Health Phys* 60:139–154, 1991.

Thrombosis and Hemostasis

Bauer KA, et al: Role of antithrombin III as a regulator of in vivo coagulation. *Semin Hematol* 28:10–18, 1991.
Dyke C, et al: The management of coagulation problems in the surgical patient. *Adv Surg* 24:229–257, 1991.
Frenkel EP: The clinical spectrum of thrombocytosis and thrombocythemia. *Am J Med Sci* 301:69–80, 1991.
Hathaway WE: Clinical aspects of antithrombin III deficiency. *Semin Hematol* 28:19–23, 1991.

Hawiger J: Adhesive interactions of platelets and their blockade. *Ann N Y Acad Sci* 614:270–278, 1991.
Hirsch DR, et al: Laboratory parameters to monitor safety and efficacy during thrombolytic therapy. *Chest* 99:113S–120S, 1991.
Thompson AR: Molecular biology of the hemophilias. *Prog Hemost Thromb* 10:175–214, 1991.
Schafer AI: Essential thrombocythemia. *Prog Hemost Thromb* 10:69–96, 1991.

AIDS

Aboulafia DM, et al: Hematologic abnormalities in AIDS. *Hematol Oncol Clin North Am* 5:195–214, 1991.
Ames ED, et al: Hodgkin's disease and AIDS. Twenty-three new cases and a review of the literature. *Hematol Oncol Clin North Am* 5:343–356, 1991.
Cohen MB, et al: Pathology of AIDS. *Immunol Ser* 44:305–322, 1989.
Curry A, et al: Opportunistic protozoan infections in human immunodeficiency virus disease: Review highlighting diagnostic and therapeutic aspects. *J Clin Pathol* 44:182–193, 1991.
Dickson DW, et al: Microglia in human disease with an emphasis on acquired immune deficiency syndrome. *Lab Invest* 64:135–156, 1991.
Golden JA: Pulmonary complications of AIDS. *Immunol Ser* 44:403–447, 1989.
Pavlakis GN, et al: Regulation of expression of human immunodeficiency virus. *New Biol* 2:20–31, 1990.
Pelstring RJ, et al: Hodgkin's disease in association with human immunodeficiency virus infection. Pathologic and immunologic features. *Cancer* 67:1865–1873, 1991.
Rao TK: Human immunodeficiency virus (HIV) associated nephropathy. *Annu Rev Med* 42:391–401, 1991.

Forensic

Little RE, et al: Sudden infant death syndrome epidemiology: A review and update. *Epidemiol Rev* 12:241–266, 1990.

Subject Index

A

B

D

E

F

H

I

J

K

L

M

N

O

P

Q

R

S

T

Author Index

A

B

C

P

Q

R

S

X

Y

Z